FOOD AND BEVERAGE CONSUMPTION AND HEALTH

OLIVE CONSUMPTION AND HEALTH

FOOD AND BEVERAGE CONSUMPTION AND HEALTH

Additional books in this series can be found on Nova's website under the Series tab.

Additional E-books in this series can be found on Nova's website under the E-book tab.

FOOD AND BEVERAGE CONSUMPTION AND HEALTH

OLIVE CONSUMPTION AND HEALTH

CONSTANTINOS A. SAVALAS
AND
SOUSSANA M. NICOLAU
EDITORS

Nova Science Publishers, Inc.
New York

For permission to use material from this book please contact us:
Telephone 631-231-7269; Fax 631-231-8175
Web Site: http://www.novapublishers.com

Library of Congress Cataloging-in-Publication Data

ISBN: 978-1-62100-774-6

Published by Nova Science Publishers, Inc. † New York

CONTENTS

PREFACE

Olive oil, which has been part of the human diet for more than 5,000 years, is almost unique among oils in that it can be consumed in the crude form without refining. This has the effect of conserving all its vitamins, essential fatty acids, and other nutrients. In addition to the fatty acid profile of olive oil, which is high in the monounsaturated oleic acid and appears to be beneficial in reducing several risk factors for coronary heart disease and certain cancers, extra virgin olive oil contains powerful antioxidants. In this book, the authors present topical research on the health benefits of olive consumption. Some of the topics discussed include dynamic rheology and sensory properties determined by inulin/extra virgin olive oil and virgin olive oil antioxidants; olive oil and postprandial lipemia.

Chapter 1 - Inulin (INL) is a functional food ingredient and extra virgin olive oil (EVOO) has interesting nutritional characteristics. This chapter investigates the effect of the addition of INL and EVOO blends at different INL:EVOO ratios (0:0, 0:60, 15:45, 30:30, 45:15, 60:0, 30:45 and 45:30) on oscillatory shear experiments, instrumental colour and sensory properties (appearance, texture and taste attributes) of fresh and frozen/thawed mashed potatoes (FMP and F/TMP respectively). To ameliorate detrimental freezing effects, mashed potatoes (MP) were formulated without and with added hydrocolloids (MPA and MPB respectively). Dynamic shear data revealed weak gel-like behaviour in the MP samples, with magnitudes of storage modulus (G') higher than those of loss modulus (G"), and a frequency-related increase mainly in elasticity. INL and EVOO addition (either alone or blended) produced softer systems as compared to 0:0 controls, although the addition of EVOO alone (0:60 ratio) produced superior softening than that of only INL (60:0 ratio). FMP and MPA samples presented more rigid structures than their F/TMP and MPB counterparts, which is associated with amylopectin retrogradation in the case of the samples subjected to a freeze/thaw cycle. Superior water-holding capacity was also observed in the case of samples with added hydrocolloids. Linear discriminant analysis (LDA) showed that the effect of the INL:EVOO ratio on sensory attributes was more significant in the F/TMP samples than in their FMP counterparts, likely due to a higher degree of oil droplet coalescence caused by freezing. In both FMP and F/TMP products, LDA indicated that ingredient taste was the attribute that best discriminated between the INL/EVOO blends used, a finding which proves that in the case of EVOO, a liquid product, textural attributes are not as significant as those of aroma and taste. Categorical principal component analysis (CATPCA) showed that in the FMP samples, the first dimension was related with rough-smooth texture and the second with mechanical texture-appearance. In the F/TMP samples, the first dimension was associated with appearance (authentic colour and uniformity) and ingredient taste attributes, whereas the second was dominated by mechanical texture (consistency and adhesiveness). Ingredient taste, consistency and adhesiveness were the sensory attributes that showed a superior internal consistency (higher Cronbach alpha coefficient) in both FMP and F/TMP samples.

Chapter 2 - Ageing, usually defined as the progressive loss of function accompanied by decreasing fertility and increasing mortality, has important social and scientific impact. In the last years interest in this process has been growing as they have grown the theories that try to explain this process. One of the most widely accepted is the free radical theory which defends that free radicals produced at the mitochondria damage all biological tissues and lead to the ageing phenotype. In fact, there is a direct relationship between accumulation of oxidative damage produced by reactive oxygen species and the physiological alterations associated with ageing. Nutrition has been related to ageing mainly at the level of caloric restriction and supplementation with antioxidants. In recent years a new approach relates the dietary fat type to mitochondrial and their sensitivity to experiencing oxidative stress because membranes adapt their lipid composition in response to dietary fat. The fatty acid composition of mitochondrial membranes affects in a direct way the properties of these membranes such as fluidity and permeability, which determines its susceptibility to oxidation, thus affects the susceptibility to oxidative stress-related phenomena. Olive oil modifies the structure, and consequently the features, of mitochondrial membranes, positively affecting the way and intensity in which different organs would age. When dietary fat is mainly olive oil a better general state at the mitochondrial function level is found, with a lower reactive oxygen species production at the mitochondrial electron transport chain level and finally with a delay in the occurrence of the ageing phenotype. In summary, the intake throughout life of virgin olive oil provides a healthier ageing.

Chapter 3 - The Mediterranean diet is associated with reduced risk of atherosclerosis, cardiovascular disease, and certain types of cancer and this has partially been explained by the consumption of virgin olive oil (VOO). Historically, the healthful properties of VOO were attributed to a high proportion of monounsaturated fatty acids, namely oleic acid, which represents 60–80% of the fatty acids present in virgin olive oil. In addition, virgin olive oil contains minor, yet significant phenolic components that other seed oils lack. Hydrophilic phenols are the most abundant natural antioxidants of VOO, in which, however, tocopherols and carotenes are also present. The prevalent classes of hydrophilic phenols found in VOO are complex phenols such as ligstroside aglycon and the dialdehydic form of elenolic acid linked to tyrosol, oleuropein aglycon and the dialdehydic form of elenolic acid linked to hydroxytyrosol. Simple phenols such as phenolic alcohols, (hydroxytyrosol, tyrosol) phenolic acids, (vanillic, caffeic, p-coumaric and ferullic acid) flavonoids, (luteolin, apigenin) and lignans, (pinoresinol, 1-acetoxypinoresinol) are present in olive oil at lower concentrations. The qualitative and quantitative composition of VOO phenols is strongly affected by the agronomic and technological conditions of production such as olive cultivar, degree of ripeness olive fruit, processing and storage conditions of the oil. A median of total phenols content of 300 ppm (as gallic acid) is reported, although the above individual phenols ranged widely (100-400 ppm). Those compounds are important for the sensory quality and storage life of VOO. Specifically ‘sweet’, ‘fruity’ and ‘bitter’ taste correlated with low, moderate and high amounts of phenolic compounds respectively. Bitterness is a common and desirable attribute of virgin olive oil flavour when present at low to moderate intensity. The stability of VOO is influenced by their concentration and type of phenols. Tocopherols are the major group of hydrophobic antioxidants occurring in VOO. Nearly 95% of the total tocopherols content is α-tocopherol, which exhibits the highest biological activity. The antioxidant activity is dependent on both concentration and lipid system factors, such as hydroperoxides concentration, metals presence, temperature, and singlet oxygen presence e.g. Natural concentration of α–tocopherol, varies between 100-400 ppm. These compounds are included in the designation of vitamin E and correlated with preventive action against reactive oxygen species (ROS) in biological systems such as plasma, membranes, and tissues.

Chapter 4 - The postprandial lipid period takes place after the intake of food, involves the metabolic processes that occur following the ingestion of a meal containing fat, and it is characterized by a considerable increase in plasma triglyceride levels. An impaired metabolism of postprandial triglyceride-rich lipoproteins (TRL), comprising chylomicrons, very-low-density lipoproteins (VLDL) and their remnants, is believed to contribute to the onset and development of atherosclerosis. Recent research has pointed out that these particles are highly atherogenic because, in contrast to low-density lipoproteins, can penetrate into the intima and be taken up by macrophages without need for prior oxidation, leading to the initiation of atherogenesis. The atherogenicity of TRL depends on their lipid composition, which is, in turn, influenced by the composition of dietary fats. The intake of oleic-acid rich oils, like olive oil, have been shown to modulate the production of postprandial TRL and their subsequent metabolism and it is likely that both the fatty acid and minor component compositions of the oil may have a role. The postprandial triglyceride response seems to be dependent mainly upon the triglyceride molecular species composition and not on the minor components. However, the unsaponifiable components of virgin olive oil and pomace olive oil can have important effects on the uptake of postprandial TRL by macrophages and other cells involved in the processes related to the development of atherosclerosis.

Chapter 5 - Over the past thirty years the knowledge of the nutritional properties of olive oil has deeply improved and olive oil is presently considered as a basic element of the "Mediterranean diet". Olive oil contains important nutrients, such as essential and monounsaturated fatty acids in addition to other particular compounds useful in a healthy diet. The quality of olive oil depends on several aspects such oxidation stability, absence of contaminants (pesticides, solvents or adulterants), nutritional values expressed as the amount of saturated fatty acids, monounsaturated and polyunsaturated fats, presence of phytosterols, vitamins and natural antioxidants. For these reasons, olive oil is one of the most expensive and is often object of frauds involving replacement of high-cost ingredients with lower grade and cheaper substitutes. For example, adulteration of virgin olive oil with different seed oils, such as hazelnut and almond oils, represents a serious problem for regulatory agencies, oil suppliers, and consumers. Moreover, in addition to economic implications, adulteration is a serious health problem related to the possible presence of carcinogenic mycotoxins. Further, many seeds, such as hazelnut (Corylus avellana L.) and peanuts, are among the major food allergens in the dried fruit shell. The presence of protein residues of hazelnut oil used for adulteration can trigger allergic reactions in the respiratory tract such as oral allergy syndrome (OAS), rhinoconjunctivitis or, in severe cases, anaphylactic shock. Adulterated olive oil becomes a source of hidden allergens very dangerous to the health of consumers. Another potential health hazard can be represented from the exposure of consumers to oxidized oils since the oxidation mechanism occurring during processing and storage can have effects on palatability, nutritional quality, and toxicity. This chapter resumes the use of an analytical technique based on a new type of ion source, Matrix-Assisted Laser

Desorption/Ionization (MALDI) coupled to a time-of-flight mass spectrometer (TOF-MS) analyzer for the comprehensive assessment of olive oil quality in terms of absence of contaminants, adulterants and oxidation processes. The main advantages of MALDI-TOF-MS in comparison to other analytical methods consist of a fast and easy sample preparation and no need for analyte derivatization.

Chapter 6 - The genus *Olea L.* is represented in the Mediterranean region by the species *Olea europaea L.* with two varieties, *O. europaea* var. *sylvestris* (wild olive), which forms part of the natural vegetation, and *O. europaea* var. *europaea*, cultivated primarily for olive and oil production. Nowadays, Andalusia (Spain) is the world's leading olive-oil-producing region. Due to its great land cover extensions and to the high flower production, high levels of olive pollen are detected in the air of southern Spain during springtime, being the most abundant pollen type and causing severe pollinosis problems among population. This fact, together with the considerable economic importance, makes the study of olive-pollen characteristics over this area of a high relevance. Olive-pollen season in south Spain runs from April to June, being the timing and severity of the pollen curve highly controlled by weather conditions. This work represents a paper review on the olive pollen studies, paying special attention to its relationship with meteorological parameters and the usefulness of back-trajectory analysis, due to they provide information about synoptic conditions responsible for high pollen counts, the origin of airborne pollen, and the type of pollen transport (local or regional). With the present review we sought 1) to determine potential pollen sources, 2) to describe pollen transport dynamic and 3) to clarify the real contribution of the different olive-growing areas to airborne pollen counts in Cordoba province.

Chapter 7 - Frying is one of the most widely spread culinary methods in developed countries, whether in home, institutional, or industrial cooking. Frying is also a means of preserving food. Frying oils are subjected to various alterations such as hydrolysis and thermal oxidation during deep frying, which generate a large number of compounds due to high temperature. As frying oil becomes part of the food being fried, the quality of frying oil is of a great importance due to absorption of those compounds into the food during frying, thereby affecting the quality of the final products. Therefore, frying oil must have high oxidative stability during long-term use. Each vegetable oil has a characteristic stability against oxidation depending on the fatty acid composition and the content and composition of antioxidants and other minor components. Minor lipid components such as certain types of phytosterols, phenolic compounds and tocopherols play an important role in vegetable oil stability, both during frying operations and in the oxidative stability of the fried products. Substantial quantities of refined olive oil and refined olive-pomace oil are produced every year; therefore, they can be alternative frying oil for industrial applications. From a nutritional stand-point in particular, the low amount of saturated fatty acids and the high amount of oleic acid in olive oil are important advantages. Therefore, frying with olive oil can offer possibilities of lowering fat intake and improving the quality of fat actually consumed, which are important in preventing cardiovascular and other diseases.

Chapter 8 - Olive oil, which has been part of the human diet for more than 5000 years, is almost unique among oils in that it can be consumed in the crude form without refining. This has the effect of conserving all its vitamins, essential fatty acids, and other nutrients. In addition to the fatty acid profile of olive oil, which is high in the monounsaturated oleic acid and appears to be beneficial in reducing several risk factors for coronary heart disease and certain cancers, extra virgin olive oil contains powerful antioxidants. In this connection, the incidence of degenerative pathologies, including those in which the excessive free radical formation has been suggested, is very low in the Mediterranean area, where the diet is rich in antioxidant compounds. Among such antioxidants, the contribution of olive oil phenolics is currently under active investigation, since they affords considerable protection against cancer (colon, breast, and skin), coronary heart disease, and ageing by inhibiting oxidative stress. This chapter focuses on antioxidant role and additional biological actions of olive oil phenolics.

Chapter 9 - Traceability/product tracing has been defined by the *Codex Alimentarius Commission* as the ability to follow the movement of a food through specified stage(s) of its production, processing, and distribution [CODEX, 2006]. The development of food traceability systems is becoming more demanding once consumers and producers are seeking for more notable foods with high quality guarantee. Consumers are interested in choosing what they are eating based on nutrition value, food safety and products' origin guarantee. As a consequence, food traceability is required by consumers and government organizations because it is a significant component of food and human safety. The European Union regulation allows the application of the following geographical indications to a food product: protected designation of origin (PDO), protected geographical indication (PGI), and traditional specialities guaranteed (TSG). An olive oil with a PDO designation demands precise definitions of several parameters such as the olive cultivar used for the oil production, cultivar geographical origin, olive orchards agronomic practice, technology used for olive oil production, and oil organoleptic characteristics. Nowadays, these parameters are defined by legislation, and are considered for olive oil certification purposes. Because chemical analyses *per se* are not sufficient to verify olive oil authenticity, DNA markers, which have already been used for olive cultivars fingerprinting, are increasingly being applied to solve food traceability and provenance issues. Nowadays, DNA analysis with molecular markers has opened way to understand complex organism's genome. Nevertheless, it is presently being applied in a vast number of areas, where food traceability is going to have a preeminent positioning. This chapter addresses recent advances concerning traceability of olive oils, aspects related to the DNA fingerprinting application in the olive oil production chain, and problems related to the DNA extraction methods and molecular marker choices.

Chapter 10 - In the marketing literature, authors have favored the study of "country of origin" concept, and less attention was given to the "region of origin", and the question of the combined use of the two concepts was neglected. The general goal of this research is to investigate whether the two concepts are distinct or in interaction. The results of an empirical study involving French consumers of olive oil show that the indication of the name of the "region", in addition to that of the "country", has a positive effect on the consumer choice.

Chapter 11 - During the last decades there is an increasing interest of people for the benefits of the Mediterranean diet, since, from many years ago, it was known that citizens from the Mediterranean countries suffered less from cardiovascular diseases, compared to others from Northern European countries and USA. Since olive oil has a dominant role in the Mediterranean diet, most of the papers during the last years were focused on the beneficial compounds of olive oil for health, as well as on their protective properties for heart and other human organs. Throughout the history, olive leaves have been exploited for the prevention, or the treatment, of hypertension, carcinogenesis, diabetes, atherosclerosis and many other traditional therapeutic uses. The most 'famous' and abundant component of olive oil is oleuropein, which is the bitter substance that has antioxidant and anti-inflammatory properties. Apart from these beneficial properties of oleuropein, other very important effects for human organism are the increase of high density lipoprotein (HDL) (good cholesterol), as well as the decrease of bad cholesterol (LDL) and blood pressure. Other very important compounds of olive oil are those of oleic acid, linoleic acid, elenolic acid, hydroxytyrosol, tyrosol, caffeic acid, ferulic acid, o-coumaric acid, gallic acid, benzoic acid e.t.c. For example, oleic acid has been associated with a reduced risk of human cancer and cardiovascular diseases. However, the benefits of olive oil consumption on human health can be ascribed not only to the elevated oleic acid content, but also to the antioxidant, antidiabetic and other properties of its minor components, such as polyphenols, and especially hydroxytyrosol, which is present in high concentrations in the extra virgin olive oil. The concentration of polyphenols in the extra virgin olive oil depends on genotype, location, latitude, climate, ripening stage, irrigation, density of planting, storage conditions of olive oil, and other agronomic and technological factors. Therefore, with the correct management of the previous factors it can be achieved the maximum concentration of polyphenols, leading to the best quality of the extra virgin olive oil, and of course, to the maximum benefit for human health. The beneficial properties for human health of the most important olive oil compounds, as well as of the compounds found in olive leaves, are presented and discussed under the most recent research findings.

Chapter 12 - It is well established that food is not considered to be mere nutritional components for maintaining human life. There are a broad number of studies reporting that many foods may provide a health benefit beyond basic nutrition. Within this context, extra virgin olive oil (EVOO) has been related to the prevention of some types of cancers and the reduced risk of coronary heart diseases. This is mainly due to its high concentration of a broad variety of phenolic compounds, such as phenyl ethyl alcohols (tyrosol, hydroxytyrosol), phenolic acids (4-hydroxybenzoic acid, 3,4-dihydroxybenzoic acid, gallic acid, vanillic acid, ferulic acid, caffeic acid), flavonoids (apigenin, luteolin), secoiridoids (oleuropein and ligstroside aglycons) and lignans [(+)-pinoresinol, (+)-acetoxypinoresinol)]. In the human organism these polyphenols are metabolized and form different compounds. Thus the study of their properties is highly important with regards to understanding their functionality. The aglycones can be absorbed from the mall intestine; however, most polyphenols are in the form of esters, glycosides, or polymers that cannot be absorbed in their native form. Thus, these compounds must be hydrolyzed by intestinal enzymes or by colonic microflora in order to be absorbed. During the course of absorption, polyphenols are conjugated in the small intestine and later in the liver, through methylation, sulfation, and glucuronidation reactions. In the blood, polyphenols are conjugated derivatives bound to albumin. They penetrate into tissues where they are metabolized and then eliminated in urine and bile. For example, hydroxytyrosol shows strong antioxidant activity. In spite of this compound's great absorption capacity in the human body, its bioavailability is low. It is reported in the literature that the oleuropeins are not absorbed in the small intestine, but instead, quickly degradated in the large intestine to yield hydroxytyrosol.

In: Olive Consumption and Health
Editors: C. A. Savalas and S. M. Nicolau

ISBN: 978-1-62100-774-6

Chapter 1

DYNAMIC RHEOLOGY AND SENSORY PROPERTIES DETERMINED BY INULIN/EXTRA VIRGIN OLIVE OIL BLENDS IN MASHED POTATOES: EFFECTS OF HYDROCOLLOIDS ADDITION AND FREEZE/THAW

***María José Jiménez*[1]*, Wenceslao Canet*[2] *and María Dolores Alvarez*[2,*]**

[1]USAS, Service Unit of Sensory Analysis
[2]Department of Characterization, Quality and Food Safety,
Institute of Food Science, Technology and Nutrition (ICTAN)-CSIC,
José Antonio Novais no. 10, Ciudad Universitaria, 28040 Madrid, Spain

ABSTRACT

Inulin (INL) is a functional food ingredient and extra virgin olive oil (EVOO) has interesting nutritional characteristics. This chapter investigates the effect of the addition of INL and EVOO blends at different INL:EVOO ratios (0:0, 0:60, 15:45, 30:30, 45:15, 60:0, 30:45 and 45:30) on oscillatory shear experiments, instrumental colour and sensory properties (appearance, texture and taste attributes) of fresh and frozen/thawed mashed potatoes (FMP and F/TMP respectively). To ameliorate detrimental freezing effects, mashed potatoes (MP) were formulated without and with added hydrocolloids (MPA and MPB respectively). Dynamic shear data revealed weak gel-like behaviour in the MP samples, with magnitudes of storage modulus (G') higher than those of loss modulus (G''), and a frequency-related increase mainly in elasticity. INL and EVOO addition (either alone or blended) produced softer systems as compared to 0:0 controls, although the addition of EVOO alone (0:60 ratio) produced superior softening than that of only INL (60:0 ratio). FMP and MPA samples presented more rigid structures than their F/TMP and MPB counterparts, which is associated with amylopectin retrogradation in the case of the samples subjected to a freeze/thaw cycle. Superior water-holding capacity was

* E-mail: mayoyes@ictan.csic.es.

also observed in the case of samples with added hydrocolloids. Linear discriminant analysis (LDA) showed that the effect of the INL:EVOO ratio on sensory attributes was more significant in the F/TMP samples than in their FMP counterparts, likely due to a higher degree of oil droplet coalescence caused by freezing. In both FMP and F/TMP products, LDA indicated that *ingredient taste* was the attribute that best discriminated between the INL/EVOO blends used, a finding which proves that in the case of EVOO, a liquid product, textural attributes are not as significant as those of aroma and taste. Categorical principal component analysis (CATPCA) showed that in the FMP samples, the first dimension was related with rough-smooth texture and the second with mechanical texture-appearance. In the F/TMP samples, the first dimension was associated with appearance (*authentic colour* and *uniformity*) and *ingredient taste* attributes, whereas the second was dominated by mechanical texture (*consistency* and *adhesiveness*). *Ingredient taste*, *consistency* and *adhesiveness* were the sensory attributes that showed a superior internal consistency (higher Cronbach alpha coefficient) in both FMP and F/TMP samples.

Keywords: Prebiotic; Extra virgin olive oil; Puréed cooked potatoes; Descriptive analysis; Viscoelasticity; Freeze/thaw

INTRODUCTION

Considering the high competitiveness of today's markets, food products that are launched to the market place should be aligned with consumers' preferences as much as possible [1]. Functional product development provides an opportunity to contribute to the improvement of food quality and consumer health and well-being [2]. A common approach employed in the food industry to develop these kinds of added-value foods involves the addition of a healthy component. It is important to know to what extent this new component modifies the product, affecting its sensory properties. In the case of macromolecules such as polysaccharides or proteins, changes in composition can affect product structure in particular, modifying both rheological behaviour and perceived texture [3].

Inulin (INL) is of interest for the development of healthy products because it simultaneously responds to a variety of consumer demands: it is fibre-enriched, prebiotic, low fat and low sugar [4]. As a dietary fibre, INL passes through the digestive tract largely undigested. In the colon, it acts as a prebiotic because it is selectively fermented by the beneficial flora, stimulates their growth, and reinforces its action against putrefactive microorganisms [5]. The addition of INL to different foods has aimed to supplement them to increase fibre ingestion, in amounts that oscillate between 3 and 6 g per portion, or to assure its bifidogenic nature, adding 3-8 g per portion [6].

Olive oil has gained the interest of consumers because of its multiple culinary applications and nutritional content (high content of oleic acid and balance between monounsatured and polyunsaturated fatty acids) and its content of minor compounds (polyphenols and tocopherols that have antioxidant properties and volatile compounds that bestow an oil its unique flavour) [7]. On November 2004, the US Federal Drug Administration (FDA) permitted a claim on olive oil labels concerning: "the benefits on the risk of coronary heart disease of eating about two tablespoons (23 g) of olive oil daily, because of the monounsaturated fat (MUFA) in olive oil" [8]. These properties might fulfill consumer expectations regarding healthier, more nutritious, more flavourful, and more natural food even in countries outside the Mediterranean region where most olive oil is consumed [9]. The Int. Olive Council (IOC) defines extra virgin olive oil (EVOO) as the commercial grade for olive oil that has been extracted by physical processes alone, without the use of solvents or refining agents. The absence of refining processes helps EVOO to preserve its delicate aroma and nutritional properties that distinguish it from other edible oils [10].

Texture is one of the most important factors determining the quality/liking of food. Others are appearance, flavour, comprising taste and smell, and nutritional aspects. However, from a nutritional point of view it is the product composition and its digestibility that primarily matters. For these reasons food scientists and nutritionists like to be able to control the relation between product composition and sensory/texture perception [11].

In frozen vegetables, health quality, nutritional quality and aspects of sensory quality like colour and texture can be objectively assessed and controlled [12]. As the stimulus in texture perception is predominantly mechanical in nature, many instrumental methods are geared to determining rheological characteristics of the food product [13]. However, this does not guarantee matching the sensory perceived texture that only can be sensed and measured by the human being. Sensory research involves the study of texture perception using sensory panels and required input from e.g. psychology and neurophysiology [14].

A number of studies deal with the perception of semisolid mashed potatoes (MP) sensory attributes by using conventional techniques such as descriptive quantitative analysis (QDA) adapted from Adams et al. [15], and considering the evaluation of appearance, texture and taste attributes. The addition of xanthan gum (XG) clearly improved the taste of the MP subjected to a freeze/thaw cycle (F/TMP), whereas addition of amidated low methoxyl pectin at higher concentrations ($\geq$ 4.5 g kg^{-1}) produced an unpleasant taste [16]. Analogously, panellists scored both FMP and F/TMP samples with added dairy proteins unacceptable as regards pleasantness to taste [17]. In turn, in F/TMP samples, increased fibrousness was related to the addition of sodium caseinate, whereas improved creaminess was associated with XG addition [18]. In EVOO-enriched MP, panellists found that increasing yellowness improved the colour of the product, since the flesh of Kennebec potatoes is white and MP without added other ingredients look rather pale [19].

MPs behave like a high-volume-fraction dispersion, so that the addition of INL (extra dry matter) would be expected to result in a firmer product. There is little information on the sensory characteristics of INL and EVOO and how they are affected by possible interactions with other ingredients, like different kinds of hydrocolloids or starch. A complicating factor is that ingredients mostly affect several texture/sensory attributes at the same time [11]. EVOO is a liquid product, and therefore, upon addition of EVOO, the systems would be expected to be softer whatever the concentration used. This chapter was focused on the possibility of optimising MP formulation complying with an improved nutritional value and at the same time to gain more insights into the rheological and sensory properties of such systems.

The aim of this chapter was therefore: (1) to examine the effect of adding INL/EVOO blends at different INL:EVOO ratios on viscoelastic and sensory properties of FMP and F/TMP samples formulated without and with added hydrocolloids (designated MPA and MPB, respectively); (2) to use LDA to investigate the possibility of objective discrimination among the different performance conditions of MP samples on the basis of descriptive sensory properties; and (3) to reduce the number of sensory properties by means of linear combinations of these, using PCA. The reliability of the sensory attributes is also discussed in some detail.

MATERIALS AND METHODS

Materials and Preparation of MP Samples

The potatoes used were tubers (cv Kennebec) from Aguilar de Campoo (Burgos, Spain). INL (Orafti®HP, BENEO-Orafti, Tienen, Belgium) was a 'long-chain' INL with a degree of polymerisation, DP > 23 and purity of 99.5% (producer's data). EVOO (Carbonell, Sevilla, Spain) was chosen for addition to MP. Kappa-carrageenan (κ-C) (GENULACTA carrageenan type LP-60) and xanthan gum (XG) (Keltrol F [E]) were donated by Premium Ingredients, S.L. (Girona, Spain). I/EVOO blends were added to the samples at five different INL:EVOO ratios (15 g kg^{-1} (INL)/45 g kg^{-1} (EVOO), 15:45; 30 g kg^{-1} (INL)/30 g kg^{-1} (EVOO), 30:30; 45 g kg^{-1} (INL)/15 g kg^{-1} (EVOO), 45:15; 30 g kg^{-1} (INL)/45 g kg^{-1} (EVOO), 30:45; 45 g kg^{-1} (INL)/30 g kg^{-1} (EVOO), 45:30). Samples without added ingredients (0:0 control), with 60 g kg^{-1} added EVOO alone (0:60) and with 60 g kg^{-1} added INL alone (60:0) were also prepared for each type of MP and processing conditions. In this way, the effect of adding ingredients (0:0 vs. 0:60/15:45/30:30/45:15/60:0 or vs. 30:45/45:30), the effect of the variation of INL:EVOO ratio at a fixed total concentration (0:60/15:45/30:30/45:15/60:0) and the effect of either adding EVOO at a fixed INL concentration (30:30/30:45 or 45:15/45:30) or adding INL at a fixed EVOO content (15:45/30:45 or 30:30/45:30) can be analysed.

Tubers were manually washed, peeled and diced. MP samples were prepared in ~2000-g batches from 1185 g of potatoes, 450 mL of semi-skimmed in-bottle sterilised milk (fat content, 15.5 g kg^{-1}), 300 mL of water, 15 g of salt (NaCl) and the corresponding EVOO concentration (0-60 g kg^{-1}) using a TM 31 food processor (Vorwerk España, M.S.L., S.C., Madrid, Spain). INL (0-60 g kg^{-1}) was previously dissolved in 750 mL of water and milk at 70 °C for 15 min, agitating with a magnetic stirrer at 600 r.p.m. MP were prepared without and with added κ-C and XG (MPA and MPB samples, respectively). In the latter case, hydrocolloids (each at 1.5 g kg^{-1}) were added to the rest of ingredients in the form of a dry powder. The ingredients were first heated to 90 °C (17 °C min^{-1}) and kept at 90 °C for 30 min (blade speed: 40 r.p.m.) [20, 21]. Shearing was performed with a propeller. The amount of evaporated liquid was determined by weighing the ingredients before and after the first cooking and then replaced by adding milk. Next, all the ingredients were cooked for an additional 5 min at 90 °C. The mash was ground for 40 s (blade speed: 1200 r.p.m.) and 20 s (blade speed: 2600 r.p.m.), and then homogenised immediately through a stainless steel sieve (diameter: 1.5 mm). Two batches were continuously being prepared and blended and half of each fresh blend (FMP samples) was analysed immediately whilst the other half was subjected to a freeze/thaw cycle (F/TMP samples). Each MP composition was prepared twice but in different weeks to assure the appropriate experiment randomization.

Freezing, Thawing and Heating Processes

Following their preparation, MP samples were placed on flat freezing and microwave thawing trays and then frozen by forced convection with liquid nitrogen vapour in an Instron programmable chamber (model 3119-05, −70/+250 °C) at −60 °C until their thermal centres reached −24 °C [22]. After freezing, the samples were packed in polyethylene plastic bags, sealed under light vacuum (–0.05 MPa) on a Multivac packing machine (Sepp Haggenmüller KG, Wolfertschwenden, Germany), and placed in a domestic freezer for storage at −24 °C. Packed frozen samples with the plastic bags perforated were then thawed in a Samsung M1712N microwave oven (Samsung Electronics S.A., Madrid, Spain) by heating for 20 min at an output power rating of 600 W. After thawing, the temperature reached at the product thermal centre was measured in all cases (+85 ± 3 °C). Samples were brought to 55 °C by placing them in a Hetofrig CB60VS water-bath (Heto Lab Equipment A/S, Birker∅d, Denmark). The sample testing temperature was maintained at 55 °C as this is the preferred temperature for consumption of MP [19-23].

Rheological Characterisation: Oscillatory Dynamic Tests

A Bohlin CVR 50 controlled stress rheometer (Bohlin Instruments Ltd., Cirencester, UK) was used to conduct small amplitude oscillatory shear (SAOS) experiments using a plate-plate sensor system with a 2 mm gap (PP40, 40 mm) and a solvent trap to minimise moisture loss during tests. After loading the sample, there was a 5-min waiting period to allow the sample to recover and reach 55 °C. Temperature control at 55 °C was achieved with a Peltier Plate system (-40 to +180 °C; Bohlin Instruments). In order to determine the linear viscoelastic (LVE) region, the first stress sweeps were run at a constant frequency (ω) of 1 rad s^{-1} over a shear stress range of 3-300 Pa. The LVE range was limited to that amplitude range for which the complex modulus (G^*) was constant [24]. Loss tangent ($\tan\delta = G''/G'$), storage modulus (G', Pa) and loss modulus (G'', Pa) values were also registered within the LVE region. The G' represents the non-dissipative component of mechanical properties and is characteristic of elasticity, while G'' represents the dissipative component of the mechanical properties and is characteristic of viscous flow [25]. Next three frequency sweeps were performed over the ω range of 0.1-100 rad s^{-1}, and again the $\tan\delta$, G' and G'' values were registered at 1 rad s^{-1}. Given that the appearance of the data on logarithmic data was nearly linear, a power law model was used to characterise the frequency dependence of both moduli [24, 26], from the following equations:

$$G' = G_0' \cdot \omega^{n'}$$

$$G'' = G_0'' \cdot \omega^{n''}$$

Where G_0' and G_0'' are elastic and viscous moduli at 1 rad s^{-1} respectively, and exponents n' and n'' denote the influence degree of ω on both moduli.

As a new sample was used each time for the dynamic tests, the resulting values were average values of the four determinations.

Table 1. Composition and processing of the samples studied with codes used for their identification

INL ($g\ kg^{-1}$)	EVOO ($g\ kg^{-1}$)	κ-C + XG ($g\ kg^{-1}$)	Processing	Sample code
0	0	-	Fresh	FMPA-0:0
0	60	-	Fresh	FMPA-0:60
15	45	-	Fresh	FMPA-15:45
30	30	-	Fresh	FMPA-30:30
45	15	-	Fresh	FMPA-45:15
60	0	-	Fresh	FMPA-60:0
30	45	-	Fresh	FMPA-30:45
45	30	-	Fresh	FMPA-45:30
0	0	1.5 + 1.5	Fresh	FMPB-0:0
0	60	1.5 + 1.5	Fresh	FMPB-0:60
15	45	1.5 + 1.5	Fresh	FMPB-15:45
30	30	1.5 + 1.5	Fresh	FMPB-30:30
45	15	1.5 + 1.5	Fresh	FMPB-45:15
60	0	1.5 + 1.5	Fresh	FMPB-60:0
30	45	1.5 + 1.5	Fresh	FMPB-30:45
45	30	1.5 + 1.5	Fresh	FMPB-45:30
0	0	-	Frozen/thawed	F/TMPA-0:0
0	60	-	Frozen/thawed	F/TMPA-0:60
15	45	-	Frozen/thawed	F/TMPA-15:45
30	30	-	Frozen/thawed	F/TMPA-30:30
45	15	-	Frozen/thawed	F/TMPA-45:15
60	0	-	Frozen/thawed	F/TMPA-60:0
30	45	-	Frozen/thawed	F/TMPA-30:45
45	30	-	Frozen/thawed	F/TMPA-45:30
0	0	1.5 + 1.5	Frozen/thawed	F/TMPB-0:0
0	60	1.5 + 1.5	Frozen/thawed	F/TMPB-15:45
15	45	1.5 + 1.5	Frozen/thawed	F/TMPB-30:30
30	30	1.5 + 1.5	Frozen/thawed	F/TMPB-45:15
45	15	1.5 + 1.5	Frozen/thawed	F/TMPB-60:0
60	0	1.5 + 1.5	Frozen/thawed	F/TMPB-0:60
30	45	1.5 + 1.5	Frozen/thawed	F/TMPB-30:45
45	30	1.5 + 1.5	Frozen/thawed	F/TMPB-45:30

Colour Measurements

The colour of the MP samples in the pots was measured using a HunterLab model D25 (Reston, VA, USA) colour difference meter fitted with a 5-cm-diameter aperture. Results were expressed in accordance with the CIELAB system with reference to illuminant D65 and a visual angle of 10°. The parameters determined were L^* ($L^* = 0$ [black] and $L^* = 100$ [white]), a^* ($-a^*$ = greenness and $+a^*$ = redness), b^* ($-b^*$ = blueness and $+b^*$ = yellowness), C^* chroma (saturation) and H^* hue, as defined by the following equations:

$C^* = (a^{*2} + b^{*2})^{1/2} \quad H^* = \arctan (b^* / a^*)$

The colour was expressed as L^*/b^*, i.e. the white/ yellow ratio [17]. The total colour difference (ΔE^*) between the fresh control made without either added hydrocolloids or ingredients and the rest of the MP samples was calculated as follows:

$$\Delta E^* = \left[\left(\frac{L_n^* - L_1^*}{K_L\, S_L} \right)^2 + \left(\frac{C_n^* - C_1^*}{K_C\, S_C} \right)^2 + \left(\frac{H_n^* - H_1^*}{K_H\, S_H} \right)^2 \right]^{1/2}$$

Where L_1^*, C_1^* and H_1^* are the reference (fresh sample) colour parameter values and S_L = 1.0, $S_C = 1 + 0.045C_1^*$ and $S_H = 1 + 0.015C_1^*$. K_L, K_C, and K_H are parametric factors and vary with the experimental conditions. All were given a fixed unit value for the combination of our specific reference conditions [20].

Sensory Analysis

Samples were subjected to a quantitative descriptive analysis (QDA) adapted for each product [15]. Sensory evaluation was conducted by an eight-member panel with 9 years'specific training in potato purées [16-23]. Each sample was tested twice and average scores calculated, so that each sample was tested sixteen times in all. Panellists were asked to evaluate samples for appearance [authentic colour (Aucol), off-colours (Offcol), shine (Shi) and uniformity (Unicol)], texture [consistency (Con), adhesiveness (Adh), creaminess (Cre) and fibrousness (Fib)], and taste [sweetness (Swe), authentic taste (Autas), off-taste (Offtas) and ingredient taste (Ingtas)]. Scores were awarded on a scale of 1–5, in which 1 indicated total absence of the sensory attribute and 5 a very definite attribute.

Samples were evaluated, in duplicate, in morning sessions (11:00 a.m.-1:00 p.m.). Daily for 64 days, assessors were given one sample (about 50 g), for scoring the sensory attributes of the 32 total samples (FMPA, FMPB, F/TMPA and F/TMPB products with added 0:0, 0:60, 15:45, 30:30, 45:15, 60:0, 30:45 and 45:30 ratios). The corresponding controls (FMPA-0:0, FMPB-0:0, F/TMPA-0:0 or F/TMPB-0:0 samples) were used for reference together with the evaluated sample every day. All the samples were served in white plastic vessels at a temperature of 55 ± 1 °C, which was reached and kept constant by placing the product in a Hetofrig CB60VS (Heto Lab Equipment A/S, Birkerød, Denmark) water bath prior to testing.

Statistical Analysis

A three-way ANOVA with interactions was applied to evaluate how (INL + EVOO) blend, presence or absence of hydrocolloids and performance or not of a freeze/thaw cycle affected the oscillatory rheological properties and characteristics derived, and the colour of the MP. Minimum significant differences were calculated using Fisher's least significant difference (LSD) tests with a 99% confidence interval for the comparison of instrumental parameters.

Sensory attributes from the quantitative descriptive analysis (QDA) (discrete values) were subjected to Friedman two-factor ranked analysis of variance ($k = 16$ and $N = 8$; FMP and F/TMP samples were analysed separately), and where differences existed between samples a regular Wilcoxon signed rank test was used to pinpoint them [27]. As recommended by the ISO 8587 [28], the Friedman test was considered to establish the statistical significance of the differences that the panellists might detect between samples. Linear discriminant analysis (LDA) was performed on the FMP and F/TMP samples considered separately ($n = 128$) to determine variability across the different sensory attribute scores in terms of addition of hydrocolloids and (INL + EVOO) blend.

In the case of highly correlated data, typical of sets of food-quality measurements, Principal component analysis (PCA) may be utilised to reduce the data set into a smaller number of principal components that explain *most* of the inter-relationships among the variables in the data. In the situation where some or all of the variables are categorical, rather than 'standard' PCA, the more appropriate technique is categorical principal component analysis (CATPCA). CATPCA analyses were conducted on the FMP and F/TMP samples considered separately ($n = 128$) to investigate the interdependence of the sensory attributes via identification of new, uncorrelated variables.

Analogously, the Cronbach's coefficient α was used as reliability test [29], which was performed on the FMP and F/TMP samples considered separately ($n = 128$) to establish the levels of reability of the scores for each sensory property evaluated. All the mentioned analyses were performed using SPSS 19.0 software (SPSS, Inc., Chicago, IL, USA).

RESULTS AND DISCUSSION

Dynamic Rheological Properties

The common tests performed using small-amplitude oscillatory shear analyses are stress sweeps (for controlled stress rheometers), frequency sweeps, time sweeps, and temperature sweeps [30]. To better understand the structural changes that took place in the INL-EVOO-based MP structures, the influence of frequency in their viscoelastic properties was studied at 55 °C. Prior to the measurement of the mechanical spectra, it was necessary to determine the LVE region (i.e. the range in which G' and G'' are independent of the stress/strain of the oscillation) [31]. As a general rule for solutions and gels, G' departs from linearity sooner than G''; therefore, to determine the LVE region, the component elastic was measured at a constant frequency of 0.16 Hz. The length of the LVE region varied with the composition of the samples, especially with the presence or absence of hydrocolloids and the performance or not of a freeze/thaw cycle, but in all the samples, a strain amplitude lower than 0.5% was comprised within the LVE region. Thus, frequency sweeps were performed at <0.5%. As an example, Figure 1 shows the stress sweeps of three FMPA samples. Dynamic curves of storage modulus G' (elastic component) are presented as functions of strain γ over four decades of strain. Above the LVE limit, G' decreased rapidly in all samples, indicating that the structure was highly prone to deformation. This is an appropriate test for analysing the gel character ($G' > G''$) of samples, since as long as the strain amplitudes are below the limiting value (γ_{max}) the G^* [measurement of the overall resistance (elastic and viscous)] pattern has a plateau value, indicating that the gel structure is stable under these conditions [32].

The frequency dependence of *G'* and *G"* (mechanical spectra) of the different INL-EVOO-based MP samples before and after the freeze/thaw cycle is shown in Figure 2.

A material that is frequency independent over a large time scale range is solid-like; a true gel is such a material. In contrast, strong frequency dependence suggest a material structure with molecular entanglements that behaves more like a solid at higher frequencies and more like a liquid at lower frequencies [33]. The difference between the strong (true) gel and the weak gel can be established using mechanical spectroscopy [32, 34]. In the former, the molecular rearrangements within the network are reduced over the time scales analysed; *G'* is higher than *G"* and almost independent of ω (low and similar *n'* and *n"* parameters).

In this chapter, the mechanical spectra revealed the existence of soft gels, with values of *G'* higher than values of *G"* and with a weak dependence with frequency throughout the frequency range measured (Figure 2). Such behaviour has been reported elsewhere in tomato and vegetable purée-based baby foods [35, 36]. In each food, the rheological behaviour is directly related to its formulation; the conformational changes experienced by potato starch were largely responsible for the predominantly elastic behaviour of the systems. However, significant differences were found between the viscoelastic properties and rheological characteristics recorded for MP made under different conditions. It is then observed that the rheology of these mixtures is governed by a continuous phase (amylose/amylopectin matrix), and eventually modify by the presence of INL/EVOO blends. In FMPA, FMPB and F/TMPB products (Figures 2a, 2b, 2d, respectively), the sample with no (INL+EVOO) blends exhibited greater elasticity than those with added INL/EVOO content. This indicates a shift in the viscoelastic behaviour of the samples with added INL:EVOO ratios towards more viscous-like products. In F/TMPA systems (Figure 2c), the sample with 60 g kg^{-1} added INL had significantly higher *G'* value than the 0:0 control. González-Tomás et al. [31] reported that by adding 7.5% of long-chain INL to low-fat starch-based custard desserts they obtained viscoelastic properties similar to the whole-milk sample.

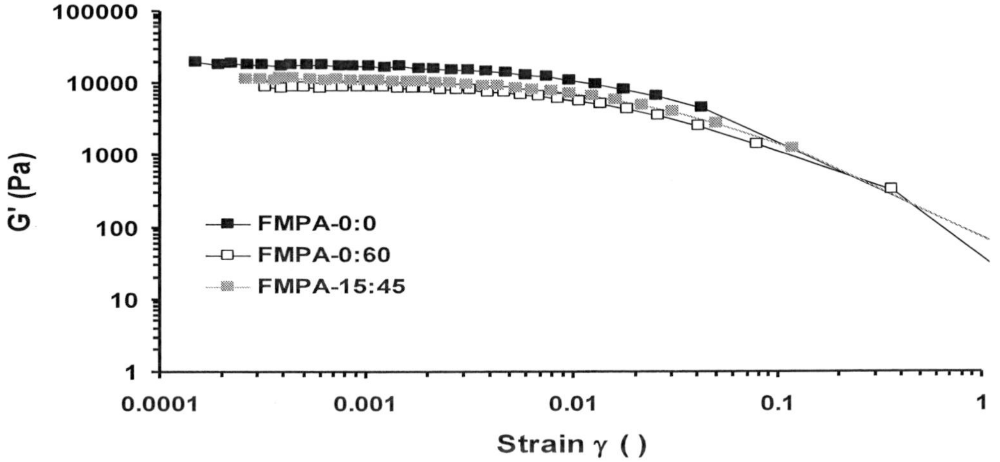

Figure 1. Stress sweeps of three freshly prepared mashed potatoes without added hydrocolloids and with added INL:EVOO ratios of 0:0, 0:60 and 15:45.

Frozen/thawed counterparts exhibited lower elasticity (Figures 2c, 2d). In contrast, Navarro et al. [24] found higher *G*' values in slowly frozen corn starch pastes compared with unfrozen and with quickly frozen samples. The slowly frozen starch systems showed also lower resistance to the applied stress despite their higher rigidity. The effect of freezing rate was explained due to the fact that the slow decrease in temperature gave amylose molecules higher opportunity to align and to release water trapped within the amylose network, favouring amylose retrogradation. In addition, slower freezing rates favoured large ice crystal formation, which distorted the system structure and contributed to thickening of the amylose network. In this chapter, both XG and κ-C are added to the MP to ameliorate the detrimental effects (syneresis, amylose retrogradation and rheological changes) of a freeze/thaw cycle [21]. Analoguosly, the addition of small amounts of XG to white sauces made with starches from different botanical sources significantly improved freeze/thaw stability [37]. According to the latter authors, this was probably due to XG interaction with solubilised amylose, reducing amylose-amylose interactions and therefore the extent of retrogradation. However, it was also reported that XG does not prevent ice recrystallisation or amylopectin retrogradation [38]; the fact that XG fails to prevent the latter is attributed to the fact that the gum acts outside the starch granule while amylopectin retrogradation takes place in the granule. Therefore, the decrease in the *G*' and *G*" values detected in the F/TMP samples as compared to their FMP counterparts could be attributed to amylopectin retrogradation associated with the freeze/thaw cycle.

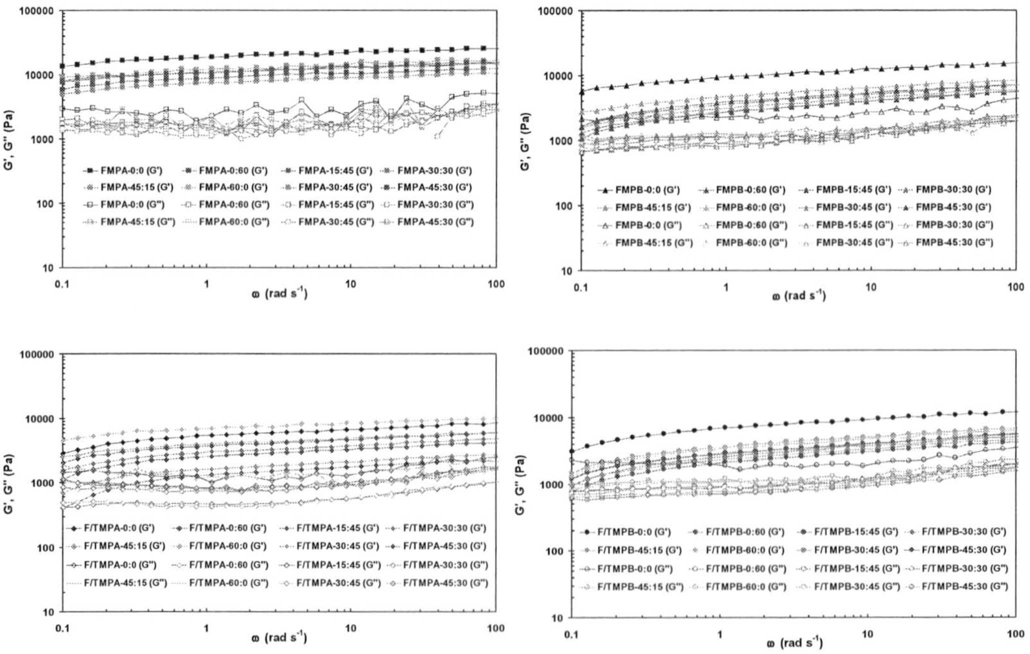

Figure 2. Dynamic properties, storage modulus (*G*', Pa) and loss modulus (*G*", Pa) versus frequency (rad s^{-1}) for fresh (FMP) and frozen/thawed mashed (F/TMP) potatoes with added different INL:EVOO ratios (0:0, 0:60: 15:45, 30:30, 45:15, 60:0, 30:45 and 45:30). (a) FMP without added hydrocolloids (FMPA). (b) FMP with added hydrocolloids (FMPB). (c) F/TMP without added hydrocolloids (F/TMPA). (d) F/TMP with added hydrocolloids (F/TMPB).

Moreover, both FMPA and F/TMPA samples were more elastic and presented a significantly higher magnitude of *G*' than the samples with added hydrocolloids. The storage modulus of the matrix is attenuated by the presence of κ-C and XG, the effect being stronger after a freeze/thaw cycle. Note as in FMPA samples (Figure 2a), some oscillation in *G*" data may be appreciated, which could indicate a significant effect of slippage on viscosity in freshly prepared MP samples formulated without added hydrocolloids. In contrast, hydrocolloids addition attenuated the differences in the loss modulus of the MP samples made with added INL:EVOO ratios (Figures 2b and d). Rodríguez-Hernández and Tecante [39] found that xanthan exerted a greater effect on *G*", while *i*-carrageenan exerted a greater effect on *G*'. This result could be attributed to the fact that XG does not form gels and therefore its presence has a greater impact on the viscose rather than on the elastic response.

In turn, Table 2 shows the results of three-way ANOVA for dynamic rheological properties (tanδ, *G*' and *G*") and rheological characteristics (*G*'/*G*" and slopes of storage and loss moduli (*n*' and *n*", respectively)) with INL:EVOO ratio, hydrocolloid addition and a freeze/thaw cycle as the main effects. For the confidence level of 99% ($P < 0.01$), significant differences were found between means due to INL:EVOO ratio and hydrocolloid addition for all the dynamic properties and rheological characteristics, whereas only nonsignificant differences were found between means due to a freeze/thaw cycle for *n*". The average value of the *G*'/*G*" ratio was close to 5 for the MPA and FMP samples and nearly 3 for the MPB and F/TMP ones, supporting that the fresh product without added hydrocolloids behaves like a stronger gel structure (Figure 2a). On the other hand, the samples with higher INL content (ratios 45:15 and 60:0) presented higher *G*'/*G*" ratio values, although these values were similar to that of the control without added ingredients. However, samples with higher EVOO concentrations (ratios 0:60 and 30:45) had lower *G*'/*G*" ratio values. This result is to be expected as increasing concentrations of liquid oil are added to the product, increasing the oil-phase volume fraction. In oil-in-water emulsions, the extent of the linear region decreased with increasing oil-phase volume fraction from 20 to 40% v/v [40]. For their part, Dickinson and Chen [41] suggested that oil/water emulsions may undergo a behaviour transition from predominantly entropic behaviour to predominantly enthalpic behaviour, with increasing oil-phase volume fraction.

In order to rationalise these results, it may be thought that the amylose/amylopectin constitutes a matrix, in which INL crystallites and oil droplets would act as filler particles. This speculation is in agreement with the microstructure observed in INL-EVOO-based MP samples [42], where amylose/amylopectin forms a rigid matrix in which INL particles are trapped. Moreover, in this framework, INL crystallites should be regarded as inactive fillers, as they contribute negatively to the viscosity of continuous phase (somehow inhibiting the cross-linking between amylose/amylopectin chains, and hence weakening the polysaccharide matrix). This behaviour is typical of gels filled with deformable particles [43]. According to the latter authors, in gels containing deformable particles, the linear decrease in *G*' in line with increasing volume fractions is due to particle compliance under stress or to particle separation from the matrix, thereby causing gel weakening. Zimeri and Kokini [44] also observed the presence of INL crystals, by optical microscopy, which were immersed in the continuous phase in samples with 5% long-chain INL. They postulated that these crystals may be the result of recrystallisation or decreased INL solubility due to cooling the hot dispersions. In turn, Bayarri et al. [45] observed by SEM, the presence of some INL aggregates embedded in the continuous matrix of starch-dairy systems, which were attributed to recrystallisation mechanism.

The influence of particle-matrix interactions was also studied by van Vliet [46] who found that a linear decrease in gel strength accompanied by an increase in volume fractions only occurred with non-interacting gel materials. This finding was attributed to the formation of aqueous boundary layers around each particle so that there was no adhesion between the particle and the matrix. As stress is applied to the system, small amounts of water may be released from the INL crystallites, thus forming an aqueous boundary layer around them. This layer would reduce any interactions with the amylose/amylopectin matrix and lead to the formation of weak points in the gelatinised starch gel. Consequently, when these gels suffer small deformations, they behave as if filled with particles with the rheological properties of water.

Table 2. Effects of INL:EVOO ratio, hydrocolloid addition and a freeze/thaw cycle on viscoelastic properties, rheological characteristics and colour parameters of MP samples

Source	tanδ	G' (Pa)	G'' (Pa)	G'/G''	n'	n''	L*/b*	ΔE*
Main effects:								
A: INL:EVOO ratio								
0:0	0.24_{e}	10144.00_{a}	1974.00_{a}	4.66_{a}	0.127_{e}	0.077_{f}	9.94_{b}	1.28_{g}
0:60	0.32_{a}	3848.31_{f}	914.22_{de}	3.65_{e}	0.166_{a}	0.121_{a}	5.57_{f}	8.02_{a}
15:45	0.28_{bc}	4806.69_{e}	1019.92_{cd}	3.97_{bc}	0.159_{b}	0.113_{bc}	6.12_{e}	5.90_{b}
30:30	0.29_{bc}	5205.44_{d}	1126.56_{c}	3.95_{cd}	0.151_{c}	0.106_{cd}	6.80_{d}	4.38_{c}
45:15	0.26_{de}	5932.12_{c}	1266.54_{b}	4.45_{a}	0.135_{d}	0.085_{e}	8.03_{c}	2.80_{f}
60:0	0.25_{e}	6303.31_{b}	1276.99_{b}	4.65_{a}	0.137_{d}	0.087_{e}	13.09_{a}	3.06_{e}
30:45	0.30_{b}	3580.25_{f}	874.36_{e}	3.71_{de}	0.157_{b}	0.114_{b}	6.10_{e}	5.74_{b}
45:30	0.27_{cd}	5085.56_{de}	1086.20_{c}	4.19_{b}	0.148_{c}	0.010_{d}	6.87_{d}	3.96_{d}
P values	<0.001	<0.001	<0.001	<0.001	<0.001	<0.001	<0.001	<0.001
LSD (99%)	*0.019*	*364.929*	*122.532*	*0.239*	*0.009*	*0.008*	*0.088*	*0.200*
B: Hydrocolloid addition								
Without κ-C and XG	0.22_{b}	7379.97_{a}	1229.07_{a}	5.14_{a}	0.112_{b}	0.082_{b}	8.13_{a}	3.45_{b}
With κ-C and XG	0.33_{a}	3846.45_{b}	1155.63_{b}	3.16_{b}	0.183_{a}	0.118_{a}	7.50_{b}	5.33_{a}
P values	<0.001	<0.001	0.0014	<0.001	<0.001	<0.001	<0.001	<0.001
LSD (99%)	*0.010*	*182.465*	*61.266*	*0.120*	*0.004*	*0.004*	*0.044*	*0.100*
C: A Freeze/thaw cycle								
Fresh	0.24_{b}	7728.97_{a}	1470.31_{a}	4.84_{a}	0.132_{b}	0.100_{a}	7.90_{a}	4.57_{a}
Frozen/thawed	0.31_{a}	3497.45_{b}	914.39_{b}	3.47_{b}	0.163_{a}	0.100_{a}	7.73_{b}	4.22_{b}
P values	<0.001	<0.001	<0.001	<0.001	<0.001	0.972	<0.001	<0.001
LSD (99%)	*0.010*	*182.465*	*61.266*	*0.120*	*0.004*	*0.004*	*0.044*	*0.100*
Interactions								
AB	<0.001	<0.001	<0.001	<0.001	<0.001	<0.001	<0.001	<0.001
AC	<0.001	<0.001	<0.001	<0.001	<0.001	<0.001	<0.001	<0.001
BC	<0.001	<0.001	<0.001	<0.001	<0.001	<0.001	<0.001	<0.001

INL, inulin; EVOO, extra virgen olive oil; κ-C, kappa-carrageenan; XG, xanthan gum. $_{abcdefg}$Different lower case letters in the same column and factor studied indicate significant diferences ($P < 0.01$).

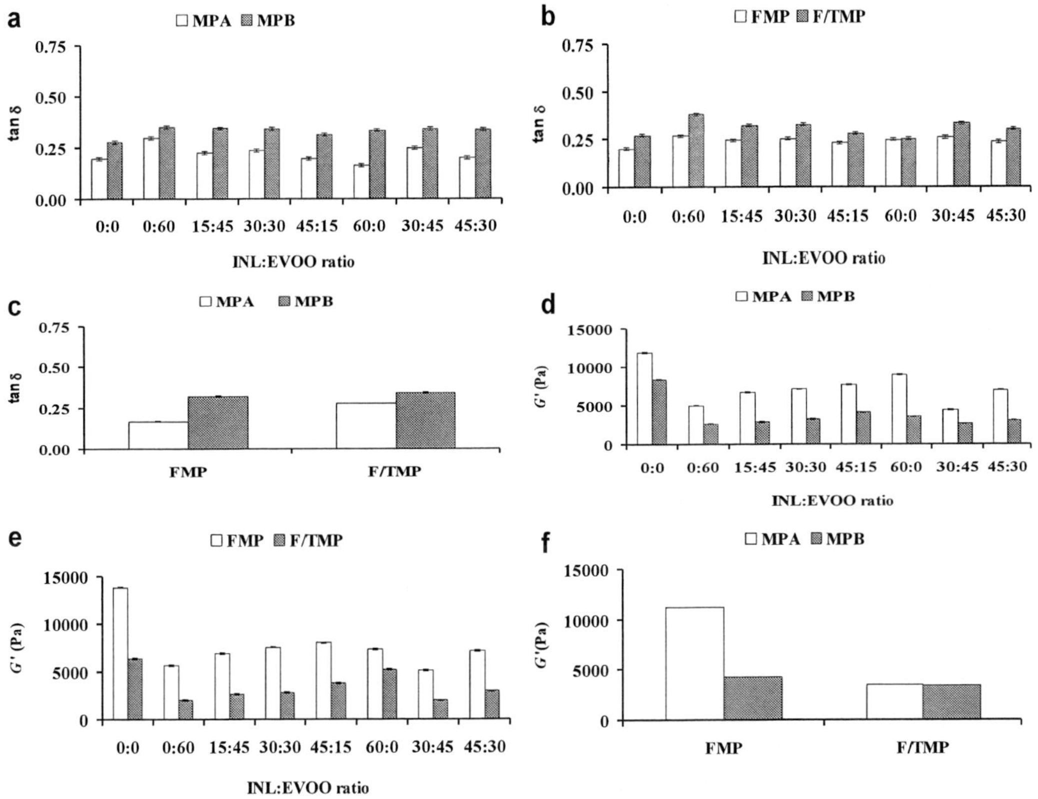

Figure 3. Rheological properties of MP samples: (a), (b), (c) loss tangent; (d), (e), (f) storage modulus. MPA: mashed potatoes without added hydrocolloids; MPB: mashed potatoes with added hydrocolloids; FMP: fresh mashed potatoes; F/TMP: mashed potatoes subjected to a freeze/thaw cycle; INL: inulin; EVOO: extra virgin olive oil.

In turn, Table 2 shows that the magnitudes of the resulting straight lines were small, and in all cases *n*'' values were lower than *n*' values, showing that *G*' was more frequency-dependent than *G*'' (Figure 2). The higher *n*' and *n*'' values were obtained for samples containing 60 g kg^{-1} EVOO, indicating that these systems possessed networks which were transient in time and involved specific interactions between denser and less flexible particles, such as droplet aggregates.The MP samples presented here contain either Na^+, from salt incorporation, or Ca^{2+} ions, proceeding mainly from added milk. One of the possible effects of Ca^{2+} ions is the formation of droplet aggregates through some Ca^{2+}-mediated bridging, as suggested by Sosa-Herrera et al. [47]. These aggregates could further disturb the formation of the polysaccharide matrix.

In addition, the three binary interactions between factors had a significant effect on all the dynamic properties and rheological characteristics, meaning that the effect of the INL:EVOO ratio on the rheological properties was dependent on the presence or absence of hydrocolloids and the performance or not of a freeze/thaw cycle. Graphs of the dynamic functions with different binary interactions are shown in Figures 3 and 4. The graph of variation in the tanδ value based on the INL:EVOO ratio for both MPA and MPB samples (Figure 3a) shows that, in all cases, tanδ was lower in the MPA than in the MPB samples. Therefore, the latter samples were softer because of XG-water interactions, which caused a decrease in starch-alone viscosity, confirming previous findings [26]. All the MPB samples had significantly higher tanδ values than the 0:0 control. As a result, addition of INL and/or EVOO (either alone or blended) produced softer, liquid-like systems. Note that the presence of hydrocolloids in the systems rendered the effect of the variation of the INL:EVOO ratio on the viscoelasticity in the MPB samples less appreciable. In the MPA products, the lowest tanδ value with respect to 0:0 control was recorded at a ratio of 60:0, indicating that in these systems the addition of INL alone gave rise to an improvement of solid character. This reinforcement of the structure could be attributed to the exclusion effect of the starch, which would lead to the formation of aggregates containing INL crystals [45].

The INL:EVOO ratio-dependent variation in tanδ value in both FMP and F/TMP samples is shown in Figure 3b. Except at a ratio of 60:0, FMP samples showed significantly lower tanδ values than their F/TMP counterparts; this could be ascribed to phase separation caused by retrogradation of the starch occurring in the frozen/thawed MPA systems [48]. In the F/TMP products, the variation of the INL:EVOO ratio at a fixed total concentration (60 g kg^{-1}) showed that when EVOO decreased and INL increased (0:60, 15:45 and 30:30 ratios) the products behaved like more solid systems, although there were nonsignificant differences in the loss tangent values of the samples with added 60:0 and 0:0 ratios (Figure 3b). Guggisberg et al. [49] observed that firmness and creaminess of low-fat set yogurt increased with both INL and fat content but the highest level of INL considered (4%) was not enough to imitate the whole-milk yogurt. In the FMP systems, all samples with added ingredients had significantly higher tanδ values than 0:0 control. In turn, the processing-dependent variation in tanδ value for MPA and MPB samples is shown in Figure 3c. A freeze/thaw cycle did not significantly affect sample viscoelasticity in the MPB samples but significantly increased it in MPA ones, corroborating the ability of κ-C and XG to provide freeze/thaw stability [21, 22, 26]. This fact was probably due to hydrocolloid interaction with solubilised amylose, reducing amylose-amylose interactions and therefore the extent of retrogradation [37].

The graph of variation in the G' value based on the INL:EVOO ratio for both MPA and MPB samples (Figure 3d) shows that, in all cases, elasticity was lower in the MPB than in the MPA samples. The probable explanation lies in the XG-water interactions that take place in the samples containing hydrocolloids [20, 21]. MPB samples occlude a great amount of water, which results in less shear thinning [42]. All the other samples (both MPA and MPB) had significantly lower values of G' with respect to 0:0 control. In both MPA and MPB products, the decrease in G' with respect to 0:0 ratio samples was greater when either 0:60 or 30:45 ratios were added, again indicating that addition of higher EVOO content caused more softening. At a fixed total concentration (60 g kg^{-1}), the elasticity increased linearly with increasing INL and decreasing EVOO concentrations. In the MPA products and at a fixed total concentration, the lowest and highest G' values were registered in samples with added 0:60 and 60:0, respectively. Also, at a fixed EVOO concentration, MPA sample elasticity decreased with INL content (15:45 vs. 30:45), whereas at a fixed INL concentration, elasticity significantly decreased with increasing EVOO concentration (30:30 vs. 30:45 and 45:15 vs. 45:30). These results suggest that EVOO was a more significant factor in the decrease in elasticity of the systems than INL.

FMP samples showed significantly higher G' values than their F/TMP counterparts (Figure 3e), which is ascribed to starch retrogradation occurring in the MPA samples subjected to a freeze/thaw cycle. In both FMP and F/TMP products, the variation of the INL:EVOO ratio at a fixed total concentration showed that when EVOO decreased and INL increased (0:60, 15:45, 30:30, 45:15 and 60:0 ratios or 30:45 and 45:30 ratios) the products behaved like more solid systems. This result is likely related to the formation of small insoluble INL particles. Such small particles can be produced by controlling heating and cooling of the dissolved INL to induce nucleation and thus small insoluble crystal formation [50]. Franck and De Leenheer [51] reported that at a high concentration (>15% for long-chain INL), INL forms a network composed of solid crystalline particles after shearing which confers gel-like texture to it. *G*' values seem to indicate that, in the MP systems, the presence of INL at quite high concentration ($\geq$ 45 g kg^{-1}) favoured the development and manifestation of its gelling properties. A freeze/thaw cycle significantly decrease *G*' in both MPA and MPB samples but the processing had a much less significant effect on the elasticity in the systems containing hydrocolloids (Figure 3f), again confirming the freeze-thaw stability conferred by the κ-C/XG blend [20, 42].

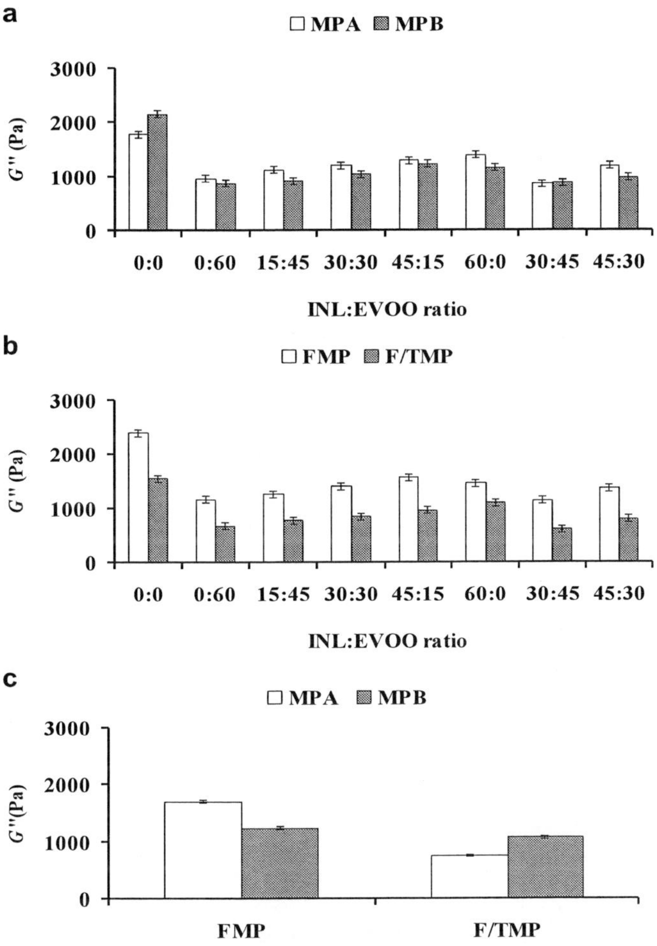

Figure 4. Rheological properties of MP samples: (a), (b), (c) loss modulus. MPA: mashed potatoes without added hydrocolloids; MPB: mashed potatoes with added hydrocolloids; FMP: fresh mashed potatoes; F/TMP: mashed potatoes subjected to a freeze/thaw cycle; INL: inulin; EVOO: extra virgin olive oil.

The variation in the *G*" values with the INL:EVOO ratio was very similar to that observed in the values of *G*' (Figure 4). The chief point of note is that differences in the viscosity of MPA samples with respect to their MPB counterparts (Figure 4a) were much less significant than those found for the elasticity (Figure 3d). On the other hand, at a ratio of 0:0, MPB samples showed significantly higher *G*" values than their MPA counterparts, again reflecting that in absence of INL/EVOO blends, xanthan exerted a greater effect on *G*" than on *G*' [21]. Analogously, a freeze/thaw cycle significantly decreased viscosity in both MPA and MPB samples, although the decrease was much less significant in the samples with added hydrocolloids (Figure 4c). This behaviour can be explained taking account that XG influenced the *G*" component more and the networks that are formed when solutions of XG are frozen and thawed are much stronger and more cohesive [52].

Instrumental Colour Measurements

Effects of INL:EVOO ratio, hydrocolloid addition and a freeze/thaw cycle on the values of the white/yellow ratio (L^*/b^*) and the total colour difference (ΔE^*) of the MP samples are also shown in Table 2. All the three main factors and their binary interactions had a significant effect on both L^*/b^* and ΔE^*. The variation in the L^*/b^* value based on INL:EVOO ratio for both MPA and MPB samples (Figure 5a) shows that in both cases, the lowest and highest L^*/b^* values were registered in the samples containing 0:60 and 60:0 ratios, respectively. Thus, addition of either EVOO alone or blended with INL produced a darker-coloured mashed potato (lower L^*/b^* ratio) than the 0:0 control. An increase in EVOO level favours either a higher L^* value (lightness) because of an increase in the overall light scattering associated with the scattering properties of fat [53], as well as a higher b^* value because of an increase in chloroplast pigment (chlorophyll and carotenoids) content. The pigment profile of the virgin olive oil comprises chlorophyll a, chlorophyll b and derivative pigments associated with the acidic medium of the oil extraction process [54]. The influence of droplet characteristics on the optical properties of coloured oil-in-water emulsions was examined [53]. The lightness (L^*) of the emulsions increased with increasing droplet concentration and decreasing droplet size. As the droplet concentration increases so does the reflectance because the droplets scatter light more effectively and hence the light beam is unable to penetrate further into the product and be absorbed.

In addition, in both MPA and MPB samples and at a fixed total concentration, L^*/b^* increased linearly with increasing and decreasing INL and EVOO contents, respectively (0:60, 15:45, 30:30, 45:15, 60:0). Unlike EVOO, INL produced a lighter-coloured mashed potato (higher L^*/b^* ratio). Commercially available INL is a spray-dried white powder which gives an opaque gel at higher concentrations when mixed properly with water [55]. In the case of INL/EVOO blends addition, except for the lowest EVOO content (60:0 ratio), all the other samples had significantly lower L^*/b^* values than the 0:0 control (Figure 5a), indicating that the darkening produced by EVOO addition is stronger than the lightening caused by INL incorporation. With regard to 0:0 control, increase yellowness caused by EVOO addition improved the product colour, as the flesh of Kennebec is too white [23, 42].

In turn, lack of colour in samples with added 60:0 ratio could be easily solved by addition of some β-carotene. Also, MPB samples had lower L^*/b^* values than MPA samples. In any case, colour parameter values of the MP samples with added 60:0 ratio indicate that the effect caused by hydrocolloid addition is weaker than the lightening produced by INL incorporation. By comparing both FMP and F/TMP samples (Figure 5b), it can be observed that at a fixed EVOO content, the increase in INL concentration did not significantly affect the colour of the MP samples (15:45 vs 30:45 and 30:30 vs 45:30); whereas at a fixed INL concentration addition of EVOO at higher concentrations considerably decreased L^*/b^* (30:30 vs 30:45 and 45:15 vs 45:30). In natural and commercial mashed potato, L^*/b^* values were lower than in the fresh controls after freezing and thawing of the samples, so that frozen-thawed were darker than fresh products [23]. Also, frozen mashed potato made from reconstituted potato flakes was darker than nonfrozen mashed potato [56].

In this study, note that the presence of EVOO significantly reduced differences in the L^*/b^* values among FMP samples and their F/TMP counterparts. As a consequence, a freeze/thaw cycle slightly decresased L^*/b^* ratio in the MPB samples but did not significantly affect it in the case of the MPA samples (Figure 5c). This is likely related to the water-holding capacity of the MPB samples, enhancing the overall light scattering of the MP.

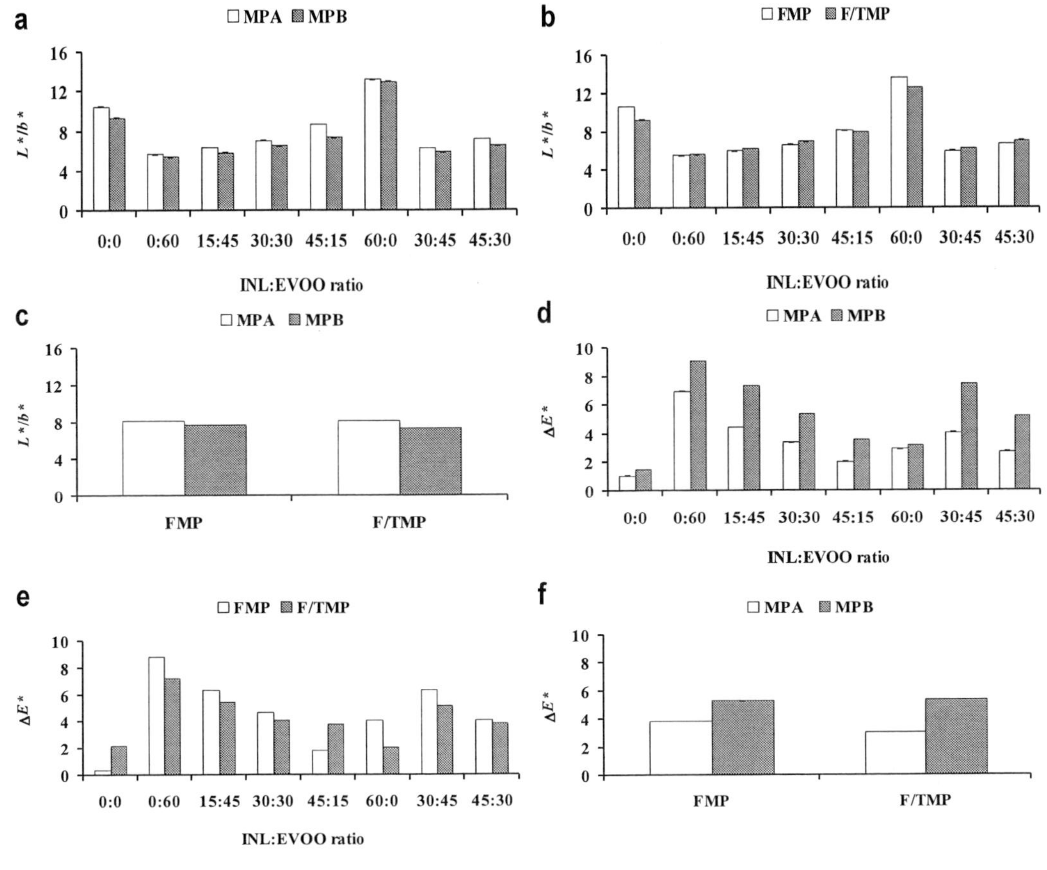

Figure 5. Instrumental colour measurements of MP samples: (a), (b), (c) white/yellow ratio; (d), (e), (f) total colour difference. MPA: mashed potatoes without added hydrocolloids; MPB: mashed potatoes with added hydrocolloids; FMP: fresh mashed potatoes; F/TMP: mashed potatoes subjected to a freeze/thaw cycle; INL: inulin; EVOO: extra virgin olive oil.

Sample colour differences with respect to the fresh INL-EVOO-free control, based on the INL:EVOO ratio for both MPA and MPB samples (Figure 5d) and for both FMP and F/TMP samples (Figure 5e), corroborates that in both cases, the highest and lowest ΔE^* values were registered in the samples containing 0:60 and 60:0 ratios, respectively. As the droplet concentration increases, more reflected light travels through the oil phase of the MP being absorbed by the pigments mentioned earlier, intensifying the colour of the MP. Moreover, in the MPB samples, there were non-significant differences between the ΔE^* values of FMP and F/TMP samples (Figure 5f).

Quantitative Descriptive Analysis (QDA)

The Friedman test showed that there were significant differences between FMP samples due to INL:EVOO ratios and hydrocolloid addition (Tables 3, 4) with regards to *authentic colour*, *shine* and *uniformity* (χ^2 = 38.99, χ^2 = 73.96 and χ^2 = 68.51, respectively; P = 0.000); *consistency*, *adhesiveness*, *creaminess* and *fibrousness* (χ^2 = 104.72, χ^2 = 106.72, χ^2 = 76.94 and χ^2 = 66.52, respectively; P = 0.000) (Table 3) and *authentic taste*, *off-taste* and *ingredient taste* (χ^2 = 72.09, χ^2 = 106.10 and χ^2 = 107.44, respectively; P = 0.000) (Table 4). The panellists found that neither INL/EVOO combinations nor hydrocolloid addition had any detectable effect on *off-colours* or *sweetness* (χ^2 = 0.00 and χ^2 = 9.96, respectively) in the FMP products. On the other hand, although there were significant differences between FMP samples with respect to *uniformity* and *off-taste*, 60 and 90% confidence intervals were needed to pinpoint them respectively, so no *uniformity* differences between ranks due to INL/EVOO blends and hydrocolloid addition were established (Table 3).

F/TMP samples (Tables 5, 6) presented significant differences in terms of *authentic colour*, *shine* and *uniformity* (χ^2 = 91.89, χ^2 = 51.37 and χ^2 = 44.63, respectively; P = 0.000); *consistency*, *adhesiveness*, *creaminess* and *fibrousness* (χ^2 = 106.34, χ^2 = 106.10, χ^2 = 78.20 and χ^2 = 49.86, respectively; P = 0.000) (Table 5) and *sweetness*, *authentic taste*, *off-taste* and *ingredient taste* (χ^2 = 35.88, χ^2 = 45.66, χ^2 = 30 and χ^2 = 108.438, respectively; P = 0.000) (Table 6). No INL:EVOO ratio or hydrocolloid addition effect on *off-colours* (χ^2 = 0.00) was detected by the panellists in the F/TMP products. However, although there were significant differences between F/TMP samples regarding *fibrousness*, *sweetness* and *authentic taste*, again a 90% confidence interval was needed to pinpoint them. In the case of F/TMP products, a 60% confidence interval was also needed to pinpoint the significant differences between F/TMP samples with respect to *uniformity* or *off-taste*, and therefore differences produced by INL/EVOO blends and hydrocolloid addition were not established for these attributes (Table 6).

Figures 6 and 7 show radar plots constructed to represent perceived sensory attributes. As far as sensory attributes describing appearance in FMP samples are concerned (Figure 6a), panellists gave FMPB-0:60, FMPA-15:45 and FMPB-30:45 samples higher scores for *authentic colour* than the rest of the samples, although only FMPA-0:0, FMPA-45:15, FMPA-60:0 and FMPB-60:0 differences were significant (Table 3), matching the results of instrumental colour measurements. Obviously, the colour of the ingredients used influences the colour of the product. INL is a white powder and when added alone produced a lighter-coloured mashed potato as indicated above. In INL-enriched dairy desserts, the average chain length of the added INL significantly affected brightness values but no other parameter.

Samples with long-chain INL were the lightest in colour [57], corroborating these findings. Conversely, it has been found that INL did not affect the colour values of low-fat ice cream [58], and the addition of oligofructose to dairy drinks did not affect the L^*, a^* and b^* values [59]. In contrast, sensory analysis indicated that adding $\geqslant$ 45 g kg^{-1} of EVOO significantly improved colour due to the yellowness conferred by the oil. The panellists found that increasing yellowness is desirable since, as mentioned above, the flesh of Kennebec potatoes is white and these MP without other added ingredients look rather pale. In the case of *shine*, the panellists found a significant difference between the FMPA-0:60 sample, which scored highest, and FMPA-0:0 and FMPB-0:0 controls, neither of which contained any EVOO (Figure 6a). Note that in the case of *uniformity* the panellists also identified FMPA-0:0 and FMPA-60:0 samples as having lower scores (Table 3) than all the other FMP samples. This could be ascribed to a lack of hydrocolloid-water interactions in the absence of XG, as well as to the absence of oil droplets, detected by the panellists.

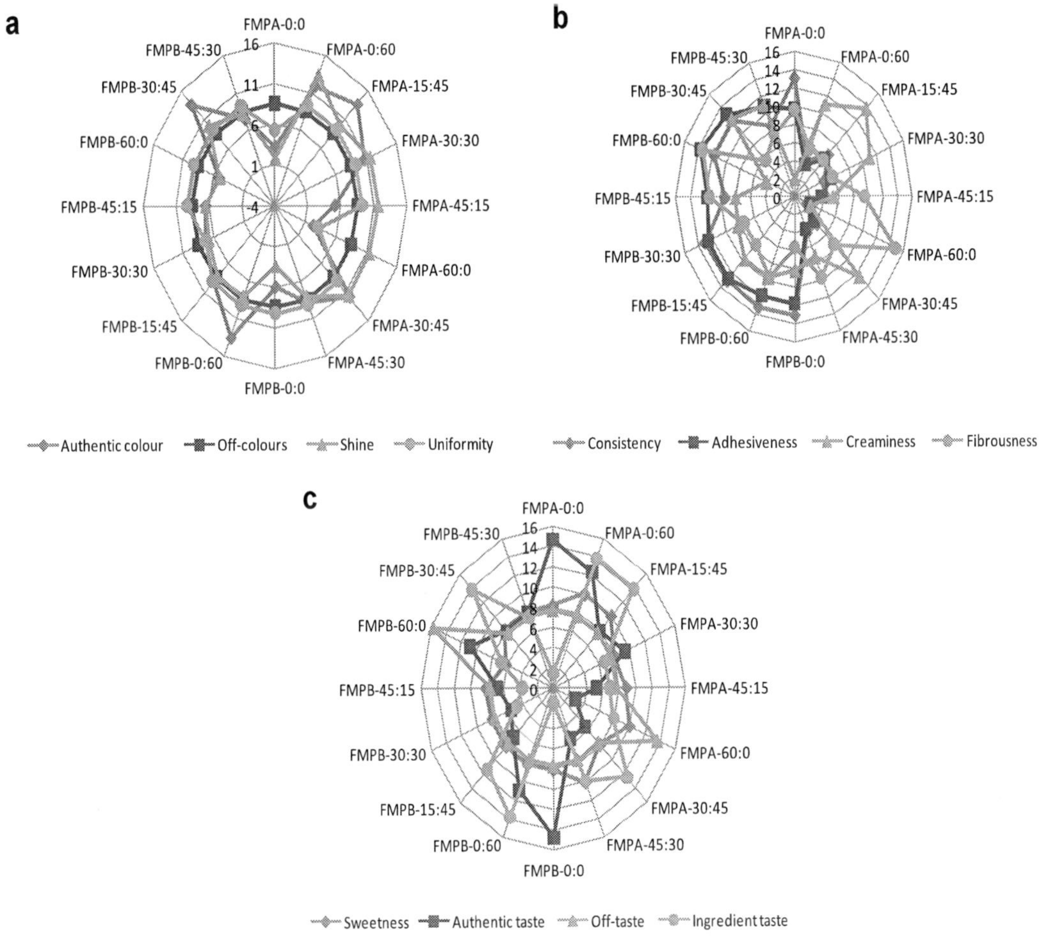

Figure 6. Sensory attributes as functions of INL:EVOO ratio in FMP samples: (a) appearance sensory attributes; (b) texture sensory attributes; (c) taste sensory attributes. Identification of system notation in Table 1. INL: inulin; EVOO: extra virgin olive oil.

Table 3. Effects of INL:EVOO ratio and hydrocolloid addition on mean ranks of sensory appearance and texture attributes for FMP samples

Sample code	Authentic colour	Off-colours	Shine	Uniformity	Consistency	Adhesiveness	Creaminess	Fibrousness
FMPA-0:0	$3.25*_{c}$	8.50	1.88_{c}	5.25*	13.00_{a}	$9.62*_{abcd}$	$2.00*_{c}$	$9.50*_{ab}$
FMPB-0:0	6.00_{abc}	8.50	3.38_{b}	9.25	13.00_{a}	11.75_{abc}	8.12_{abc}	5.62_{b}
FMPA-0:60	11.88_{ab}	8.50	$13.38*_{a}$	9.25	$4.25*_{bc}$	$3.75*_{cd}$	11.00_{ab}	$5.62*_{b}$
FMPB-0:60	13.62_{a}	8.50	8.25_{abc}	9.25	13.00_{a}	11.75_{abc}	9.62_{abc}	9.50_{ab}
FMPA-15:45	$13.62*_{a}$	8.50	10.00_{abc}	9.25	$6.50*_{abc}$	$5.75*_{abcd}$	$13.62*_{a}$	5.62_{b}
FMPB-15:45	9.12_{abc}	8.50	8.25_{abc}	9.25	13.00_{a}	12.75_{ab}	9.62_{abc}	7.50_{ab}
FMPA-30:30	$10.62*_{abc}$	8.50	11.50_{ab}	9.25	$4.25*_{bc}$	$5.25*_{bcd}$	$11.00*_{ab}$	5.62_{b}
FMPB-30:30	7.38_{abc}	8.50	6.75_{abc}	7.38	13.00_{a}	12.62_{ab}	8.38_{abc}	7.50_{ab}
FMPA-45:15	5.00_{bc}	8.50	$11.62*_{ab}$	9.25	$4.25*_{bc}$	$3.75*_{cd}$	$5.25*_{abc}$	9.50_{ab}
FMPB-45:15	6.38_{abc}	8.50	6.50_{abc}	9.25	9.50_{abc}	11.75_{abc}	8.12_{abc}	11.50_{ab}
FMPA-60:0	$2.25*_{c}$	8.50	$11.38*_{ab}$	3.12*	$1.75*_{c}$	$2.25*_{d}$	$2.38*_{c}$	14.88_{a}
FMPB-60:0	5.00_{bc}	8.50	5.00_{abc}	9.25	11.75_{ab}	13.75_{a}	4.12_{bc}	13.38_{ab}
FMPA-30:45	11.88_{ab}	8.50	11.62_{ab}	9.25	$4.25*_{bc}$	$3.75*_{cd}$	12.50_{ab}	7.50_{ab}
FMPB-30:45	13.62_{a}	8.50	10.00_{abc}	9.25	11.88_{ab}	12.88_{ab}	12.12_{ab}	5.62_{b}
FMPA-45:30	8.88_{abc}	8.50	8.25_{abc}	9.25	$4.25*_{bc}$	$3.88*_{cd}$	$7.12*_{abc}$	$9.62*_{ab}$
FMPB-45:30	7.50_{abc}	8.50	8.25_{abc}	9.25	8.38_{abc}	10.75_{abc}	11.00_{ab}	7.50_{ab}
χ^2 value	38.99	0.00	73.96	68.51	104.72	106.72	76.94	66.52
P value	0.000	1.000	0.000	0.000	0.000	0.000	0.000	0.000

a-d For each sensory attribute mean ranks without the same letter are significantly different ($P < 0.05$). *For each sensory attribute and for the same.

INL: EVOO ratio mean ranks between FMPA samples and their FMPB counterparts are significantly different ($P < 0.05$); FMPA: fresh mashed potatoes without added hydrocolloids; FMPB: fresh mashed potatoes with added hydrocolloids. INL, inulin; EVOO, extra virgin olive oil.

Table 4. Effects of INL:EVOO ratio and hydrocolloid addition on mean ranks of sensory taste attributes for FMP samples

Sample code	Sweetness	Authentic taste	Off-taste†	Ingredient taste
FMPA-0:0	8.12	14.62_a	7.62_b	1.50_d
FMPB-0:0	8.12	14.75_a	7.62_b	1.50_d
FMPA-0:60	10.00	12.38_{ab}	7.62_b	13.75_a
FMPB-0:60	8.12	10.88_{abc}	7.62_b	13.75_a
FMPA-15:45	10.00	8.00_{abc}	7.62_b	$13.75*_a$
FMPB-15:45	8.12	6.88_{abc}	7.62_b	11.25_{abc}
FMPA-30:30	8.12	$9.38*_{abc}$	7.62_b	6.75_{abcd}
FMPB-30:30	8.00	5.52_{abc}	7.62_b	4.75_{bcd}
FMPA-45:15	8.88	5.25_{bc}	7.62_b	$6.75*_{abcd}$
FMPB-45:15	8.12	6.75_{abc}	7.62_b	3.75_{cd}
FMPA-60:0	10.00*	$2.88*_c$	13.62_{ab}	7.88_{abcd}
FMPB-60:0	6.12	10.88_{abc}	15.62_a	6.75_{abcd}
FMPA-30:45	8.00	$5.38*_{bc}$	7.62_b	12.50_{ab}
FMPB-30:45	8.12	8.00_{abc}	7.62_b	13.75_a
FMPA-45:30	10.12	$5.38*_{bc}$	7.62_b	$10.00*_{abc}$
FMPB-45:30	8.00	8.00_{abc}	7.62_b	7.62_{abcd}
χ^2 value	9.96	72.09	106.10	107.44
P value	0.822	0.000	0.000	0.000

$_{a\text{-}d}$ For each sensory attribute mean ranks without the same letter are significantly different ($P < 0.05$). † For *off-taste* mean ranks without the same letter are significantly different ($P < 0.10$). * For each sensory attribute and for the same INL:EVOO ratio mean ranks between FMPA samples and their FMPB counterparts are significantly different ($P < 0.05$); FMPA: fresh mashed potatoes without added hydrocolloids; FMPB: fresh mashed potatoes with added hydrocolloids; INL, inulin; EVOO, extra virgin olive oil.

As can be seen from the sensory appearance attributes (Figure 7a) of the F/TMP samples, F/TMPA-60:0 had the lowest score for *authentic colour* (Table 5)and sample F/TMPB-45:15 scored the highest, though differences with F/TMPA-0:60, F/TMPB-0:60, F/TMPA-15:45, F/TMPB-15:45, F/TMPA-30:30, F/TMPB-30:30, F/TMPA-45:15, F/TMPA-30:45, F/TMPB-30:45, F/TMPA-45:30 and F/TMPB-45:30 samples were nonsignificant. It is obvious that the presence of EVOO, even at the lowest level, masked the lightening effect caused by INL incorporation, suggesting that panellists only detected loss of colour when samples with added INL alone were subjected to a freeze/thaw cycle. In the case of *shine*, the panellists distinguished a marked difference between the F/TMPB-0:0 control, which obtained the lowest score, and the F/TMPA-0:60 and F/TMPB-30:45 samples with the highest scores (although differences between F/TMPA-0:60 and F/TMPB-30:45 samples were nonsignificant).

With regards to the sensory texture attributes of FMP samples (Figure 6b, Table 3), in the case of *consistency* the panellists gave significantly higher scores to samples FMPA-0:0, FMPB-0:0, FMPB-0:60, FMPB-15:45 and FMPB-30:30 than to all the other samples (except for FMPA-15:45, FMPB-45:15, FMPB-60:0, FMPB-30:45 and FMPB45:30 samples). FMPA-60:0 scored lowest for this texture attribute. Therefore, the sensory panel indicated that 60 g kg^{-1} INL provided superior softening in FMP samples than 60 g kg^{-1} EVOO. Note that except for both controls, all the FMPB samples had higher scores for *consistency* than their FMPA counterparts. Conversely, both FMPA and F/TMPA samples were more elastic, with a significantly higher magnitude of *G'* than their counterparts with added hydrocolloids. A previous study showed that in MP samples, κ-C provided the appropriate texture, while XG imparted creaminess to the product, which was associated with an increase in the number of XG-water interactions [21]. The effect of κ-C on the thickening of the product was ascribed to the interaction of κ-C with denatured milk protein, while XG exhibited a considerably greater capacity (even at very low concentration) to retain water than κ-C. Therefore, it would appear that panellists were more sensitive to the effect of carrageenan in the products with added hydrocolloids, whereas rheological measurements would seem to measure the water holding capacity conferred by the gum. In the case of *adhesiveness* (Table 3), the panellists distinguished significant differences between the FMPB-60:0 sample, which scored the highest, and FMPA-0:60, FMPA-30:30, FMPA-45:15, FMPA-60:0, FMPA-30:45 and FMPA-45:30 samples, which obtained lower scores, possible because they did not contain hydrocolloids, thus confirming previous findings [16, 19, 21]. This fact is mainly ascribed to the absence of κ-C, indicating that *adhesiveness* is also affected by the gelling properties of the carrageenan.

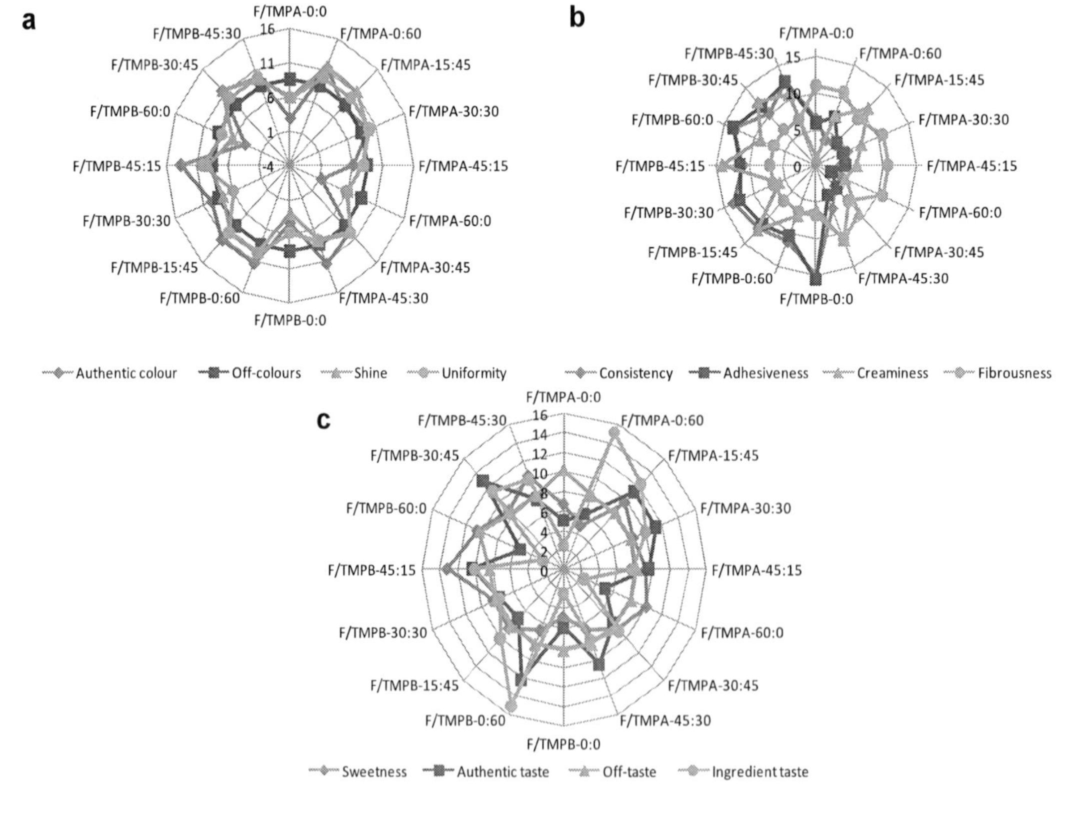

Figure 7. Sensory attributes as functions of INL:EVOO ratio in F/TMP samples: (a) appearance sensory attributes; (b) texture sensory attributes; (c) taste sensory attributes. Identification of system notation in Table 1. INL: inulin; EVOO: extra virgin olive oil.

For *creaminess* (Figure 6b), panellists distinguished a significant difference between the FMPA-0:0 control and the FMPA-60:0 sample with added INL alone, both of which had a lower score, and the FMPA-0:60, FMPA-15:45, FMPA-30:30, FMPA-30:45, FMPB-30:45 and FMPB-45:30 samples, which presented a softer mouthfeel. Therefore, by adding EVOO to FMP samples at concentrations $\geq$ 30 g kg^{-1}, either individually or blended with INL, increased their *creaminess* compared with the control without added ingredients or the product with added INL alone. In the experiments referred to in this chapter, panellists gave the FMPA-60:0 sample the highest score for *fibrousness*, although only the differences between this score and those for FMPB-0:0, FMPA-0:60, FMPA-15:45, FMPA-30:30 and FMPB-30:45 were significant (Table 3). An extensive description of creaminess, based on discussions with consumers, includes a range of sensations typically associated with fat content, such as a full sweet taste, compact smoothness, not rough, not dry, with a velvety (not oily) coating [11]. In various studies it has been shown that creaminess is strongly related to other sensory characteristics, such as the $\eta_{app,50}$ which was a principal factor influencing creaminess in MP with added XG, mainly at concentrations up to 1.5 g kg^{-1} [17]. For only dairy products a combination of thickness and smoothness was sufficient to predict creaminess reasonably well [60]. However, for other products creaminess was less well explained [61] indicating that other factors are also important, like for instance, fat content [62, 63]. Creaminess is negatively affected by texture attributes such as roughness [64, 65], and heterogeneous mouthfeel [64, 66]. On the other hand, in dairy desserts, the addition of long-chain INL gave rise to a low-fat product with the same thickness intensity as the full-fat sample [45], though less creamy, rougher and with more mouth coating, which was attributed by the latter authors to aggregate formation characterised by a rough outline.

In the F/TMP samples (Figure 7b, Table 5), panellists scored the F/TMPB-0:0 control higher for *consistency* and *adhesiveness* than any of the other samples, matching the results of oscillatory properties (Figure 2d). Furthermore, differences between F/TMPB-0:0 and the rest of the frozen/thawed samples with added hydrocolloids (F/TMPB samples) were nonsignificant for both *consistency* and *adhesiveness*, irrespective of the INL:EVOO ratio. A previous study showed that INL concentrations were responsible for minor difference in most rheological properties, firmness and overall acceptability of MP samples, whereas the addition of κ-C and XG resulted in the main differences between samples [26]. As the effect of INL on the thickening of the product was limited, the addition of small amounts of κ-C and XG to MP samples significantly improved freeze/thaw stability, confirming previous findings [21]. On the other hand, this result confirms that in the case of olive oil, a liquid product, textural attributes are not as significant as those of aroma and taste [9]. Panellists scored sample F/TMPB-45:15 the highest for *creaminess*, although only the differences between the score for this sample, and those for F/TMPA-0:0 control and F/TMPA-60:0, which had the highest INL concentrations, were significant (Table 5). Long-chain INL is used as a fat replacer in several dairy products [45] due to its ability to act as a fat mimetic or fat replacer, based on its capacity to form microcrystals, which interact with each other, forming small aggregates that occlude a great amount of water and that may ultimately agglomerate into a gel network [4, 49, 55]. However, the fat mimetic capacity of INL depends not only on the chain length, but also on the concentration of added INL [67]. Long-chain INL has been used in low-fat yogurts as a fat replacer where it was shown to significantly improve creaminess, mouthfeel, and smoothness [68, 69]. The addition of long-chain INL also improved creaminess and consistency of low-fat custards [70] and mimicked those of full-fat custard

[71]. Probably, INL at 45 g kg^{-1} enhanced creaminess in the F/TMPB samples thanks to the lubricating and coating properties either of the gum or the oil. In the case of *fibrousness* (Figure 7b, Table 5), the most important point to note is that panellists perceived greater *fibrousness* in the F/TMPA samples than in all their F/TMPB counterparts. Therefore, it was obvious that the assessors associated decreased *fibrousness* with the presence of hydrocolloids retarding starch retrogradation [37].

As regards the sensory taste attributes (Figure 6c, Table 4) of the FMP samples, in the case of *authentic taste*, the panellists noted that the FMPA-0:0 and FMPB-0:0 controls, which had the highest scores, differed significantly from the FMPA-45:15, FMPA-60:0, FMPA-30:45 and FMPA-45:30 samples, which scored the lowest. Panellists considered that MP without added ingredients produced an unpleasant taste in the mouth due to an excessively strong potato flavour. In addition, panellists scored the sample with added hydrocolloids and added INL alone, i.e. FMPB-60:0, significantly higher for *off-taste* than the rest of the samples. Analogously, increasing INL concentration by up to 6% significantly reduced the overall acceptability of all the FMPA, FMPB, F/TMPA and F/TMPB samples [26]. Panellists found that the addition of 6% INL gave the F/TMPB samples an unfamiliar taste and odour, despite the fact that differences between scores for both F/TMPA and F/TMPB samples were nonsignificant. Although INL has been considered to have a bland neutral taste without any off-flavour or aftertaste [72], its effect on the flavour of vanilla dairy desserts may be different from the effect of fat. The obvious influence of INL on sweetness and vanilla flavour intensity in skimmed milk samples with lower starch concentrations suggests a faster flavour release in these systems [71]. Conversely, samples FMPA-0:60, FMPB-0:60, FMPA-15:45 and FMPB-30:45 scored highest for *ingredient taste* (Table 4). Panellists ascribed these differences to an aromatic note detected in the MP samples with added EVOO at the highest concentrations. EVOO must have an acidity below 0.8% (like oleic acid) and a flavour that results purely from the fruit's metabolism, which yields fruity, bitter, and pungent characteristics, with no defects (a fusty, musty, winey, or rancid taste) [9]. Volatile compounds stimulate the olfactory receptors causing the perception of the whole aroma of the virgin olive oil [73]. The sensory characteristics of 22 EVOOs from California, Italy, Spain, Chile, and Australia were compared using a generic descriptive analysis [9]. With the exception of "thick" and "citrus", all sensory attributes were significantly different among the oils. Spanish EVOOs were characterised by their tropical fruit, herb, mint, floral, bitter, and pungent attributes. The effects of fat on odour and flavour attributes may be related to the flavour-releasing properties of fat. In sixteen virgin olive oils, volatile and phenolic compounds have been related to olfactory and gustative properties respectively [74]. The volatile composition revealed several correlations with olfactory attributes perceived by sensory analysis: the sum of aldehydes C_6 was correlated with the orthosonal perception of fruity olive and the retrosanal odour of almond.

F/TMPB-45:15 scored highest among the F/TMP products (Figure 7c, Table 6), as regards *sweetness*, whereas F/TMPB-0:0 and F/TMPA-0:60 samples had the lowest scores for this taste attribute. This indicates that, as expected, INL addition increased the sugariness of the F/TMP samples because of its higher total soluble solid content (TSS). In both MPA and MPB samples, the highest TSS values corresponded to samples with added INL alone (60:0 ratio) and were higher in the MPB samples, which is logical as two polysaccharides were also added to these MP samples [42]. Supplementation with INL introduced more reducing sugars and led to increased total carbohydrate content [75].

Table 5. Effects of INL: EVOO ratio and hydrocolloid addition on mean ranks of sensory appearance and texture attributes for F/TMP samples

Sample code	Authentic colour	Off-colours	Shine	Uniformity	Consistency	Adhesiveness	Creaminess	Fibrousness†
F/TMPA-0:0	2.88_{c}	8.50	6.00^{*}_{ab}	5.88	6.50^{*}_{bc}	5.88^{*}_{bcd}	1.12^{*}_{c}	10.88^{*}_{a}
F/TMPB-0:0	4.50_{bc}	8.50	3.00_{b}	5.88	15.00_{a}	15.62_{a}	6.00_{abc}	6.88_{b}
F/TMPA-0:60	11.38_{ab}	8.50	11.62_{a}	9.88	3.88^{*}_{c}	7.25^{*}_{abcd}	7.38_{abc}	10.88^{*}_{a}
F/TMPB-0:60	11.38_{ab}	8.50	9.62_{ab}	9.88	11.25_{abc}	10.38_{abcd}	7.38_{abc}	6.88_{b}
F/TMPA-15:45	8.00^{*}_{abc}	8.50	11.25_{ab}	9.88	3.88^{*}_{c}	4.38^{*}_{cd}	11.00_{ab}	8.88_{ab}
F/TMPB-15:45	11.38_{ab}	8.50	9.62_{ab}	9.88	12.25_{abc}	11.38_{abc}	12.50_{ab}	6.88_{b}
F/TMPA-30:30	9.62_{abc}	8.50	9.62_{ab}	9.88*	5.12^{*}_{bc}	4.38^{*}_{cd}	7.38_{abc}	10.88^{*}_{a}
F/TMPB-30:30	9.62_{abc}	8.50	7.75_{ab}	5.88	13.38_{ab}	12.38_{abc}	6.00_{abc}	6.88_{b}
F/TMPA-45:15	6.25^{*}_{abc}	8.50	7.75_{ab}	7.88	3.88^{*}_{c}	4.38^{*}_{cd}	6.12^{*}_{abc}	10.88^{*}_{a}
F/TMPB-45:15	13.50_{a}	8.50	9.25_{ab}	9.88	11.12_{abc}	11.38_{abc}	14.25_{a}	6.88_{b}
F/TMPA-60:0	1.38^{*}_{c}	8.50	6.00_{ab}	5.88	3.88^{*}_{c}	2.50^{*}_{d}	4.75^{*}_{bc}	10.88^{*}_{a}
F/TMPB-60:0	3.88_{bc}	8.50	6.00_{ab}	7.88	13.38_{ab}	13.50_{ab}	9.00_{abc}	6.88_{b}
F/TMPA-30:45	9.75_{abc}	8.50	9.62_{ab}	9.88	3.88^{*}_{c}	4.38^{*}_{cd}	9.12^{*}_{abc}	6.88_{b}
F/TMPB-30:45	11.38_{ab}	8.50	11.50_{a}	9.88	10.00_{abc}	11.50_{abc}	12.38_{ab}	6.88_{b}
F/TMPA-45:30	11.38_{ab}	8.50	7.75_{ab}	7.88	6.25^{*}_{bc}	4.38^{*}_{cd}	11.00_{ab}	10.88^{*}_{a}
F/TMPB-45:30	9.75_{abc}	8.50	9.62_{ab}	9.88	12.38_{ab}	12.38_{abc}	10.62_{ab}	6.88_{b}
χ^2 value	91.89	0.00	51.37	44.63	106.34	106.10	78.20	49.86
P value	0.000	1.000	0.000	0.000	0.000	0.000	0.000	0.000

$_{a\text{-}d}$ For each sensory attribute mean ranks without the same letter are significantly different ($P < 0.05$).

† For *fibrousness* mean ranks without the same letter are significantly different ($P < 0.10$).

* For each sensory attribute and for the same INL:EVOO ratio mean ranks between F/TMPA samples and their F/TMPB counterparts are significantly different ($P < 0.05$); F/TMPA: frozen/thawed mashed potatoes without hydrocolloids; F/TMPB: frozen/thawed mashed potatoes with added hydrocolloids. INL, inulin; EVOO: extra virgin olive oil.

Table 6. Effects of INL:EVOO ratio and hydrocolloid addition on mean ranks of sensory taste attributes for F/TMP samples

Sample code	Sweetness†	Authentic taste†	Off-taste	Ingredient taste
F/TMPA-0:0	6.75_{ab}	5.00_{e}	10.25	2.50_{b}
F/TMPB-0:0	4.88_{b}	6.00_{de}	8.25	2.50_{b}
F/TMPA-0:60	4.88_{b}	$6.12*_{de}$	8.25	15.12_{a}
F/TMPB-0:60	6.75_{ab}	12.25_{a}	8.25	15.12_{a}
F/TMPA-15:45	9.75_{ab}	$11.25*_{ab}$	8.25	$12.38*_{a}$
F/TMPB-15:45	8.62_{ab}	7.12_{cde}	8.25	10.00_{ab}
F/TMPA-30:30	8.50_{ab}	$11.25*_{ab}$	8.25	$10.00*_{ab}$
F/TMPB-30:30	8.50_{ab}	7.75_{bcde}	8.25	7.75_{ab}
F/TMPA-45:15	$9.25*_{ab}$	9.62_{abcd}	8.25	$7.75*_{ab}$
F/TMPB-45:15	13.12_{a}	10.25_{abc}	8.25	10.00_{ab}
F/TMPA-60:0	10.12_{ab}	5.12_{e}	8.25	2.50_{b}
F/TMPB-60:0	10.50_{ab}	5.25_{e}	10.25	2.50_{b}
F/TMPA-30:45	8.62_{ab}	$7.88*_{bcde}$	8.25	$8.88*_{ab}$
F/TMPB-30:45	8.62_{ab}	12.75_{a}	8.25	11.25_{a}
F/TMPA-45:30	$6.75*_{ab}$	$10.62*_{abc}$	8.25	$7.75*_{ab}$
F/TMPB-45:30	10.38_{ab}	7.75_{bcde}	8.25	10.00_{ab}
χ^2 value	35.88	45.66	30.00	108.38
P value	0.002	0.000	0.012	0.000

$_{a\text{-}d}$ For each sensory attribute mean ranks without the same letter are significantly different ($P < 0.05$).

† For *sweetness* and *authentic taste* mean ranks without the same letter are significantly different ($P < 0.10$).

* For each sensory attribute and for the same INL:EVOO ratio mean ranks between F/TMPA sample and its F/TMPB counterpart are significantly different ($P < 0.05$); F/TMPA: frozen/thawed mashed potatoes without added hydrocolloids; F/TMPB: frozen/thawed mashed potatoes with added hydrocolloids. INL, inulin; EVOO, extra virgin olive oil.

Similar results were obtained by Castro et al. [59] in dairy drinks with added olifructose and by González-Tomás et al. [57] and Villegas et al. [67] in dairy drinks with added INL. Panellists scored F/TMPB-0:60, F/TMPA-15:45, F/TMPA-30:30, F/TMPA-45:15, F/TMPB-45:15, F/TMPB-30:45 and F/TMPA-45:30 samples higher for *authentic taste* than the F/TMPA-0:0 and F/TMPB-0:0 controls (Table 6). A freeze/thaw cycle clearly mitigated the strong potato flavour detected in the fresh controls (Table 4). Panellists gave F/TMPA-0:60 and F/TMPB-0:60 samples the highest score for *ingredient taste* (Figure 7c), although only the differences between scores for these samples and those for samples without added EVOO (F/TMPA-0:0, F/TMPB-0:0, F/TMPA-60:0 and F/TMPB-60:0 samples) were significant. This means that a freeze/thaw cycle did not affect the aroma and taste attributes of EVOO.

Linear Discriminat Analysis (LDA)

To sum up, the Friedman test confirms significant variability among the sensory attributes of MP samples under the different experimental conditions. The purpose of the application of LDA analyses was to focus on the possible objective discrimination between the different ingredients added to MP samples on the basis of the sensory attributes considered in the QDA. LDA analyses were designed to develop a small number of functions with which to discriminate among the different performance conditions of MP based on linear combinations of eleven sensory attributes. In the LDA analyses, one colour attribute (*off-colours*) was rejected for the model as its variance was zero.

Table 7 summarises the generation of the discriminant functions for the four different LDA analyses performed on the FMP and F/TMP samples considered separately (n = 128), and using hydrocolloid addition and INL:EVOO ratio as discriminating factors respectively. Only significant discriminating functions are shown. The relative percentages of variance accounting for discriminating function 1 were clearly higher in all the analyses. For LDAs using hydrocolloid addition as discriminating factor, note that function 1 is good alone, with 100% relative percentages in both FMP and F/TMP samples.

In turn, when considering INL:EVOO ratio as discriminating factor, function 1 had the highest relative percentage (> 90%) for the F/TMP samples, and canonical correlation of 0.97. This evidences that detection of the effect of the INL:EVOO ratio by the panellists was more significant in the samples that had been subjected to a freeze/thaw cycle. As shown above, mechanical spectra confirmed some structural changes occurring in the MP samples after a freeze/thaw cycle as a consequence of amylopectin retrogradation process. In addition, it has been reported that in F/TMPA samples with added oil the structural damage caused by freezing enabled the oil droplets to come close enough together to aggregate, while in the F/TMPB ones with added κ-C and XG and oil, the XG is adsorbed onto the surface of the droplets, enhancing stability against flocculation and coalescence and forming a white film as observed by scanning electron microscopy [76].

Table 7. Summary of the discriminant analysis results for each discriminating factor used in FMP and F/TMP samples

Discriminant function	Eigenvalue	Relative percentage	Canonical correlation	*P* value
Discriminating factor: hydrocolloid addition				
FMP samples				
1	3.50	100	0.88	0.000
F/TMP samples				
1	6.26	100	0.93	0.000
Discriminating factor: INL:EVOO ratio				
FMP samples				
1	14.83	67.4	0.97	0.000
2	5.50	25.0	0.92	0.000
3	1.18	5.4	0.74	0.000
4	0.31	1.4	0.48	0.017
F/TMP samples				
1	18.53	90.90	0.97	0.000
2	1.19	5.80	0.74	0.000
3	0.35	1.70	0.51	0.011

FMP: fresh mashed potatoes; F/TMP: frozen/thawed mashed potatoes; INL, inulin; EVOO, extra virgin olive oil.

Table 8. Standardised discriminant function coefficients for the four LDA analyses carried out in the FMP and F/TMP samples using different discriminat factors

Independent variables	Discriminant function			
	1	2	1	2
D Discriminating factor: hydrocolloid addition				
	FMP samples		F/TMP samples	
Authentic colour	-0.29	-	-0.25	-
Shine	0.31	-	0.14	-
Uniformity	0.18	-	-0.07	-
Consistency	0.39	-	**0.97**	-
Adhesiveness	**0.98**	-	0.48	-
Creaminess	**0.41**	-	0.23	-
Fibrousness	0.07	-	-0.16	-
Sweetness	0.10	-	0.28	-
Authentic taste	-0.33	-	-0.08	-
Off-taste	0.35	-	0.19	-
Ingredient taste	-0.04	-	**0.65**	-
Discriminating factor: INL:EVOO ratio				
	FMP samples		F/TMP samples	
Authentic colour	0.15	-0.29	0.16	-0.06
Shine	-0.21	-0.11	-0.18	0.51
Uniformity	-0.27	0.38	**0.28**	0.16
Consistency	0.25	-0.21	-0.01	0.25
Adhesiveness	-0.04	0.02	-0.12	**-0.90**
Creaminess	0.63	-0.14	0.12	**1.05**
Fibrousness	**0.74**	**0.51**	0.19	0.07
Sweetness	0.16	0.09	0.03	0.30
Authentic taste	0.05	-0.10	-0.03	0.28
Off-taste	0.35	**0.95**	-0.21	0.01
Ingredient taste	**1.25**	-0.03	**1.00**	-0.32

FMP: fresh mashed potatoes; F/TMP: frozen/thawed mashed potatoes; INL, inulin; EVOO, extra virgin olive oil.

In general oil retention from an emulsion was found to increase with decreasing stability of the emulsions towards coalescence, either due to lowering the adsorb amount of protein at the oil water interface [77], adapting the composition of the adsorbed layer [78] or by partial coalescence [79]. For reversible aggregating emulsions this lead to increased sensations of fat-related texture attributes. It resulted in higher ratings for a group of viscosity-related attributes as thickness, creaminess, and fatiness and lower ratings for a group of friction related attributes as roughness, dryness and astringency [78, 79]. Therefore, a higher degree of coalescence before intake could justify that the panellists had increased sensory perception of the INL:EVOO ratio in the samples subjected to a freeze/thaw cycle.

Table 8 shows the standardised coefficients of the functions used to discriminate among the different levels of the discriminating factor used in the LDA. The relative magnitude of the coefficients in this table shows how the sensory attributes are used to discriminate among the groups. In the case of the only discriminant function 1 extracted by the LDA in which the addition of hydrocolloids is the discriminating factor for the FMP samples, *adhesiveness* is the sensory attribute that best separates samples without and with added hydrocolloids (FMPA and FMPB samples, respectively). Also, in the case of discriminant function 1 where hydrocolloid addition is the discriminating factor for the F/TMP samples, first *consistency* and then *ingredient taste* are the variables that best separate the samples without and with added hydrocolloids (F/TMPA and F/TMPB samples, respectively).

In the case of the LDA using INL:EVOO ratio as a discriminating factor in the FMP samples, for the first discriminant function *ingredient taste* is clearly the sensory attribute that best separates the eight levels of INL/EVOO blends added to MP, whereas for the second function first *off-taste* and then *fibrousness* are the attributes that best separate the levels of INL:EVOO ratio. Also in the case of discriminant function 1 (more significant) extracted by the LDA using the INL:EVOO ratio as a discriminating factor, again *ingredient taste* is the sensory attribute which best separate the eight INL:EVOO ratios in the F/TMP samples, while for the second function first *creaminess* and then *adhesiveness* are the attributes that best separate the levels of of INL/EVOO blends.

Table 9. Group centroids for the LDA analysis carried out in FMP and F/TMP samples using INL:EVOO ratio as discriminant factor

	FMP samples		F/TMP samples	
Group centroids	1	2	1	2
INL:EVOO ratio				
0:0	-8.09	-0.50	-7.08	-1.74
0:60	3.70	-1.44	4.86	-1.44
15:45	3.02	-1.33	2.81	0.73
30:30	-1.68	-1.06	1.50	0.61
45:15	-2.47	0.37	1.22	-0.63
60:0	1.65	5.79	-6.86	1.39
30:45	3.31	-1.48	2.07	0.61
45:30	0.56	-0.35	1.48	0.48

FMP: fresh mashed potatoes; F/TMP: frozen/thawed mashed potatoes; INL, inulin; EVOO, extra virgin olive oil.

Table 9 shows the group centriods and Figure 8 shows the projections of the observations onto the two axes extracted by the LDA using the INL:EVOO ratio as a discriminating factor in the FMP and F/TMP samples each considered separately. As expected from the high relative percentages of the discriminant functions 1, mainly in the F/TMP samples, the target effect is better defined by the function 1, while there is more overlap in the case of the function 2.

In the case of LDA using FMP samples (Figure 8a), centroid values show that the first function discriminates mainly between 0:0 control and the rest of the samples, (it separates them by more than 6 units; Table 9). This result is clearly due to that the panellists scored both FMPA and FMPB samples with added 0:0 ratio higher for *autenthic taste* (Figure 6c; Table 4) due to the strong potato taste detected in the samples without other ingredients added. The FMPA samples with a 0:0 addition ratio also scored quite high for *fibrousness*—in this case influenced by the low *creaminess* detected in the samples without either κ-C and XG or other ingredients added. The most obvious discrimination was between 0:0 control and samples containing 60 g kg^{-1} added EVOO alone and those containing 45 g kg^{-1} added EVOO and 15 and 30 g kg^{-1} added INL respectively, which received the highest *ingredient taste* scores (Table 4) due to their high oil content and the lowest *fibrousness* scores (Table 3). Note that discrimination between 0:60, 15:45, and 30:45 ratios was quite poor (Figure 8a), partially due to the similar *ingredient taste* scores given by the panellists to the samples containing these three INL/EVOO blends. It turned out to be insufficient to know in detail the chemical composition of the product and the threshold values of these components for taste and odour perception [11]. Both the bitter taste and the trigeminal sensation of pungency stimulate the taste receptors and the trigeminal nerve [9]; those sensory properties have been associated with phenolic compounds present in EVOO [7]. Also, the structure of the food product appeared to be a main factor in determining taste and odour perception [80]. High fat custards produced less sensation of dryness and roughness, more sensations of flavour, and more sensations of creamy and fatty mouth and after feel than their zero-fat containing counterparts [81]. Addition of extra virgin olive oil in increasing concentrations enhanced the sensory quality of MP in terms of reduced granularity, denseness, cohesiveness, adhesiveness and fibrousness, and increased homogeneity, ease of swallowing and palate coating [76]. In turn, presence of EVOO in MP significantly increased the overall acceptability of the product which was ascribed by the panellists chiefly to lubricating and coating properties conferred by the oil [42]. It is clear that many sensory attributes cannot be related to a single physical property in a single way [11].

For the FMP samples, centroid values show that the second function only discriminates between samples with 60 g kg^{-1} added INL alone and the rest (Table 9, Figure 8a). This ties up with the fact that the addition of INL at 60 g kg^{-1} produced an unpleasant and unfamiliar taste as evidenced by the higher *off-taste* scores (Figure 6c, Table 4) awarded to these samples. In addition, this result is also due to that the panellists scored the FMP samples with added 60:0 ratio higher for *fibrousness* (Table 3) due to the sandy texture detected in the samples with higher INL contents. Concerning this observation, González-Tomás et al. [57] investigated how adding INL of different average chain lengths (long-chain, native, and short-chain INL) at a concentration of 7.5% (wt/wt) would affect the physicochemical and sensory characteristics of starch-based dairy desserts formulated with either skim or whole milk. The results showed that the effect of adding 7.5% INL of different average chain length can give rise to products with different rheological behaviour and different sensory characteristics. The skim milk sample with long-chain INL and the whole milk sample without INL were perceived to have the same creaminess and consistency intensity, but addition of long-chain INL also increased roughness intensity and, consequently, the sensory quality was negatively affected.This effect could be due to small crystals or crystal aggregates of long-chain INL in the product that influence the sensory characteristics of the samples [42]. Some authors have reported on the particle size of INL crystals [45], whereas others have discussed the effects that adding different sized particles may have on the sensory characteristics of dairy matrices. Hebette et al. [50] described the complex melting and crystalline behaviour of an aqueous suspension of INL crystallites. They observed the presence of 8-like shaped INL crystallites with particle size from 5 to 20 μm by optical microscopy. Kim et al. [82] also found differences in INL particle sizes between low shearing, high shearing, and thermally induced gels. The average particle size of INL crystals varied from 30 μm for low-shear induced gel to approximately 2 μm for thermally induced gels. Therefore, INL crystals with a particle size from 2 to 30 μm could be expected in the FMP samples. According to this information, the increase in *fibrousness* perceived for FMP samples with added long-chain INL alone could be explained by the presence of INL crystals, confirming previous findings [26, 42].

In the case of F/TMP samples (Figure 8b), function 1 discriminates clearly between 0:0 control and samples with 60 g kg^{-1} added I alone, and the rest. Again, this is chiefly due to the lower *ingredient taste* scores given by the panellists to the samples without added EVOO. Centroid values (Table 9) show that function 1 discriminates less between samples with addition ratios of 15:45, 30:30, 45:15, 30:45 and 45:30 but more between these and the 0:60 ratio. Taking the F/TMP samples separately, function 2 also discriminates clearly between samples with addition ratios of 0:0 and 60:0, and the rest. This is explained by the fact that the F/TMP samples with added EVOO at highest concentrations scored higher for *creaminess* and lower for *adhesiveness*. Fat is a well-known enhancer of creaminess sensations [81], which covers oral tissue with a coating therefore reducing the friction between food and oral tissue. Starch break-down and the resulting loss in viscosity allow fat droplets to migrate from the bulk of the bolus to the surface where it provides additional lubrication [83].

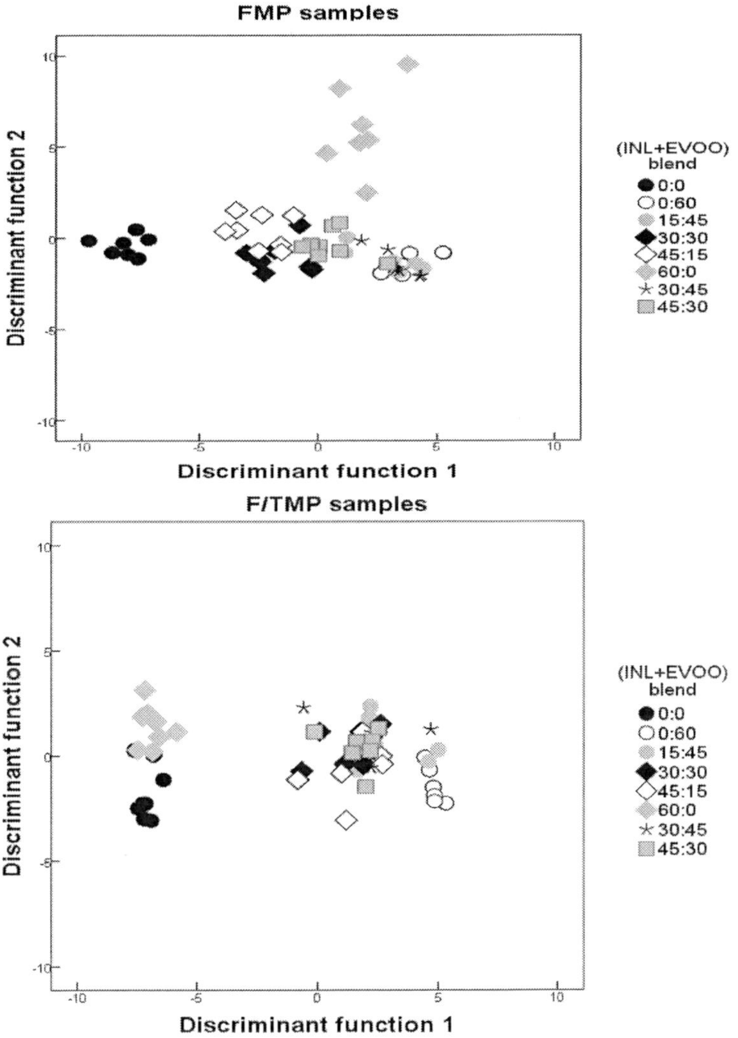

Figure 8. Plot of observations on the two principal axes obtained via LDA based on the INL:EVOO ratio used as discriminating factor for: (a) FMP samples; (b) F/TMP samples; INL: inulin; EVOO: extra virgin olive oil.

Categorical Principal Components Analysis (CATPCA)

Table 10 shows the components extracted in each CATPCA analysis [FMP and F/TMP subgroups considered separately (n = 128)] for eleven sensory attributes with eigenvalues greater than unity (Kaiser's rule) [84]. Analogously, in the CATPCA analyses, one colour attribute (*off-colours*) was rejected for the model as its variance was zero.

For the FMP samples, CATPCA revealed that three principal components (PC-1 to PC-3) explained almost 70% of the variance between the data, although the first two components explained 56% of the total variance. In turn, for the F/TMP samples, four principal components (PC-1 to PC-4) explained almost 74% of the variance between the data, but the first two components explained only 44% of the total variance. Table 11 shows the rotated varimax PC loadings. The loading for each scored sensory attribute represents its relative contribution to a principal component. Sensory attributes with the highest loadings for each PC are marked in boldface, indicating that this PC is dominated by these particular attributes and, therefore the meaning of each component.

Figure 9 shows the projection of the scored sensory attributes on the rotated space defined by the first, second and third factorial axes for both the FMP and F/TMP samples. Total variation explained in Figure 9a is 69.2%, whereas total variation explained in Figure 9b is lower (59%). When the eleven sensory attributes were taken into account for the FMP samples, the first PC, which explains 28.55% of the total variance (Table 10), presents positive and quite high correlations, in descending order, with *creaminess* and *authentic colour* (Table 11). This first PC also presents negative and relatively high correlation with *fibrousness* (Figure 9a). This means that the greater either the *creaminess* or the *authentic colour*, the lower the *fibrousness* of the FMP samples. This is logical as *fibrousness* is a geometrical textural attribute reflecting the graininess perceived during preparation of the sample in the mouth prior to swallowing [20], whereas creaminess is a complex sensory attribute that is often considered an indicator of high, premium-quality and is critical for consumer acceptance of many food products [85].

Despite the fact that *creaminess* is a sensory characteristic highly coveted in a wide range of food products, it has not been clearly defined. Recently, it was defined as the combined perception of fat, smoothness and thickness by Bayarri et al. [45]. Creaminess mainly depends on the microstructure, on some surface properties, as well as on certain interactions between texture attributes and some flavours [86]. Certainly, FMP samples with added EVOO, either alone or blended with INL, scored highest for *creaminess* and presented softer mouthfeel, promoting positive effect on the *authentic colour* of the resulting products by increasing yellowness. PC-1 integrates *fibrousness*, one geometrical attribute, and *creaminess*, both associated with the arrangement of particles in the product, and surface roughness or smoothness properties of MP texture according to Szczesniak [87]. Hence, component 1 may be identified mainly with geometrical textural attributes which serve as an index of the *creaminess/fibrousness* of the FMP samples. Analogously, De Wijk et al. [81], using a trained panel, developed a set of sensory attributes to describe flavour, odour, mouthfeel and afterfeel of commercial vanilla custard desserts. Two main sensory dimensions were recognised in the resulting sensory space, one running from melting to thick and another one running from rough to creamy/fatty. Similar information was obtained from a group of consumers that described the perceptible differences on texture of eight samples of commercial vanilla dairy desserts of different brands by means of Free Choice Profile. In this case the first dimension was related with thick-fluid attributes and the second one with rough-smooth texture [88].

PC-2 (which explains over 27% of the total variance) was positively weighted by *consistency* and *adhesiveness* and negatively dominated by *shine* and *ingredient taste* (Table 11). This means that when the assessors detected more mechanical strength in the FMP products, they detected poorer *shine* and *EVOO taste*. In the FMP samples, component 2 was mainly a contrast between mechanical texture attributes (*consistency*, *adhesiveness*) and appearance and taste ones (*shine*, *ingredient taste*), acting as an index of the mechanical behaviour and the *shine* associated with particularly fat-related flavours. PC-3 was negatively weighted by *sweetness*. Therefore, this sensory taste attribute was unrelated to any other of the scored sensory attributes. On the other hand, intercorrelated sensory attributes with nearly equal loadings are assumed to represent some redundancy. *Consistency* and *adhesiveness* had nearly equal loadings.

Table 10. Total variation explained by the categorical principal components (CATPCA) under the two CATPCA analyses carried out

	FMP samples		F/TMP samples	
Component	**Eigenvalue**	**Percent of variance**	**Eigenvalue**	**Percent of variance**
PC-1	3.14	28.55	2.63	23.95
PC-2	3.00	27.32	2.22	20.16
PC-3	1.47	13.37	1.64	14.87
PC-4	-	-	1.63	14.85

FMP: fresh mashed potatoes; F/TMP: mashed potatoes subjected to a freeze/thaw cycle.

Table 11. Rotated varimax principal components (PC) loadings of the sensory attributes

Sensory attribute	FMP samples			F/TMP samples			
	PC-1	PC-2	PC-3	PC-1	PC-2	PC-3	PC-4
Authentic colour (Aucol)	**0.788***	-0.223	0.268	**0.777**	0.184	0.343	0.208
Shine (Shi)	0.158	**-0.842**	0.151	0.407	-0.244	0.635	-0.172
Uniformity (Unicol)	0.662	0.157	0.366	**0.726**	-0.095	-0.240	0.039
Consistency (Con)	0.206	**0.823**	0.223	0.006	**0.938**	-0.080	0.063
Adhesivenes (Adh)	0.151	**0.749**	0.308	0.024	**0.909**	-0.069	0.054
Creaminess (Cre)	**0.876**	-0.110	-0.136	0.672	0.260	0.088	-0.327
Fibrousness (Fib)	**-0.747**	-0.049	0.374	-0.094	-0.544	-0.264	0.565
Sweetness (Swe)	0.108	-0.222	**-0.869**	-0.094	-0.104	-0.029	**-0.830**
Authentic taste (Autas)	0.079	-0.620	0.286	0.506	0.066	0.047	0.658
Off-taste (Offtas)	-0.684	-0.183	0.054	0.023	-0.042	**-0.875**	-0.054
Ingredient taste (Ingtas)	0.427	**-0.707**	0.314	**0.782**	-0.168	0.448	0.038

* The highest PC loadings for each factor are in boldface; FMP: fresh mashed potatoes; F/TMP: mashed potatoes subjected to a freeze/thaw cycle.

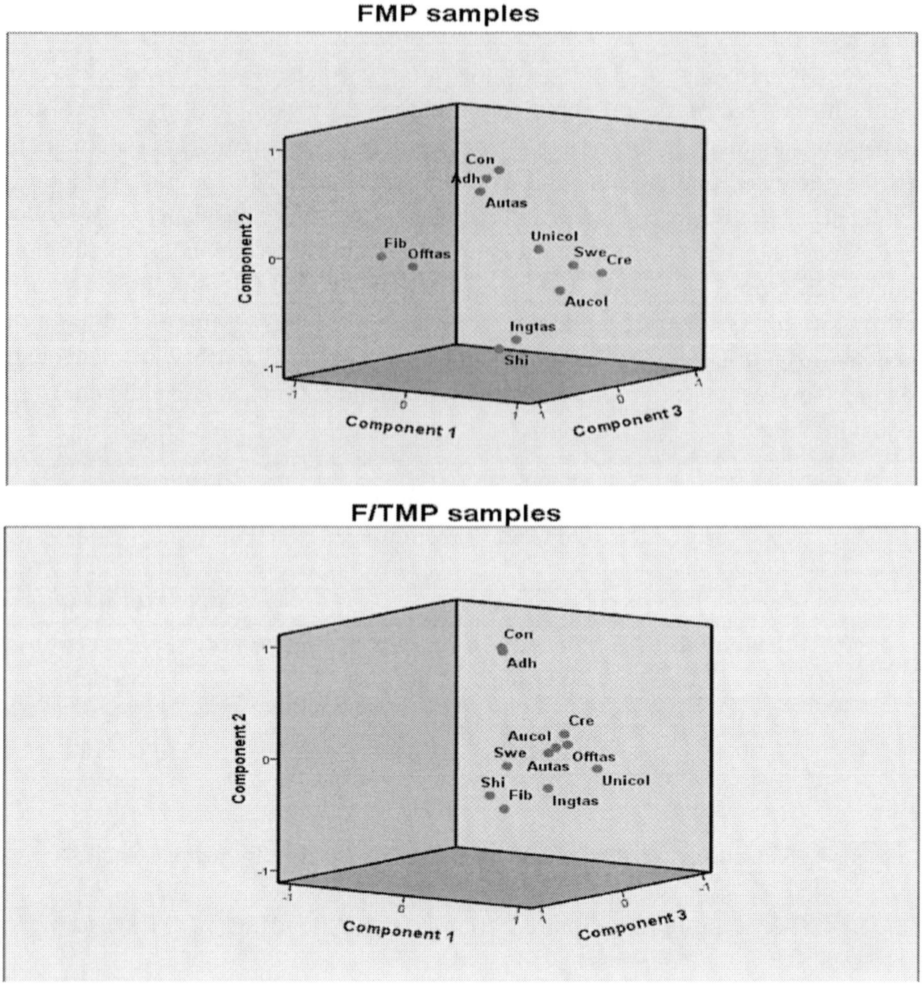

Figure 9. Plot for the first three principal components from categorical principal components analysis (CATPCA) carried out for: (a) FMP samples; (b) F/TMP samples; INL: inulin; EVOO: extra virgin olive oil.

In the case of the F/TMP samples (Figure 9b, Table 11), PC-1 (which explains over 24% of the total variance, Table 10) was positively weighted by *authentic colour*, *uniformity* and *ingredient taste*. The greater the addition of EVOO with respect to the frozen/thawed 0:0 control, the more intensive either the colour or the fat-related flavours. All the three loadings are positive and two variables are sensory appearance attributes. Therefore, component 1 may be interpreted as a representation of the presence of EVOO affecting either the colour or the taste of the F/TMP samples. It is worth noting that by considering the F/TMP samples separately, PC-2 is dominated by the same sensory texture attributes than in the case of their FMP counterparts (Table 11). Again, *consistency* and *adhesiveness* positive and highly weighted component 2, which may be identified chiefly with mechanical texture attributes. PC-3 and PC-4 presented a negative correlation with *off-taste* and *sweetness* respectively, indicating the absence of any relationship between these taste attributes and those well correlated under the first principal components plane (PC-1 and PC-2), and showing that any effect of *off-taste* or *sweet taste* detected in the product was not significant for the appearance and texture perceived in the same.

Reliability Analysis

Two or more items measuring the same thing for the same individual may not have exactly the same value. However, repeated measurements of a series of individuals will show some agreement or consistency [89]. In order to establish the levels of agreement between assessors, we used a reliability test. The reliability of the scores for each sensory property evaluated was tested by means of Cronbach's alpha coefficient [α] [29] (Table 12), based on the average inter-item correlations between its measures. The coefficient α is a measure of the internal consistency within the group of assessors (panel). Again, the colour attribute *off-colours* was discarded in the analysis as its variance was zero.

It is a widely accepted rule that α should be at least 0.70 in order to demonstrate consistence in the sub-items and know that the items are measuring the same construct [84]. The results obtained in the FMP samples showed a very good internal consistency for *ingredient taste*, *adhesiveness*, *consistency*, *off-taste* and *authentic colour* (Cronbach's α = 0.989, 0.979, 0.975, 0.959 and 0.945, in that order, respectively). Conversely, the assessors showed a very poor internal consistency for *sweetness* (Cronbach's α = -0.529). In turn, the results obtained in the F/TMP samples showed a very acceptable internal consistency for *off-taste*, *ingredient taste*, *consistency*, *adhesiveness*, *authentic colour* and *creaminess* (Cronbach's α = 1.000, 0.994, 0.979, 0.976, 0.960 and 0.948, in that order, respectively). However, again assessors showed a poorer internal consistency for *sweetness* (Cronbach's α = 0.657). Therefore, *ingredient taste*, *consistency* and *adhesiveness* were the three sensory attributes that showed a superior internal consistency in both FMP and F/TMP samples. The relatively low internal consistency detected for *sweetness* suggests that more training in the use of this taste attribute might be needed.

Table 12. Reliability analyses for FMP and F/TMP samples

Sensory attribute	**Cronbach's alpha coefficient**	
	FMP samples	F/TMP samples
Authentic colour	0.945	0.960
Shine	0.912	0.816
Uniformity	0.934	0.797
Consistency	0.975	0.979
Adhesiveness	0.979	0.976
Creaminess	0.931	0.948
Fibrousness	0.898	0.839
Sweetness	-0.529	0.657
Authentic taste	0.919	0.755
Off-taste	0.959	1.000
Ingredient taste	0.989	0.994

When a panel member is discarded a change is produced in the Cronbach alpha coefficient value. By studying this variation (data not shown), it is possible to determine the homogeneity of the judgments made by each panellists for each attribute. Thus, a decrease in the Cronbach coefficient indicates that the assessor is very homogeneous whereas an increase in the α value would indicate that the contrary is true. It was found that in the FMP samples, assessors 3 and 7 were the least homogeneous in their scores for the taste attributes *off-taste* and *ingredient taste*, whereas assessors 2, 4, 6 and 8 were the most homogeneous for all the sensory attributes. In turn, in the F/TMP samples, panellists 2 and 6 were the least homogeneous for all the sensory attributes, except for *sweetness*, while panellists 3 and 7 were the most homogeneous for all the sensory attributes.

CONCLUSION

The rheology of mashed potatoes is governed by a continuous phase (amylose/amylopectin matrix), which is eventually modified by the presence of INL/EVOO blends. In FMPA, FMPB and F/TMPB products, samples with no (INL+EVOO) blends exhibited greater elasticity than those with added INL/EVOO content. This indicates a shift in the viscoelastic behaviour of the samples with added INL:EVOO ratios towards more viscous-like products. INL crystallites and oil droplets should be regarded as inactive filler particles. The decrease in the G' and G'' values detected in the F/TMP samples as compared to their FMP counterparts is attributed to amylopectin retrogradation associated with the freeze/thaw cycle. However, the presence of hydrocolloids significantly improved freeze/thaw stability and mitigated the effect of INL:EVOO ratio variations on the viscoelasticity of the mashed potatoes. With respect to 0:0 controls, the addition of INL alone produced the lightest-coloured mashed potatoes (higher L^*/b^* ratio), whereas EVOO addition alone caused samples to darken (higher colour difference (ΔE^*)). When INL/EVOO blends were added, the darkening produced by EVOO addition was stronger than the lightening caused by INL incorporation. With regard to 0:0 controls, increasing yellowness due to the presence of EVOO improved product colour, as the flesh of Kennebec potatoes is too white.

In FMP samples considered separately, LDA showed that the most obvious discrimination was between 0:0 control and samples containing 0:60, 15:45 and 30:45 ratios, which is mainly ascribed to the fact that the samples containing higher EVOO concentrations received higher *ingredient taste* scores due to an aromatic note and fat-related flavours detected by the panellists. In F/TMP samples considered separately, LDA showed that the sensory characteristics of the product with an added 60:0 ratio were similar to those of the product without added ingredients, which is mainly attributed to the fact that the samples without added EVOO received higher and lower *adhesiveness* and *creaminess* scores respectively. Panellists also scored the F/TMP samples with an added 0:60 ratio higher than the rest for *ingredient taste*, indicating that a freeze/thaw cycle did not affect the aroma and taste attributes of the extra virgin olive oil.

CATPCA of the FMP samples, considered separately, showed that component 1 served as a *creaminess/fibrousness* index of the product in response to increased lubricating and coating properties produced by the presence of EVOO, whereas when the F/TMP samples were analysed separately, the first principal component served as an index of *authentic colour*, *uniformity* and *ingredient taste* in response to improved yellowness and flavour-releasing properties of the EVOO. The results obtained were highly consistent (Cronbach alpha coefficient) for all the sensory attributes except *sweetness*. The addition of either INL or EVOO at 30 g kg^{-1} is strongly recommended in order to achieve an increase in the daily intake of soluble fibre and monounsaturated fat (MUFA) while at the same time improving the sensory quality of the resulting products. The information obtained may be of great interest in designing mashed potatoes with nutritional and sensory characteristics that meet consumer demands.

Acknowledgments

The authors wish to thank the Spanish Ministry of Science and Innovation for financial support (AGL2007-62851). The authors also thank Laura Barrios (SGAI-CSIC) for assistance with non-parametric statistical tests.

References

[1] Van Trijp, H. C. M., Punter, P. H., Mickartz, F., & Kruithof, L. (2007). The quest for the ideal product: comparing different methods and approaches. *Food Quality and Preference*, *18*, 729-740.

[2] Hasler, C. M. (1998). Functional foods: their role in disease prevention and health promotion. *Food Technology*, *52* (11), 63-70.

[3] Arcia, P. L., Costell, E., & Tárrega, A. (2010). Thickness suitability of prebiotic dairy desserts: relationship with rheological properties. *Food Research International*, *43*, 2409-2416.

[4] Arcia, P. L., Costell, E., & Tárrega, A. (2011). Inulin blend as prebiotic and fat replacer in dairy desserts : optimization by response surface methodology. *Journal of Dairy Science*, *94* (5), 2192-2200.

[5] Roberfroid, M. B., Van Loo, J., & Gibson, G. (1998). The bifidogenic nature of chicory inulin and its hydrolysis products. *Journal of Nutrition*, *128*, 11-19.

[6] Coussement, P. A. A. (1999). Inulin and oligofructose: safe intakes and legal status. *Journal of Nutrition*, *129* (7S), 1412S-1417S.

[7] Bendini, A., Cerretani, L., Carrasco-Pancorbo, A., Gómez-Caravaca, A. A., Segura-Carretero, A., Fernández-Gutiérrez, A., & Lercker, G. (2007) Phenolic molecules in virgin olive oils: a survey of their sensory properties, health effects, antioxidant activity and analytical methods. An overview of the last decade. *Molecules*, *12*, 1679-1719.

[8] US Food and Drug Administration. Press Release P04-100. November 1, 2004. http://www.fda.gov/bbs/topics/news/2004/NEW01129.htlm. Accessed on April 14, 2010.

[9] Delgado, C., & Guinard, J.-X. (2011). Sensory properties of californian and imported extra virgin olive oils. *Journal of Food Science*, *76* (3), S170–S176.

[10] Boskou, D., Blekas, G., & Tsimidou, M. (2006). Olive oil composition. In D. Boskou (Ed.), *Olive oil: Chemistry and Technology, Vol. 4* (pp. 41-72), Champaign: AOCS Press.

[11] van Vliet, T., van Aken, A., de Jongh, H. H. J., & Hamer, R. J. (2009). Colloidal aspects of texture perception. *Advances in Colloid and Interface Science, 150*, 27-40.

[12] Canet, W., & Alvarez, M. D. (2006). Quality and safety of frozen vegetables. In S. Da-Wen (Ed.), *Handbook of Frozen Food Processing and Packaging* (pp. 377-415), London/New York: Boca Raton: CRC Taylor & Francis Group.

[13] Wilkinson, C., Dijksterhuis, G. B., & Minekus, M. (2000). From food structure to texture. *Trends in Food Science and Technology, 11*, 442-450.

[14] van Vliet, T. (2002). On the relation between texture perception and fundamental mechanical parameters for liquids and time dependent solids. *Food Quality and Preference, 13*, 227-236.

[15] Adams, M. J, Bedford, L. V., & Geering, J. (1981). *QAV – a Method for the Sensory Appraisal of Quality Processed Vegetable Varieties. Technical Memorandum 278.* The Campden Food Preservation Research Association, Chipping, Campden, Gloucestershire, UK, pp 7-29.

[16] Canet, W., Fernández, C., & Alvarez, M. D. (2011). Functionality of amidated low methoxyl pectin and xanthan gum blends on the texture and color of mashed potatoes. *Journal of Food Process and Engineering, 34*, 746-776.

[17] Fernández, C., Alvarez, M. D., & Canet, W. (2008). Steady shear and yield stress of fresh and frozen/thawed mashed potatoes: effect of biopolymers addition. *Food Hydrocolloids, 22*, 1381-1395.

[18] Fernández, C., Canet, W., & Alvarez, M. D. (2010). Rheological properties and sensory attributes of mashed potatoes made with mixtures of sodium caseinate and xanthan gum. In C. S. Hollingworth (Ed.), *Food Hydrocolloids: Characteristics, Properties and Structures* (pp. 81–117), New York: Nova Science Publishers, Inc.

[19] Alvarez, M. D., Fernández, C., & Canet, W. (2011). Flow behaviour and sensory properties of extra virgin olive oil-enriched mashed potatoes: influence of cryoprotectants and freezing. In N. Benkeblia, & Pedreschi, F. (Eds.), *Food 5* (*Special Issue 1*) United Kingdom: Global Science Books (GBS).

[20] Alvarez, M. D., Canet, W., & Fernández, C. (2008). Effect of addition of cryoprotectants on the mechanical properties, colour and sensory attributes of fresh and frozen/thawed mashed potatoes. *European Food Research and Technology, 226*, 1525-1544.

[21] Alvarez, M. D., Fernández, C., & Canet, W. (2009). Enhancement of freezing stability in mashed potatoes by the incorporation of kappa-carrageenan and xanthan gum blends. *Journal of the Science of Food and Agriculture, 89*, 2115-2127.

[22] Fernández, C., Canet, W., & Alvarez, M. D. (2009). Quality of mashed potatoes: effect of adding blends of kappa-carrageenan and xanthan gum. *European Food Research and Technology, 229*, 205-222.

[23] Alvarez, M. D., Canet, W., & Fernández, C. (2005). Effect of freezing/thawing conditions and long-term frozen storage on the quality of mashed potatoes. *Journal of the Science of Food and Agriculture, 85*, 2327–2340.

[24] Navarro, A. S., Martino, M. N., & Zaritzky, N. E. (1997). Correlation between transient rotational viscometry and a dynamic oscillatory test for viscoelastic starch based systems. *Journal of Texture Studies*, *28*, 365-385.

[25] Mohamed, A., & Xu, J. (2003). Effect of ionic strength and pH on the thermal and rheological properties of soy protein-amylopectin blend. *Food Chemistry*, *83*, 227-236.

[26] Alvarez, M. D., Fernández, C., Solas, M. T., & Canet, W. (2011). Viscoelasticity and microstructure of inulin-enriched mashed potatoes: influence of freezing and cryoprotectants. *Journal of Food Engineering*, *102*, 66-76.

[27] O'Mahony, M. (1986). Additional nonparametric tests. In S. R. Tannenbaum, & P. Walstra (Eds.), *Statistical methods and procedures* (pp. 303–365). New York: Marcel Dekker Inc.

[28] ISO 8587. (2006). *Sensory Analysis. Methodology-Ranking*. International Organization for Standardization, Genève, Switzerland.

[29] Cronbach, L. (1951). Coefficient alpha and the internal structure of tests. *Psychometrica*, *16*, 297–334.

[30] Tunick, M. H. (2011). Small-strain dynamic rheology of food protein networks. *Journal of Agriculture and Food Chemistry*, *59*, 1481-1486.

[31] González-Tomás, L., Coll-Marqués, J., & Costell, E. (2008). Viscoelasticity of inulin-starch-based dairy systems. Influence of inulin average chain length. *Food Hydrocolloids*, *22*, 1372–1380.

[32] Campo-Deaño, L., Tovar, C. A., & Borderías, J. (2010). Effect of several cryoprotectants on the physicochemical and rheological properties of suwari gels from frozen squid surimi made by two methods. *Journal of Food Engineering*, *97*, 457-464.

[33] Kaur, L., Singh, J., McCarthy, O. J., & Singh, H. (2007). Physico-chemical, rheological and structural properties of fractionated potato starches. *Journal of Food Engineering*, *82*, 383–394.

[34] Clark, A. H., & Ross-Murphy, S. B. (1987). Structural and mechanical properties of biopolymer gels. *Advances in Polymer Science*, *83*, 57-192.

[35] Rao, M. A., & Cooley, H. J. (1992). Rheology of tomato pastes in steady and dynamic shear. *Journal of Texture Studies*, *23*, 415–425.

[36] Ahmed, J., & Ramaswamy, H.S. (2006). Viscoelastic properties of sweet potato puree infant food. *Journal of Food Engineering*, *74*, 376–382.

[37] Arocas, A., Sanz, T., & Fiszman, S. M. (2009). Improving effect of xanthan and locust bean gums on the freeze-thaw stability of white sauces made with different native starches. *Food Hydrocolloids*, *23*, 2478-2484.

[38] Ferrero, C., Martino, M. N., & Zaritzky, N. E. (1994). Corn starch–xanthan gum interaction and its effect on the stability during storage of frozen gelatinized suspensions. *Starch*, *46*(8), 300–308.

[39] Rodríguez-Hernández, A. I., & Tecante, A. (1999). Dynamic viscoelastic behavior of gellan-i-carrageenan and gellan-xanthan gels. *Food Hydrocolloids*, *13*, 59–64.

[40] Sun, C., & Gunasekaran, S. (2009). Effects of protein concentration and oil-phase volume fraction on the stability and rheology of menhaden oil-in-water emulsions stabilized by whey protein isolate with xanthan gum. *Food Hydrocolloids*, *23*, 165-174.

[41] Dickinson, E., & Chen, J. S. (1999). Heat-set whey protein emulsion gels: Role of active and inactive filler particles. *Journal of Dispersion, Science and Technology*, *20*, 197–213.

[42] Alvarez, M. D., Fernández, C., Olivares, M. D., & Canet, W. (2010). Rheological behaviour and functionality of inulin-extra virgen olive oil-based mashed potatoes. *International Journal of Food Science and Technology*, *45*, 2108-2118.

[43] Jampen, S., Britt, I. J., Yada, S., & Tung, M. A. (2001). Rheological properties of gellan gels containing filler particles. *Journal of Food Science*, *66*, 289–293.

[44] Zimeri, J. E., & Kokini, J. L. (2003). Morphological characterization of the phase behaviour of inulin-waxy maize starch systems in high moisture environments. *Carbohydrate Polymers*, *52*, 225-236.

[45] Bayarri, S., González-Tomás, L., Hernando, I., Lluch, M. A., & Costell, E. (2011). Texture perceived on inulin-enriched low-fat semisolid dairy desserts. Rheological and structural basis. *Journal of Texture Studies*, *42*, 174-184.

[46] van Vliet, T. (1988). Rheological properties of filled gels: Influence of filler matrix interaction. *Colloid and Polymer Science*, *266*, 518-524.

[47] Sosa-Herrera, M. G., Berli, C. L. A., & Martínez-Padilla, L. P. (2008). Physocochemical and rheological properties of oil-in-water emulsions prepared with sodium caseinate/gelan gum mixtures. *Food Hydrocolloids*, *22*, 934-942.

[48] Eliasson, A. C., & Kim, H. R. (1992). Changes in rheological properties of hydroxypropyl potato starch pastes during freeze-thaw treatments I. A rheological approach for evaluation of freeze-thaw stability. *Journal of Texture Studies*, *23*, 279-295.

[49] Guggisberg, D., Cuthbert-Steven, J., Piccinali, P., Bütikofer, U., & Eberhard, P. (2009). Rheological, microstructural and sensory characterization of low-fat and whole milk set yogurt as influenced by inulin addition. *International Dairy Journal*, *19*, 107-115.

[50] Hébette, C. L. M., Delcour, J. A., Koch, M. H. J., Booten, K., Kleppinger, R., Mischenkod, N., & Reynaers, H. (1998). Complex melting of semi-crystalline chicory (*Cichoriumintybus L.*) root inulin. *Carbohydrate Research*, *310*, 65–75.

[51] Franck, A., & De Leeheer, L. (2005). Inulin In A. Steinbüchel, & S. Ki Ehee (Eds.), *Polysaccharides and Polyamides in the Food Industry*, (pp. 281-322), Weinheim: Wiley-VCH Verlag GmbH & Co. KGaA.

[52] Giannouli, P., & Morris, E. R. (2003). Cryogelation of xanthan. *Food Hydrocolloids*, 17, 495-501.

[53] Chantrapornchai, W., Clydesdale, F., & McClements, D. J. (1999). Influence of droplet characteristics on the optical properties of colored oil-in-water emulsions. *Colloids and Surfaces A*, *155*, 373-382.

[54] Criado, M. N., Romero, M. P., Casanovas, M., & Motilva, M. J. (2008). Pigment profile and colour of monovarietal virgin olive oils from Arbequina cultivar obtained during two consecutive crop seasons. *Food Chemistry*, *110*, 873-880.

[55] Bot, A., Erle, U., Vreeker, R., & Agterof, W. (2004). Influence of crystallisation conditions on the large deformation rheology of inulin gels. *Food Hydrocolloids*, *18*, 547-556.

[56] O'Leary, E., Gormley, T. R., Butler, F., & Shilton, N. (2000). The effect of freeze-chilling on the quality of ready-meal components. *Lebensmittel-Wissenschaft und-Technologie*, *33*, 217–224.

[57] González-Tomás, L., Bayarri, S., & Costell, E. (2009). Inulin-enriched dairy desserts: physicochemical and sensory aspects. *Journal of Dairy Science*, *92*, 4188-4199.

[58] Akalin, A. S., Karagözlü, C., & Ünal, G. (2008). Rheological properties of reduced-fat and low-fat ice cream containing whey protein isolate and inulin. *European Food Research and Technology*, *227* (3), 889-895.

[59] Castro, F. P., Cunha, T. M., Barreto, P. L. M., Amboni, R. D. M. C., & Prudêncio, E. S. (2009). Effect of oligofructose incorporation on the properties of fermented probiotic lactic beverages. *International Journal of Dairy Technology*, *62* (1), 68-74.

[60] Kokini, J. L., & Cussler, E. L. (1983). Predicting the texture of liquid and melting semi-solid foods. *Journal of Food Science*, *48* (4), 1221-1225.

[61] Cussler, E. L., Kokini, J. L., Weinheimer, R. L., & Moskowitz, H. R. (1979). Food texture in mouth. *Food Technology*, *33* (10), 89-92.

[62] Frost, M. B., Dijksterhuis, G., & Martens, M. (2001). Sensory perception of fat in milk. *Food Quality and Preference*, *12* (5-7), 327-336.

[63] Kilkast, D., & Clegg, S. (2002). Sensory perception of creaminess and its relationship with food structure. *Food Quality and Preference*, *13* (7, 8), 609-623.

[64] de Wijk, R. A., Terpstra, M. E. J., Janssen, A. M., Prinz, J. F. (2006). Perceived creaminess of semi-solid foods. *Trends in Food Science & Technology*, *17*, 412-422.

[65] de Wijk, R. A., Prinz, J. F., & Janssen, A. M. (2006). Explaining perceived oral texture of starch-based custard desserts. *Food Hydrocolloids*, *20*, 24-34.

[66] Jellema, R. H., Janssen, A. M., Terpstra, M. E. J., De Wijk, R. A., & Smilde, A. K. (2005). *Journal of Chemometrics*, *19*, 191-200.

[67] Villegas, B., Carbonell, I., & Costell, E. (2007). Inulin milk beverages: sensory differences in thickness and creaminess using r-index analysis of the ranking data. *Journal of Sensory Studies*, *22*, 377-393.

[68] Kip, P., Meyer, D., & Jellema, R. H. (2006). Inulins improve sensoric and textural properties of low-fat yoghurts. *International Dairy Journal*, *16*, 1098-1103.

[69] Modzelewska-Kapituła, M., & Kłębukowska, L. (2009). Investigation of the potential for using inulin HPX as a fat replacer in yoghurt production. *International Journal of Dairy Technology*, *62*, 209-214.

[70] Lobato, L. P., Grossmann, M. V. E., & Benassi, M. T. (2009). Inulin addition in starch-based dairy desserts: Instrumental texture and sensory aspects. *Food Science and Technology International*, *15*, 317-323.

[71] Tárrega, A., & Costell, E. (2006). Effect of inulin addition on rheological and sensory properties of fat-free starch-based dairy desserts. *International Dairy Journal*, *16*, 1104-1112.

[72] Franck, A. (2002). Technological functionality of inulin and oligofructose. *British Journal of Nutrition*, *2*, 287–291.

[73] Angerosa, F., Servili, M., Selvaggini, R., Taticchi, A., Esposto, S., & Montedoro, G. (2004). Volatile compounds in virgen olive oil: occurrence and their relationship with the quality. *Journal of Chromatography A*, *1054* (1), 17-31.

[74] Cerretani, L., Salvador, M. D., Bendini, A., & Fregapane, G. (2008). Relationship between sensory evaluation performed by Italian and Spanish official panels and volatile and phenolic profiles of virgin olive oils. *Chemosensory Perception*, *1*, 258-267.

[75] Cardarelli, H. R., Aragon-Alegro, L. C., Alegro, J. H. A., Castro, I. A. & Saad, M. I. (2008). Effect of inulin and lactobacillus paracasei on sensory and instrumental texture properties of functional chocolate mouse. *Journal of the Science of Food and Agriculture*, *88*, 1318-1324.

[76] Alvarez, M. D., Fernández, C., Jiménez, M. J., & Canet, W. (2011). Texture of extra virgin olive oil-enriched mashed potatoes: sensory, instrumental and structural relationships. *Journal of Texture Studies*, doi:10.1111/j.1745-4603.2011.00301.x

[77] Dresselhuis, D. M., Cohen Stuart, M. A., van Aken, G. A., Schipper, R. G., & de Hoog, E. H. A. (2008). Fat retention at the tongue and the role of saliva: adhesion and spreading of 'protein-poor' versus 'protein-rich' emulsions. *Journal of Colloid and Interface Science*, *321*, 21-29.

[78] Dresselhuis, D. M., de Hoog, E. H. A., Cohen Stuart, M. A., Vingerhoeds, M. H., van Aken, G. A. (2008). The occurrence of in-mouth coalescence of emulsion droplets in relation to perception of fat. *Food Hydrocolloids*, *22*, 1170-1183.

[79] Benjamins J., Vingerhoeds, M. H., Zoet, F. D., de Hoog, E. H. A., van Aken, G. A. (2009). Partial coalescence as a tool to control sensory perception of emulsions. *Food Hydrocolloids*, *23*, 101-115.

[80] Taylor, A. J. (2002). Release and transport of flavors in vivo: physicochemical, physiological, and perceptual considerations. *Comprehensive Reviews in Food Science and Food Safety*, *1*, 45-57.

[81] de Wijk, R. A., van Gemert, L. J., Terpstra, M. E. J., & Wilkison, C. L. (2003). Texture of semi-solids; sensory and instrumental measurements on vanilla custard desserts. *Food Quality and Preference*, *14*, 305-317.

[82] Kim, Y., Faqih, M. N., & Wang, S. S. (2001) Factors affecting gel formation of inulin. *Carbohydrate Polymers*, *46*, 135-145.

[83] de Wijk, R. A., & Prinz, J. F. (2007). Fatty versus creamy sensations for custard desserts, white sauces, and mayonnaises. *Food Quality and Preference*, *18*, 641-650.

[84] Ojiako, U., Ashleigh, M., Chipulu, M., & Maguire, S. (2011). Learning and teaching challenges in project management. *International Journal of Project Management*, *29*, 268-278.

[85] Antmann, G., Ares, G., Salvador, A., Varela, P., Fiszman, S. M. (2011). Exploring and explaining creaminess perception: consumers' underlying concepts. *Journal of Sensory Studies*, *26*, 40-47.

[86] Weene, H., Jellema, R. H., & De Wijk, R. A. (2005). Sensory sub-attributes of creamy mouthfeel in commercial mayonnaises, custard desserts and sauces. *Food Quality and Preference*, *16*, 163-170.

[87] Szczesniak, A. S. (2002). Texture is a sensory property. *Food Quality and Preference*, *13*, 215-225.

[88] González-Tomás, L., & Costell, E. (2006). Relation between consumer's perception of color and texture of dairy desserts and instrumental measurements using GPA. *Journal of Dairy Science*, *89,* 4511-4519.

[89] Guerrero, L., Colomer, Y., Guàrdia, M. D., Xicola, J., & Clotet, R. (2000). Consumer attitude towards store Brands. *Food Quality and Preference*, *11*, 387-395.

In: Olive Consumption and Health
Editors: C. A. Savalas and S. M. Nicolau

ISBN: 978-1-62100-774-6

Chapter 2

OLIVE OIL, MITOCHONDRIAL OXIDATIVE STRESS AND AGEING

P. Pérez-López*[1], *M. C. Ramirez-Tortosa*[2], *N. El Azem-De haro*[2], *A. González* [1], *S. Granados-Principal* [2], *M. Battino* [3] *and J. L. Quiles* [1]

[1]Institute of Nutrition and Food Technology "José Mataix Verdú". Department of Physiology. University of Granada. Granada, Spain

[2]Institute of Nutrition and Food Technology "José Mataix Verdú". Department of Biochemistry and Molecular Biology II. University of Granada, Spain

[3]Institute of Biochemistry, Faculty of Medicine, Polytechnic University of Marche, Ancona, Italy

ABSTRACT

Ageing, usually defined as the progressive loss of function accompanied by decreasing fertility and increasing mortality, has important social and scientific impact. In the last years interest in this process has been growing as they have grown the theories that try to explain this process. One of the most widely accepted is the free radical theory which defends that free radicals produced at the mitochondria damage all biological tissues and lead to the ageing phenotype. In fact, there is a direct relationship between accumulation of oxidative damage produced by reactive oxygen species and the physiological alterations associated with ageing.

Nutrition has been related to ageing mainly at the level of caloric restriction and supplementation with antioxidants. In recent years a new approach relates the dietary fat type to mitochondrial and their sensitivity to experiencing oxidative stress because membranes adapt their lipid composition in response to dietary fat. The fatty acid composition of mitochondrial membranes affects in a direct way the properties of these

* Correspondence: Institute of Nutrition and Food Technology "José Mataix Verdú",
University of Granada. Biomedical Research Center.
Health Sciences Technological Park. Lab 120.
Avenida del Conocimiento s/n, 18071-Granada, Spain
E-mail: jlquiles@ugr.es Phone: +34958241000, Ext: 20316.

membranes such as fluidity and permeability, which determines its susceptibility to oxidation, thus affects the susceptibility to oxidative stress-related phenomena.

Olive oil modifies the structure, and consequently the features, of mitochondrial membranes, positively affecting the way and intensity in which different organs would age. When dietary fat is mainly olive oil a better general state at the mitochondrial function level is found, with a lower reactive oxygen species production at the mitochondrial electron transport chain level and finally with a delay in the occurrence of the ageing phenotype. In summary, the intake throughout life of virgin olive oil provides a healthier ageing.

ABBREVATION

ADP	adenosine diphosphate
AP	apurinic/apyrimidinic
ATP	adenosine triphosphate
CCO	cytochrome c oxidase
CE	cholesterol esters
CRM	caloric restriction mimetics
CoQ	coenzyme Q
CoQ_{10}	coenzyme Q_{10}
ETC	electronic transport chain
FAD	flavin adenine dinucleotide
$FADH_2$	reduced flavine mononucleotide
H_2O_2	hydrogen peroxide
MLSP	maximum lifespan potential
mtDNA	mitochondrial DNA
mtETC	mitochondrial electron transport chain
MUFA	monounsaturated fatty acids
NAD^+	nicotinamide adenine dinucleotide
NADH	reduced nicotinamide adenine dinucleotide
$O_2^{\cdot -}$	superoxide anion
OXPHO	oxidative phosphorylation
PL	phospholipids
PUFA	polyunsaturated fatty acids
ROS	reactive oxygen species
SFA	saturated fatty acids
TG	triglycerides
Ψ_{mt}	mitochondrial membrane potential

1. INTRODUCTION

Ageing is considered an endogenous process characterized by the progressive loss of function with decreased fertility, increased mortality and augmented susceptibility to the age-related diseases (Kirkwood and Austad, 2000). Furthermore, ageing affects to all multi-celled organisms and has been described as an endogenous and progressive decline in the effectiveness of physiological processes after the reproductive phase of life (Camougrand and Rigoulet, 2001; Barja, 2002; Sohal et al., 2002, Vijg and Suh, 2005). Many hypotheses have been developed and tested to explain the aging process at the organismal, organ, cellular and molecular levels (Yin and Chen, 2005). The progressive loss of cell functions could be due to a genetic program present in all the individuals or else to the stochastic accumulation of errors in the somatic cells (Fraga, 2009; Camougrand and Rigoulet, 2001), In addition another possible triggers of the ageing process have been defined, such as accumulation of DNA mutations, free radical overproduction, cellular oxidative stress and telomere shortening (Yin and Chen, 2005). In the study of ageing is important to considerate the added difficult to separate the process itself from diseases related to ageing (Quiles et al., 2004a).

Different disciplines, from sociology to medicine, have studied the determinants of longevity (Capri, 2007; De Benedictis et al., 2001). Each species reaching a certain age at which all the individuals have died. In the case of the human, this maximum lifespan has been established at 110 to 120 years. The life expectancy is affected by genetic as well as environmental factors, in addition to the stochastic component resulting from the interaction between individual changes for survival and unpredictable events that occur over the course of a lifetime (Lai and Chan, 2011, De Benedictis et al., 2001). At present, a minimal percentage of individuals are capable of reaching this maximum life, due to a certain extent to diseases related to wrong and inadequate nutrition (Quiles et al., 2004a). In societies more advanced there are other problems. Since XVIII at present, the life expectancy has grown at a rate of approximately three months per year; however, the cost of health has also grown and previously unknown diseases have appeared, such as Alzheimer's, cardiovascular diseases, etc. So, it can be said that the average lifespan has lengthened in developed countries with respect to undeveloped ones, although the maximum duration of life appears to be the same (Halliwell and Gutteridge, 1999; Partridge and Gems, 2002; McKeown, 2009).

If ageing is deleterious for individuals and it exists all over the world, why does it happen? The answer to that question might be that ageing is the side effect of something else. Thus, the genes that delay ageing could do that by repression of the cause that generates the damage associated to ageing. Reproduction appears to be a source of this type of damage. When ageing decreases fertility is frequently reduced, as well as by the presence of punctual mutations that extent the life. Due to many genes that participate in the response to the change in nutrient levels are too involved in the reduction of ageing, food could be another source of damage. Furthermore, it is know that the reduction in the ingestion of food diminishes ageing in a variety of organisms from yeast to mammals (Masoro, 2000; Partridge and Gems, 2002).

2. Ageing Theories

The molecular basis of this age-related decline is not well understood yet, and many theories have been advanced to explain the mechanisms of ageing (Medvedev, 1990). However any "single cause" theory could explain the full complexity of this process in all living organisms (Sacher, 1980). Overall, any theory must explain, according to Sanz et al. (2006a) some characteristics of ageing: its progressive, endogenous, irreversible and deleterious effect for the individual. Sohal et al. (2002) defends that any theory should be able to:

- To explain how an organism loses the capacity of maintaining its homeostasis to the end of its life.
- To clarify the bases for the wide variations in the duration of life in the species.
- To identify the factors responsible for the extending of life by genetic mutations or through experimental variations such as caloric restriction in rodents or environmental temperature changes in poykilotherms.
- To demonstrate how variations in the factors suspected of causing senescence can alter the degree of ageing.

We can group the existing theories on ageing into two blocks: stochastic theories and genetic-evolutionary theories.

2.1. Stochastic Theories

These theories propose that a random damage accumulates over time in different biological molecules until reaching a level where the damage triggers the physiological decline known as ageing.

In 1928 Pearl enunciated the **rate-of-living theory**, based on the observation that species with high metabolic rates had shorter lives, stating that life expectancy is inversely proportional to the metabolic rate of the species. Harman (1956, 2006) explained the biochemical link between metabolism and longevity, which was unknown. He proposed the **theory of free radicals**, which becoming one of the most widely accepted theories on ageing, and it suggests that normal ageing is the result of the random damage to tissues by free radicals. Later, Harman began to focus his theory towards the mitochondria as the major source of free radicals in the organisms. Miquel (Miquel et al., 1980) was based in that to propose the **mitochondrial theory** (progressive damage to mitochondrial DNA by reactive oxygen species, ROS). As at present many ROS are known not to be free radicals, today we talk about "theory of ageing of oxidative stress" (Yu and Yang, 1996).

There is another group of stochastic theories that could be explained by theory of oxidative stress due to certain similarities with it (Halliwell and Guteridge, 1999). On the whole form the group of theories of damage accumulation, and it includes the **crossing-over theory** (the random crossing-over of proteins and DNA alter cell functioning); the **theory of the catastrophic error** (accumulation of random damage in protein synthesis); the **theory of glycosylation** (the formation of glycosylate proteins give rise to a serious disruption of cell functions); the **theory of longevity determinants** (ageing is caused by the products of metabolim and the capacity to protect oneself against such products determines the degree of ageing); the **membrane hypothesis** (damage to the cell membrane diminishes the capacity to eliminate waste products, a decreased protein synthesis, a loss of water for the cytoplasm and diminishes enzyme activity); **entropy theory** (certain mechanisms, such as the restriction of caloric intake, reducing the degree of entropy production, releasing energy more slowly and retarding molecular deterioration) (Gutierrez-Robledo, 1998).

2.2. Evolutive Theories

In the evolutive theories, such as the **theory of immediate survival**, the ageing occurs because nature selects genes which are important for immediate survival, even if they are deleterious long-term (Kirkwood and Austrad, 2000).

More than 300 hypotheses have been proposed to explain the process occurs in ageing (Medvedev, 1990). One of these is the **immunological theory** (Walford, 1969), where ageing appears because of the decreasing in the capacity of immune system to produce antibodies: as the immune response diminishes, the capacity of the system to discriminate between its constituents and foreign elements also declines, with an increase in autoimmune reactions. This theory only can be applied to the immune system, and does not rule out the possibility that these changes might be secondary to other earlier ones, such as hormonal types.

On the other hand, the **neuroendocrine theory** (Medvedev, 1990; Weinert and Timiras, 2003) is based on fact that no part of the body can act in isolation from the nervous and endocrine systems. So, if one of these is disturbed, the other systems are also affected. However, this theory is not universal because of all organisms have not neuroendocrine system but nevertheless undergo aging (Gutierrez-Robledo, 1998).

2.3. Genetic Theories

The genetic theories of aging (Finch and Ruvkun, 2001) in generally propose that aging is the continuation of the development and differentiation process encoded in the genome. This theory postulates that aging would be the late consequence of the expression of genes selected by evolution for increasing reproductive success. As the young are in change of reproduction and genetic transmission, they manifest principally the selection of beneficial genes, without take into account what occurs to these genes at later ages.

One of the theories proposed in this group was the **hypothesis of disposable soma** (Lithgow and Kirkwood, 1996), which defends that the utilization of energy over a lifetime should be used preferentially for reproduction, and suggests that among the main candidates determining the life expectancy or a species from the genetic standpoint are genes that regulate the repair and maintenance of somatic cells. According to this hypothesis, natural selection favours those genes that act in the early stages of life to permit the species reproduction, against those ones that are in charge of preserving non-germinal cells or available soma (Kirkwood and Rose, 1991; Kirkwood and Austad, 2000).

The **telomeres theory** (Olovnikov, 1973; Mikhelson, 2001) proposed that the shortening of the telomeres in each of the cycles of cell division is the factor responsible for the limitation in the proliferation of the cell cultures, the "Hayflick limit" (Hayflick and Moorehead, 1961). According this theory, ageing could be combat braking or blocking the process that shorten the telomeres.

3. Nutrition and Ageing

The impact of the diet and dietary components on ageing and age-associated degenerative diseases has been widely recognized (Tanaka, 1998; Finkel and Holbrook, 2000). From long time ago, nutrition has been linked with ageing mainly as caloric restriction studies. On the other hand, several studies have focused to antioxidant role of many substances ingested with diet and the possible supplementation with those antioxidants. A very interesting approach to the problem comes from the fact that oxidative stress is related with the fatty acid composition of biological membranes and fluids. In fact, the intake of a particular type of dietary fat affects in a direct way the fatty acids and antioxidants profiles of the body and in an indirect way the susceptibility of the organism to undergo oxidation (Mataix, 1998; Ramírez-Tortosa, 1999a, 1999b; Quiles, 1999a).

3.1. Caloric Restriction

Some observations prove that the caloric restriction affects positively longevity in several species. McCay et cols. proposed first the limited food intake in 1935 (McCay et al., 1989), and they described the increase in longevity or life spam in several species and rodents, and also observed that diseases related age appeared later. Since then, caloric restriction has been demonstrated to enhance mean life span in a wide range of species, and decreasing the development of age-related disease in rodents (Masoro, 2000; Finckel and Holbrook, 2000). Reduction of food intake by 20%-50% increases longevity in many species from yeast to nonhuman primates (Ingram et al., 2006; Everitt et al., 2010).

The more accepted hypothesis to explain this phenomenon is based on the possible oxidative stress reduction. It was observed that mice which were fed with caloric restricted diet generated less oxidative stress than those who were fed *ad limitum*, besides to having lower lipid, protein and DNA oxidation (Finckel and Holbrook, 2000, Le Couteur et al., 2011). Caloric restriction of rodents, which confers increased longevity, is also associated with reduced mitochondrial hydrogen peroxide productions, which was observed in mitochondria isolated from liver (Hagopian et al., 2005), skeletal muscle (Bevilacqua et al., 2004) and brain (Sanz et al., 2005) in calorie-restricted rats. However, when caloric restriction only affects lipids (Sanz et al., 2006b) or carbohydrates (Sanz et al., 2006c) there are not change in mitochondrial ROS production or extend longevity in mice.

In addition, caloric restriction gives rodents higher capacity to withstand different physiological stress improves thermotolerance and diminishes heat-induced damage in olds rats (Quiles et al., 2004a).

Caloric restriction can be considered an effective mechanism to act therapeutically against ageing and related diseases (Roth et al., 1999). Nevertheless, the possible use of caloric restriction as an anti-aging therapy in humans would involve practical and ethical difficulties that make it almost impossible to consider feasible or desirable (Finckel and Holbrook, 2000). Because of the difficulty in maintaining a caloric restriction diet for humans, there have been attempts to develop drugs that replicate the effects of caloric restrictions, the caloric restriction mimetics (CRM) (Ingram et al., 2006, 2004; Minor et al., 2010).

3.2. Supplementation with Antioxidant

Oxidative stress plays a very important role in the global process of aging. The free radical theory of aging hypothesizes that oxygen-derived free radicals are responsible for the age-related damage at the cellular and tissues levels. In a normal situation, exits equilibrium between oxidants, antioxidants and biomolecules, however in ageing the antioxidant capacity decreases. Thus, the possible anti-ageing therapy through the use of antioxidants is one of the alternatives to slow the process of senescence. Antioxidants are substances capable of inhibit or delay oxidation of a substrate. Endogenous antioxidant defenses are both non-enzymatic (uric acid, glutathione, nutritional factors including vitamins and phenols, etc) and enzymatic (superoxide dismutase, glutathione peroxidase, catalase, etc.). The most important source of antioxidants is provided by nutrition (Fusco et al., 2007). Nutritional antioxidants act through different mechanisms and in different compartments, but are mainly free radical scavengers (Berger, 2005):

- Neutralizing free radicals
- Reducing the peroxide concentrations and repairing oxidized membranes
- Quenching iron to decrease reactive oxygen species production
- Neutralizing reactive oxygen species via lipid metabolism, shot-chain free fatty acids and cholesteryl esters.

Vitamin C is the main water-soluble antioxidant and acts as first defense against free radicals in whole blood and plasma, and combined to α-tocopherol (the major form of vitamin E in humans) is particularly effective in inhibiting oxidation (Niki et al., 1995). Vitamin E is a lipid-soluble vitamin found in cell membranes and circulating lipoproteins that acts directly with a variety of oxygen radicals. Vitamin C promotes vitamin E regeneration (Maxwell, 1995). Carotenoids are lipid-soluble antioxidants and their supplementation improves antioxidant status and reduction of lipid peroxidation (Upritchard et al., 2003).

Antioxidant supplementation has been frequently indicated as a potential mean to improve health status and increase longevity (Harman, 1962). The possible relationship between antioxidant supplementation and longevity is due to the relationship of the latter with the rate of mitochondrial oxygen radical generation and the degree of unsaturation of membrane fatty acids (Barja, 2002).

Miquel and Economos used thiazolidine carboxylate to increase vitality and life span in mice (Miquel and Economos, 1979). The oral administration of glutathione against to age-associated decline in immune activity was described by Furukawa (Furukawa et al., 1987). Throughout the scientific development was observed the use of numerous antioxidants to counter the ageing process, as vitamins C and E, the coenzyme Q and some herbal extracts rich in flavonoids and polyphenols (Gutiérrez-Mariscal et al., 2011; Fusco et al., 2007; Halliwel and Gutteridge, 1999; Huertas et al., 1999). Coenzyme Q10 is an endogenous synthesized lipid, which transport electrons to complex III from complexes I and II and from the oxidation of fatty acids and branched-chain amino acids. Although CoQ10 is biosynthesized intracellularly, a small proportion is acquires through the diet. Results with these antioxidants were positives in terms of age-related oxidative stress attenuation, however, in relation to longevity increased only were observed positive effects in some cases

(Quiles et al., 2004b). Furthermore, coenzyme Q addition to dietary fat type modules age-related changes in mitochondrial DNA deletion and oxidative stress in rat heart (Ochoa-Herrera et al., 2001) and brain (Quiles et al., 2010). The reasons are not clear, but perhaps require a deeper understanding of the pharmacological properties of the molecules studied, particularly in relation to absorption, tissue distribution, metabolism and dosage. Also, it should consider the role of ROS on cellular signaling, so must be adjust the antioxidants dose in order to avoid changes in redox state which could alter cell function.

3.3. Fatty Acids and Ageing

In addition to ROS production, there is another constitutive characteristic of long-lived animals that links aging with oxidative stress: the degree of fatty acid unsaturation of tissue cellular membranes (Quiles et al., 2006a). Unsaturated fatty acids are the cellular macromolecules most sensitive to oxygen radical damage due to the presence of highly unstable electrons near their double bonds, and their sensitivity to lipid peroxidation is major in molecules with more number of double bonds. Thus, a low level of fatty acid unsaturation (e.g., that of oleic acid) will decrease cellular oxidative stress. Some studies show that the degree of fatty acid unsaturation of mammalian tissues is negatively correlated with maximum longevity (Pamplona et al., 2000a).

Moreover, lipid peroxidation products can produce protein covalent modifications. In this sense, lower levels of malondialdehyde-lysine and carboxymethyl-lysine protein adducts have been found both in mitochondria and tissues of the long-lived mammals and birds that display a low degree of fatty acid unsaturation (Pamplona et al., 2002). Recent studies indicate that experimentally induced decreases in liver and brain fatty acid unsaturation also lower oxidative damage in mtDNA (Pamplona et al., 2004). This will be one of the main lines to follow in this chapter.

4. The Role of Mitochondria in Ageing

Progressive loss of mitochondrial functionality is one of the common events associated with ageing. For this reason, these organelles are considered the biological clock of ageing (Salvioli et al., 2001). In fact, mitochondria have been proposed as the link between the age-dependent accumulation of oxidative damage produced by ROS and the physiological alterations associated with ageing (Van Remmen and Richardson, 2001). In this sense, several experimental studies suggest that mitochondrion is one of the main targets of the ageing process. According to Salvioli et al. (2001) this evidence includes:

- Accumulations of deletions and certain mutations of the mitochondrial DNA (mtDNA) in addition to decreased the mtDNA copy number in some tissues.
- Age-dependent decline in the activity of some enzymes in the mitochondrial electron-transport chain (mtETC).
- Greater production of free radicals, presumably as a consequence of the avove-described alterations.

- Changes in the morphology of mitochondria and collapse of the mitochondrial membrane potential (Ψ_{mt}).

Variations in the functionality of mitochondria may determine adequate or inadequate ageing, according to studies of specific population groups around the world. For example, an inherited variation in an mtDNA germ line (halogroup J) has been associated with a more adequate ageing process and to an extended life in the Italian population (De Benedictis et al., 2000). On other hand, in Japan, three mutations associated to an mtDNA germ line have been found with a high frequency in centenarians in this part of the world (Tanaka et al., 1998).

Another question is the role of mitochondria as a key element in cell-signal transduction. Thus, mitochondria may also be considered an element of control for the nuclear gene expression. In this sense, a number of adaptation or regulation proteins have been found at the mitochondrial level or are translocated to the mitochondria to cope with this role, as with Nur77/TR3, p53, PKCδ, JNK/SAPK, some caspases and several members of the bcl2 family, such as Bid, Bax or Bim (Finkel and Holbrook, 2000).

Regarding mitochondria in the ageing process, the control of apoptosis is vital. This control is frequently lost in aged cells, which in addition are more prone to suffer from oxidative stress. ROS decrease Ψ_{mt}, allowing the opening of the transition pore and the subsequent escape to the outside of calcium and other substrates. This sequence of reactions leads to apoptosis in lymphocytes as well as liver and the brain cells of aged mice (Watson et al., 2000).

5. Mitochondria as Source of Cellular Energy and Oxidative Stress

Oxidative stress theory, proposed by Denhan Harman in the fifties, (Harman, 1956) is based that reactive oxygen species, ROS, are a normal product of aerobic life and the accumulation of oxidative damage due to ROS results in changes that affect ageing. ROS and free radical react with several biological molecules inducing lipids peroxidation, oxidative changes in proteins, inactivation enzymatic, DNA alterations, etc. giving rise to what is known as ageing (Halliwell and Gutteridge, 1999).

In recent years, it has been ascertained that although ROS are produced through a large number of pathways of the aerobic metabolism, the main source of these species is the mitochondria (Lenaz, 1998; Halliwell and Gutteridge, 1999; Cadenas and Davies, 2000; Sastre et al., 2000; Salvioli et at., 2001, Van Remmen and Richardson, 2001, Vendelbo and Nair, 2011).

5.1. Mitochondrial Structure and Function

Mitochondria have two membranes, one external membrane, which is porous and another internal rich in proteins and which is a permeability barrier for ions. Both membranes are composed by lipids and proteins.

However, mitochondrial membrane is different from the rest of biological membranes since its protein content goes beyond 80% while most of biological membranes are less than 50% (Quiles, 1995). The protein complexes within the mtETC must be mentioned because of its importance and significance in the context of oxidative stress. In aerobic organisms, the mtETC produces the energy needed for life support. Basically, food is oxidized through the loss of electrons that are accepted by electronic carriers as nicotinamide adenine dinucleotide (NAD^+) and flavins (flavin mononucleotide, FMN, and flavin adenine dinucleotide, FAD). The reduced nicotinamide adenine dinucleotide (NADH) and the reduced flavins ($FMNH_2$ and $FADH_2$) are oxidized again by oxygen, producing great amounts of ATP. Oxidation occurs with small jumps in which energy is gradually released (Lenaz, 1998). The mtETC is composed mainly by 5 lipoprotein complexes (Quiles, 1995; Lenaz, 1998; Cadenas and Davies, 2000):

- Complex I or NADH dehydrogenase complex
- Complex II or succinate dehydrogenase
- Complex III or bc_1 complex
- Complex IV or cytochrome c oxidase (CCO)
- Complex V or ATPase.

The mtETC fraction that metabolises oxygen is Complex IV. Cytochrome c oxidase uses four molecules of reduced cytochrome c to remove one electron from each one and to pass them to an oxygen molecule. This tetra-electronic reduction of oxygen is not tenable in a single step but rather must be done electron by electron. Because of this gradual reduction, the protein complex must be sure that partially oxidized oxygen, highly toxic, will not leak to the medium before being transformed into water.

5.2. Mitochondria as Oxidative Stress Source

Mitochondria play a vital metabolic role by producing most of the cellular adenosine triphosphate (ATP) via oxidative phosphorylation (OXPHOS) (Tzagoloff, 1982). OXPHOS is responsible for converting energy from macronutrients (carbohydrates, fatty acids, and amino acids) to ATP through reactions by which those macronutrients are oxidized, oxygen is reduced to water, and adenosine diphosphate (ADP) is phosphorylated to ATP. More than 50 years ago, it was suggested for the first time that mitochondria might be involved in ageing (Harman, 1956). At the time, ageing was ascribed to the deleterious effects of radical oxygen species (ROS) produced by mitochondria as a result of age-related OXPHOS dysfunction (Page et al., 2010).

The product of the monovalent and bivalent reduction of oxygen are superoxide anion ($O_2^{\cdot-}$) and hydrogen peroxide (H_2O_2), respectively, which are usually produced during aerobic metabolism, mainly at the mitochondrial level (Cadenas and Davies, 2000). It has been estimated that a 1-5% of the oxygen consumed by the mitochondria is not fully reduced to water, but it is transformed to $O_2^{\cdot-}$, which is transformed to H_2O_2 spontaneously or as the result of the action of superoxide dismutase enzymes. Although CCO is the enzyme involved in the oxygen reduction, it hardly generates free radicals. The two main sites of free-radical production at the mtETC are complex I and complex III (Cadenas et al., 1977; Ksenzenko et al., 1983; Shimomura et al., 1985; Cross and Jones, 1991, Selivanov et al., 2008). This occurs when some electrons, during the pass from one complex to the other, escape and join the surrounding oxygen, generating $O_2^{\cdot -}$ (Lambert and Brand, 2009).

Other sources of ROS are located in the external mitochondrial membrane, where the desamination process of biogenic amines by monoamine oxidases produces H_2O_2 from O_2 through a bi-electronic reduction (Hauptmann et al., 1996), and in peroxisomes, where catalase exhibits both catalytic and peroxidatic activity, predestine peroxisomes to a source of oxidative stress (Angermüller et al. 2009)

The physiological level of ROS production at the mtETC depends on the metabolic state of mitochondria. At the state of mitochondrial rest (state 4), in which there is a low respiration level and no ADP availability, is associated with a high rate of ROS production, probably as a consequence of the high degree of reduction of the chain components. On the contrary, at the state 3, the active mitochondrial state, there is a high oxygen expenditure and elevated ADP availability. This state shows relatively low ROS production. In the state of anoxia (state 5), with a limitation in the oxygen delivery and absence of respiration, no ROS production is observed (Cadenas and Davies, 2000). From viewpoint of ageing, the complex I seem to be the main site for ROS production (Sanz et al., 2006a).

Several studies have found an inverse correlation between the rate of respiratory ROS production and lifespan. Barja et cols. Reported a negative correlation between ROS production of isolated heart mitochondria and MLSP in mammals and birds (Barja, 2002), which was later confirmed by Lambert et al. (Lambert et al., 2007). The mitochondrial ROS production is generally lower in longer lived species (Page et al. 2010).

5.3. Mitochondrial as Oxidative Stress Target

The sensibility of biological membranes to oxidative stress is due to the presence of a double carbon-carbon bond in the lipid tails of its phospholipids (Montine et al., 2002). Oxidative damage to membrane lipids may be directly generated by ROS as hydroxyl radicals or the superoxide anion, or indirectly by some products of lipid peroxidation such as some highly reactive aldehydes (Esterbauer et al., 1991). Oxidative damage of membrane lipids leads to its alteration and to changes in membrane fluidity and, in conclusion, alterations in membrane function (Halliwell and Gutteridge, 1999). There are several membrane proteins that are easily inactivated by oxidative stress (ATPase, ANT, COO, etc.). Damage to mitochondrial proteins, as result of direct oxidative stress or a consequence of lipid peroxidation, may lead to cross-linking, degradation and loss of function of such proteins. Moreover, this damage leads to the opening of the permeability transition pore, a key step in the process of apoptosis. Therefore, mtETC protein alteration has two consequences: one direct consequence is the loss of mitochondrial functionality, but another indirectly consequence is a rise in the ROS production (Lippe et al., 1991; Forsmark-Andree et al., 1997).

Mitochondria have their own genome, which is different in structure and organization from the nuclear genome. It is composed of a variable number of copies of identical circular double-strand DNA (up to 10 copies). It is located in the mitochondrial matrix, near specific areas of the inner mitochondrial membrane (i.e. close to the main source of ROS). Its size is small (16,5 Kb) and codifies for 13 mitochondrial proteins: seven subunits from complex I, ones from complex III, three proteins from complex IV, two from complex V (ATPase), 22trRNA and two rRNA (Lenaz, 1998; Cadenas and Davies, 2000; Van Remmen and Richardson, 2001). Mitochondrial DNA is not protected by histones, as opposed to nuclear DNA, and it has been traditionally considered of a high susceptibility to be oxidatively attacked (Richter et al., 1988). For a long time, it was considered that mitochondria did not have a system to repair damaged DNA but actually it is recognized the existence of an mtDNA repair system, which can repair the oxidative damage (i.e. damage to bases and single-strand breaks) (Bohr and Anson, 1999). The main mtDNA lesions generated by ROS are base modifications, such as the ubiquitous 8-oxoguanine (8-oxoG) lesion, although base loss and stand breaks may also occur. All of these lesions are repaired primarily by the base excision repair (BER) pathway, which is catalyzed in mammalian mitochondria, similary that occur in nuclear BER, by DNA glycosylases, apurinic/apyrimidinic (AP) endonuclease, DNA polymerase (POLγ in mitochondria) and DNA ligase. POLγ is de only polymerase present in the mitochondria (De Souza-Pinto et al., 2008; Gredilla et al., 2010; Maynard et al., 2010)

As many reports suggest, oxidative damage to mtDNA is more important from the viewpoint of ageing than that involving lipids and proteins, due to the ability of damaged mtDNA to be spread because of the division capacity of mitochondria and cells, which allows amplification of the physiological consequences of the damage. Furthermore, oxidative damage to mtDNA might be even more important than the damage to the nuclear DNA as the entire mitochondrial genome codifies for genes that are truly expressed, while the nuclear genome contains a huge amount of nontranscribed sequences (Van Remmen and Richardson, 2001). There are several ways through oxidative stress affects mtDNA, as alteration to bases, the rise in the number of deletions and the occurrence of punctual mutations. With ageing, there is an accumulation of mtDNA damage. The effects of mtDNA damage and mutations are particularly important in tissues containing post-mitotic cells, because of these cells cannot be replaced by intact ones. Therefore, it has been reported that oxidative damage to mtDNA in cardiac and neuronal tissue is inversely related to the maximum life span potential in mammals (Barja and Herrero, 2000), suggesting that such accumulation may play a role in the determination of lifespan (Gredilla et al., 2010).

Actually, a good approach to studying oxidative alterations to bases is through the analysis of 8-hydroxy-2-deoxyguanosine using liquid chromatography-tandem mass spectrometry (LC-MS/MS) in urine (Sauvain et al., 2011). Concerning DNA deletions, it has been reported that rise with ageing among a wide variety of post-mitotic tissues from several species (Yoneda et al., 1995). Moreover, the rise in the percentage of deletions has been directly correlated with oxidative damage. The "common deletion" is so called because of its frequency, which increases two- to three-fold with ageing in some tissues such as the brain (Cortopassi et al., 1992). Nonetheless, since the percentage at which the level of deletions increases does not exceed 2-3%, the physiological significance for ageing is speculative (Van Remmen and Richardon, 2001).

According to Halliwell and Gutteridge (1999), the steady state level of oxidative stress is the result of the balance between the levels of damage and the degree of repair or replacement of damaged molecules, so, in terms of balance, a net increase of oxidative stress during ageing may be found in terms of higher levels of damage or as the result of defects in the repair system. Depending on the capacity of the affected tissue to repair the damage or to replace the altered cell, tissue function will be affected in a higher or lower extent (Quiles et al., 2002b).

6. Olive Oil and Mitochondria

6.1. Dietary Fat Type and Membrane Unsaturation

One of the most important findings concerning fatty acids and ageing comes from the collaborative work between Dr. Pamplona and Dr. Barja, both in Spain. These scientists have proven through comparative studies that long-lived mammals and birds have low rates of mitochondrial ROS production and low levels of oxidative damage in their mitochondrial DNA (Pamplona et al., 2002). They also affirm that long-lived mammals and birds posses a low degree of unsaturation in their cell membranes (Sanz et al., 2006a). In conclusion, animals with higher lifespan have membrancs containing fatty acid less susceptible to lipid peroxidation. This leads to lower levels of DNA damage from lipid peroxidation and of lipoxidation-derived protein modification in such species (Pamplona et al., 1998, 1999, 2000a, 2000b, 2002, 2004; Herrero et al., 2001; Sanz et al., 2006a).

As stated above, oxidative damage to membrane lipid is extremely important in ageing. In spite of the fact that dietary lipids modulate the membrane lipid profile and peroxidation rate (Mataix et al., 2006), their effects on ageing have been only partially studied. Studies have focuses primarily on short-term treatments based on n-3 polyunsaturated fatty acids (Carrie et al., 2000). Polyunsaturated fatty acids (PUFA) from membrane phospholipids are highly sensitive to oxidation, so membranes very rich in PUFA should be more prone to oxidation; in this way, several studies have demonstrated that the inverse relationship between the degree of fatty-acid unsaturation and the lifespan is not due to a low content of unsaturated fatty acids in long-lived mammals, but mainly to redistributions between components of the polyunsaturated n-3 fatty acid series (Pamplona et al., 1998, 1999). The fatty-acid redistributions among species may be attributable to differences in the elongase and desaturase systems. As is well know, a fine control in the elongation and desaturation pathways is crucial for the maintaining of the membrane function through proper fluidity, signaling and other means (Sanz et al., 2006a).

Differences in peroxidizability between species lead to differences in oxidation at the level of lipids, DNA or protein. For example, fatty-acid differences have been confirmed between a short-lived species such as the rat (maximum lifespan potential (MLSP) = 4 years) versus a long-lived species such as the pigeon (MLSP = 35 years) in relation to lipid peroxidation and lipoxidation-derived protein modification in heart mitochondria, in the sense that the lower double bond content present in different lipids of the pigeon) were associated with a lower concentration of lipid peroxidation products *in vivo*, and a lower level of malondialdehyde-lysine protein adducts in heart mitochondria of pigeons than in rats (Pamplona et al., 1999). Therefore, the constitutive lower level of unsaturation in long-lived animals helps to protect their tissues and mitochondria against lipid peroxidation and oxidative protein modification and can be a factor contributing to their slow rate of aging.

In summary, there is a correlation between the maximum longevity of animals and the degree of unsaturation of membrane fatty acids. That correlation joins the previously stated one between the rate of mitochondrial oxygen radical generation and the maximum longevity of animals. In long-lived homeothermic vertebrates, both free-radical production and the membrane fatty-acid unsaturation are lower.

6.2. Olive Oil and Mitochondrial Oxidative Stress

The importance of a particular dietary fat profile is well known in relation to avoiding cardiovascular disease, certain types of cancer and alteration at the immunological level (Quiles et al., 2006b). Also, the dietary fatty-acid profile has been demonstrated to be important to the mitochondrial oxidative stress associated with the ageing process (Quiles et al., 2002b, 2004b, 2006a; Ochoa, 2003).

Dietary fat type influences several biochemical parameters at the mitochondrial membrane level (Mataix et al., 1998; Quiles et al., 1999a). The importance of fatty acids resides in the fact that biological membranes adapt it lipid composition to some extent in response to dietary fat (Huertas et al., 1991a; Quiles et al., 1999a; Ochoa-Herrera et al., 2001). Moreover, oxidative stress is related to biological membrane composition (Mataix, 2004). However, because there is distinct tissues this phenomenon is observed differently in several biological membranes present in the organism (Mataix et al., 1998).

Thus, humans and animals fed on olive oil based diets have membranes richer in oleic acid than those fed on sunflower oil based diets, whose membranes are richer in linoleic acid. In addition, adaptations of the electron transport system in response to dietary fat type have been widely reported (Huertas et al., 1991b; Quiles et al., 2001; Battino et al., 2002a). A polyunsaturated fat source (e.g. sunflower oil) will lead to membranes becoming more prone to oxidation than a saturated (animal fat) or a monounsaturated (e.g. olive oil) source. This has been widely demonstrated under several physiological and pathological situations using both animal and human models (Quiles et al., 1999b, 2002b; Ramírez-Tortosa et al., 1999a, 1999b; Battino et al., 2002b; Ochoa et al., 2002).

Evidences form animal studies suggest that MUFA-rich membranes are more resistant to oxidative processes, protecting the aged cell (Bello et al., 2006, Quiles et al., 2006a). Mitochondrial structure, integrity and DNA stability to oxidation were also enhanced when rats consumed a diet rich on virgin olive oil (Quiles et al., 2006c). It has been also demonstrated that the oxidative modifications produced by the ingestion of fried fats may be successfully buffered when using virgin olive oil (Battino et al., 2002b).

Traditionally the beneficial effect of olive oil on oxidation was exclusively attributed to its high oleic acid content, which is enriched in lipoproteins and cellular membranes, thereby protecting them from oxidative damage (Reaven and Witztum, 1996). Other diets are high in oleic acid, for example, oleic acid is present in pork but these fail to promote the low cardiovascular disease profiles or other beneficial trends associated with the Mediterranean diet. However, virgin olive oil contains minor components with antioxidant properties that increase its antioxidant effect, which have been widely studied (Covas et al., 2006; Bogani et al., 2007). One of these minor components is hydroxytyrosol, which come from the hydrolysis of oleuropein. Hydroxytyrosol has been demonstrated in numerous studies to have antiatherogenic properties with strong antioxidant power, and it acts as a powerful scavenger of free radicals with the superoxide anion, hydrogen peroxide, hypochlorous acid, etc. (Granados-Principal et al., 2010, 2011; Bullon et al., 2009).

7. The Study of Olive Oil, Mitochondrial Oxidative Stress and Ageing

There are several studies comparing virgin olive oil and another type of fat as the single life-long dietary fat source in rats. The results may be grouped into those related to general aspects of oxidative stress status in blood (Quiles et al., 2004b), those concerning the effects on liver mitochondrial DNA deletions and ultrastructural abnormalities (Quiles et al., 2006a), those concerning differences between mitotic and non-mitotic tissues in relation to different aspects of mitochondrial function (Quiles et al., 2002b; Ochoa et al., 2003), and those concerning changes in brain mitochondrial DNA deletions (Ochoa, 2011).

7.1. Differences between Mitotic and Non-Mitotic Tissues

In 2003, Ochoa et al. studied differences between mitotic (liver) and non-mitotic (skeletal and cardiac muscles) tissues in relation to ageing from the standpoint of mitochondrial oxidative stress and function. For this, they examined rats fed over 24 months on a diet differing in the lipid source (virgin olive oil or sunflower oil). To ageing study animal was killed at 6, 12, 18 and 24 months and liver, heart and skeletal muscle mitochondria were isolated. Regarding the fatty-acid profiles of mitochondrial membranes, they found (Ochoa et al., 2003) that the proportion of satured fatty acids (SFA) in liver did not change with age in either group, although there was a higher proportion of these fatty acids in the sunflower group at 6, 12, 18 and 24 months. Only dietary fat affected liver SFA. In heart, the sunflower group increased SFA with age. They were found differences between diets at 12 and 18 months, with animals fed on sunflower oil showing the highest levels. However, in skeletal muscle only were detected differences between groups at 6 months with the olive group registering the highest SFA proportion. The effect on age differed in the rats fed virgin olive oil having lower SFA levels at 12, 18 and 24 months. Age also affected skeletal muscle SFA. Animals fed on olive oil hag higher MUFA levels in all tissues, except for 6 months in skeletal muscle. Ageing did not affect the proportion of MUFA the same way, if not that depended on the tissue. In liver, age did not affect olive group, while in the sunflower group the rats 18 and 24 months old showed significantly lower values than in rats 12 months old. In heart, MUFA decreased in both dietary groups at 18 and 24 months with respect to 6 months. In skeletal muscle, age led to increased MUFA in both groups. The lipid source significantly affected the three tissues studied, while age was significant only for heart and muscle. For all tissues studied the proportion of PUFA proved higher in the sunflower group (except for heart at 18 months). No age effect was detected in liver. In heart, the olive group increased in PUFA at 18 and 24 months with respect to 6 and 12 months. The sunflower group showed a significant decrease at 12 months with respect to 6 and 24 months. In skeletal muscle, both groups registered a similar response, with the highest value at 18 months.

Oxidative stress in these animals was studied through the analysis of mitochondrial hydroperoxides (Ochoa et al., 2003). In liver, differences between diets were found only at 12 months, with the sunflower group reaching the highest levels. Both groups showed a significant decrease at 24 months compared with 6 and 18 months. The non-mitotic tissues increased hydroperoxide levels with age. Animals fed on sunflower oil reached higher values for all time periods except for 6 months. So, the lipid source had a direct effect only on heart and muscle hydroperoxides.

Mitochondrial function in these animals was investigated through the study of some elements of the mitochondrial electron-transport chain (Quiles et al., 2002b), namely, cytochrome b, coenzyme Q (CoQ) and the amount and activity of the complex IV (the cytochrome C oxidase system). In liver, CoQ levels for animals fed olive oil compared with sunflower oil were higher for 6 months of age and lower for 24 months. Age affected only the sunflower-oil group, with an increase in animals of 24 months of age. In heart, for both age periods, olive oil led to lower levels of CoQ than sunflower oil. In skeletal muscle, the olive-oil group registered lower levels of CoQ than did the sunflower-oil group at both ages. In terms of age, this molecule increased at 24 months for both dietary groups. Concerning cytochrome b in liver, the olive-oil group showed higher values for 6 months and lower levels for 24 months, compared with the sunflower-oil group. Age affected only the sunflower-oil group, with a sharp increase at 24 months. For heart, no differences were found between dietary treatments for 6 months of age, and higher levels were found in sunflower oil at 24 months. For skeletal muscle, both groups were similar at 6 months and the olive-oil group differed from the sunflower group at 24 months (with lower values).

Increased catalase activity is associated with a greater resistance to oxidative damage and, in this sense, catalase seems to be important in overall antioxidant enzymatic defense systems with respect to lifespan (Beckman and Ames, 1998; Brown-Borg and Rakoczy, 2000). Ochoa et al. (2003) found that another factor must be considered when catalase activity during ageing is considered, i.e., the dietary lipid source. Liver-catalase activity increased with virgin olive oil but remained unchanged with sunflower oil. In heart, both groups showed increased catalase activity with age, but this increase was higher in the olive-oil group. Finally, skeletal muscle decreased catalase activity in both dietary groups. With respect to heart, the increased activity found in olive group is important because it has been suggested that catalase can function as a major pathway for detoxification of H_2O_2 in cardiac tissue (Molina and García, 1997).

In addition, Quiles et al. (2002) have previously reported that ageing depresses cytochrome oxidase activity, the final electron acceptor at the mitochondrial electron transport chain (METC), in heart and skeletal muscle but not in liver (Quiles et al., 2002b). In parallel, the levels of other METC components such as cytochrome b increased a situation that could lead to the uncoupling of the METC and subsequently augment free-radical production. Cytochrome b enhancement is considered a marker of ageing (Kipling, 2001) and occurs at the main site of free-radical production in the METC (Lenaz, 1998). Ochoa et al. study shown that with the PUFA-rich diet, cytochrome oxidase decreased and cytochrome b increased more than with the MUFA-rich diet (Ochoa et al., 2003).

Ageing, considered as an endogenous and progressive phenomenon (Barja, 2002) leads throughout the lifespan to different disturbances in mitochondria and their components, such as mtDNA (Lee et al., 1997; Michikawa et al., 1999, Ploszaj, T. et al., 2010). These disturbances (which have a high oxidative component) have a negative impact on mitochondrial structure and function. Depending on the capacity of the affected tissue to repair the damage or to replace the altered cell, tissue function is affected to a greater or lesser extent (Quiles et al., 2002b). In this way, mitotic tissues with the ability to regenerate their cells, such as liver, appear to be able to buffer the damage, at least in part, as suggested by the lack of alterations of mitochondrial function in terms of cytochrome c oxidase activity (Quiles et al. 2002b). However, a loss in function is found in postmitotic tissues such as skeletal muscle, heart or brain, which lack de opportunity to replace damaged cells and are likely to have a less effective repair system (Souza-Pinto et al., 1999). This loss in function is reflected in the decrease in cytochrome c oxidase activity (Quiles et al., 2002b; Ochoa et al., 2003). Mitochondria from postmitotic tissues buffer the unfavorable situation by increasing in some elements of the mtETC, such as cytochrome b or polyunsaturated fatty acids. The increase in polyunsaturation could enhance membrane fluidity and CCO activity by the presence of a more polyunsaturated cardiolipin, as has been previously suggested (Huertas et al., 1991b; Quiles et al., 2001). However, both actions raise ROS production. The role of dietary fatty acids in this mechanism could reside in the building of an environment more or less prone to the generation and propagation of ROS. Moreover, dietary fat could modulate the phenomenon through variations in the antioxidant system and overall upregulate or attenuate the process. Thus, as postmitotic tissues are the most affected by ageing, the influence of diet should be particularly important in these tissues.

7.2. Studies on Fatty Acids, Oxidative Stress and Ageing in Blood

Quiles et al. (2004b) studied aspects of oxidative stress during ageing on blood and plasma, and they try to determine if the dietary manipulation affects the plasma fatty-acid profile, following the quantitative determination (mg/dl) of cholesterol esters (CE), triglycerides (TG) and phospholipids (PL) in rats fed with olive-oil or sunflower dietary fat. Although some studies suggest that fatty acids become more saturated with ageing, this being associated with a decrease in the degree of polyunsaturation (Imre et al., 2000; Ulmann et al., 1991). Most authors (e.g. Engler et al., 1998) reported lower levels of saturated fatty acids (SFA) with ageing as well as increased levels of selected PUFA, but Quiles et al. demonstrated that animals fed only on olive oil led to cholesterol esters, triglycerides and phospholipids more saturated with age, while no changes in SFA were found with age in animals fed on sunflower oil. These results paralleled net increases in all classes of PUFA for cholesterol esters, triglycerides and phospholipids for both dietary groups with ageing (except for triglycerides in the olive-oil group), which suggests that net changes in fatty acids during ageing depend to some extent on the specific dietary fat, although the general feature of increased polyunsaturation is maintained.

Consequences of the intake of PUFAn-6 or MUFA on health are well established, both those related to the effects on blood lipids and those related to oxidative stress. In this sense, it has been reported that plasma and subcelullar-membrane lipid profiles of animals fed on diets with PUFAn-6 fatty acids are associated to higher levels of oxidative stress at different levels than when animals are fed on virgin olive oil. Examples of such a situation include the performance of physical exercise (Mataix, 1998), the intake of thermally oxidized fats (Quiles et al., 2002c; Battino et al., 2002b) or the stress produced by xenobiotics such as doxorubicin (Quiles et al., 2002a; Mataix et al., 2001). How to prevent or attenuate the side effects of doxorubicin has been extensively studied to try minimizing its cardiotoxicity, causes mainly by free radical production. The use of virgin olive oil as dietary fat (8g/100g of diet) attenuates the toxic effects of doxorubicin in rats at several points in the electron transport chain and results in lower levels of peroxides in the mitochondria and microsomes of the liver (Huertas et al., 1991a). The type of dietary fat affects of doxorubicin at the level of mitochondrial free radical production, which could be important in the chemotherapeutic treatment of patients with cancer (Mataix et al., 2008).

Even under the situation of ageing, it has been demonstrated that lipid peroxidation is lower in animals fed on olive oil (Quiles et al., 2010; Ochoa et al., 2003). It has been reported that n-6 PUFA-rich diets lead to higher levels of lipid peroxidation and DNA double-strand breaks in rat tissues and blood during ageing, when compared with MUFA-based diets (Quiles et al., 2006c; Ochoa et al., 2003). However, PUFA-rich diet supplemented with antioxidant would help preserve the beneficial aspects of PUFAn-6 in health. It has been demonstrated that when n-6 PUFA diets are supplemented on coenzyme Q_{10}, the lifespan lengthens, lipid-peroxidation levels fall and higher antioxidant capacity is reached (Quiles et al., 2004a; Ochoa et al., 2007). Coenzyme Q addition to an n-6 PUFA-rich diet resembles benefits on age-related mitochondrial DNA deletion and oxidative stress of a MUFA-rich diet in rat heart (Quiles et al., 2010).

Opposing results concerning free-radical damage and ageing have been reported (Halliwell and Gutteridge, 1999). However, overall, it appears that free-radical damage (and particularly the levels of DNA damage) increased during ageing (Halliwell and Gutteridge, 1999; Chevanne et al., 2003). DNA damage in peripheral blood lymphocytes (in terms of DNA double-strand breaks) is higher with ageing, according with the free-radical theory of aging of Harman (2006). Quiles et al. fed rats lifelong with two different dietary fat sources: virgin olive oil and sunflower oil, and they found that virgin olive oil led lower levels of DNA damage and changes in the total antioxidant capacity (Quiles et al., 2004a).

7.3. Studies on Mitochondrial DNA Deletions, Oxidative Stress, and Ultrastructural Alterations in Liver

The liver is the central metabolic organ of the body; therefore dietary changes can have a major impact on ageing liver and on general health (Anantharaju et al., 2002; Quiles et al., 2002b). Moreover, the liver is critical in the protection from oxidative damage and plays a major role in the breakdown of potentially harmful lipophilic toxins (Thomas et al., 2002). Although the ageing liver appears to preserve its function relatively well (Anantharaju et al., 2002), several changes have been associated with this organ during the process of ageing. According to mitochondrial theory of ageing, the ageing process results from accumulation of mitochondrial DNA (mtDNA) damage. Growing evidence indicates the role of mtDNA mutations in elevated production of reactive oxygen species, which are proved to increase the number of mtDNA mutations (Ploszaj et al. 2010). Quiles et al. investigated possible effects on the frequency of liver mitochondrial DNA deletions, oxidative stress and mitochondrial abnormalities in liver mitochondria during ageing by following a model of feeding rats lifelong with two different dietary-fat sources (virgin olive or sunflower oils).

The study of the fatty-acid profile of mitochondrial phospholipids revealed no differences between both dietary treatments in relation to saturated fatty acids. It found a net increase in the amount of these types of fatty acids, individually as well as for total acids, with ageing (except for C24:0 in olive-oil group). MUFA were higher in animals fed on olive oil both at 6 and 24 months. Ageing increased these fatty acids in the virgin-olive-oil group. In animals fed sunflower oil, only the total amount of monounsaturated fatty acids were affected by ageing, which increased. PUFAn-6 was higher in animals fed on sunflower oil for both time periods.

Ageing led to a net increased in all studies PUFAn-6 in both dietary groups, as well as PUFAn-3, having virgin-olive-oil groups the higher content in these fatty acids, both individually and as a total. The total PUFA index showed no differences between dietary groups, but ageing resulted in an enhancement. Finally, concerning the ratio between PUFAn-3 and PUFAn-6, animals fed on sunflower oil led to an index seven-fold higher than animals fed on virgin olive oil; ageing did not alter this index. In summary, the different lipid profile of the diets was properly reflected in liver mitochondrial phospholipids of young and old animal, suggesting a proper adaptation of the rats to dietary fats (Quiles et al., 2006c).

There is substantial evidence from human and animal studies linking mtDNA deletions and ageing. Deletion frequency is affected by age, tissue of origin, species and the presence of some age-related diseases (such as Alzheimer's) and these aspects also oscillate depending on the laboratory (Kang et al., 1998). Quiles et al. found increased frequency of the so-called common deletion at the mtDNA levels in aged animals, with those fed on sunflower oil being twice as frequent as those fed on virgin olive oil (Quiles et al., 2006c). This proved that the age-related rise in mtDNA deletions can be modulated by the dietary-fat profile. A similar effect was previously demonstrated for caloric restriction (Kang et al., 1998). Also, mtDNA deletions corresponded to increased levels of oxidative stress with ageing in both dietary groups, although this increases was greater in animals fed on sunflower oil. It found that sunflower oil led to deterioration in mitochondrial structure, as suggested by the lower percentage of cristae per μm of mitochondrial contour found in old animals fed on sunflower oil compared to the young animals fed on the same oil (Quiles et al., 2006c). Additionally, animals fed on virgin olive oil had a higher number of mitochondrial cristae in both age periods. Mitochondrial circularly (the increase of which represents control loss) was higher in old animals fed on sunflower oil compared to those fed on virgin olive oil (Quiles et al., 2006a; 2006c). These results demonstrate that the age-related increase in liver mtDNA-deletion frequency is differentially modulated by the intake of different dietary fats, with virgin olive oil leading to a lower frequency of deletions than the n-6 polyunsaturated sunflower oil. On the other hand, mtDNA-deletion frequency could be correlated with mitochondrial oxidative-stress status and ultrastructural alterations.

7.4. Studies on Mitochondrial DNA Deletions, Oxidative Stress, and Ultrastructural Alterations in Heart

Life expectancy as well as the proportion of the aged population has increased over the last decades. Ageing causes many physical changes and age-related chronic diseases such as atherosclerosis, diabetes, cancer, and cardiovascular, coronary heart and neurodegenerative diseases. The prevalence of heart disease increases with age (Rosamond et al., 2008). Ageing heart has unique histological and biochemical features, so that increased apoptosis and necrosis, greater myocyte volume, and connective-tissue accumulation are frequently found in the myocardium of old animals (Kajstura et al., 1996). Heart is a postmitotic tissue that exhibits a highly aerobic metabolism due to the abundance of large mitochondria. Therefore, the physiology and bioenergetics of cardiomyocytes with age has been an important research for many years (Judge and Leeuwenburhg, 2007). Quiles et al. investigated possible benefits on age-related mitochondrial DNA deletions and oxidative stress of two different dietary-fat sources (virgin olive oil or sunflower oils) and the supplementation of sunflower oil with CoQ_{10} in rat heart (Quiles et al., 2010).

After the study of the fatty-acid profile of rat heart mitochondrial phospholipids after 6 and 24 months of the experimental dietary treatment, in relation to the ration between oleic (C18:1n-9) and linoleic (C18:2n-6) acids, the higher ratio was found both at 6 and 24 months for the virgin-olive-oil group. At 24 months, ageing increased the ratios in virgin olive and sunflower plus CoQ_{10} groups. No statistically significant difference was found between sunflower group for 6 and 24 months of age. Coenzyme Q addition to an n-6 PUFA-rich diet improved the ratio between monounsaturated and polyunsaturated acids. The different lipid profile of the diets was properly reflected in heart mitochondrial phospholipids of young and old animals, that suggests a proper adaptation of the rats to dietary fats (Quiles et al., 2010).

It has been reported that mitochondria in aged rodent cardiomyocytes have a tendency to become larger and swollen in appearance and to exhibit lower amounts of cristae (Wessells and Bodmer, 2007). In this study, no changes were found in the mitochondrial area or perimeter during ageing, which agrees with previous findings in liver (Quiles et al., 2006c). The lower density of cristae for rats fed on sunflower oil, in comparison with those fed on virgin olive oil, has also been previously described in liver mitochondrial cristae (Quiles et al., 2006c). The involvement of mitochondrial DNA (mtDNA) in the ageing process stems mainly from its location, close to the mitochondrial respiratory chain, which is the main ROS source generation, thus explaining in part its susceptibility to oxidative damage. According to several authors, complex I is probably one of the complexes most affected by ageing (Sanz et al., 2006a). Quiles et al. measured the frequency of a particular deletion in complex I, found the lower values for animals fed on virgin olive oil at both 6 and 24 months. Concerning ageing changes, sunflower and sunflower plus CoQ groups showed higher percentages at 24 months and no ageing-associated changes were found for the virgin-olive-oil group, so ageing led to higher values only for the animals fed on the n-6 PUFA-rich diet, however, sunflower plus CoQ group shown lower values than sunflower group. Previously was reported that the dietary fat type can modulate the age-related increase in the frequency of this deletion in rat liver (Quiles et al., 2006c), this study present similar results for the heart, but in addition, a positive effect of CoQ_{10} supplementation is also reported. These results demonstrate that the age-related rise in mtDNA deletions can be attenuated. Only caloric restriction has been previously demonstrated to have such a capacity in attenuating the age-related increase in mtDNA deletion frequency (Kang et al., 1998).

One of goals was to determine whether low dosages of CoQ for long time periods raise CoQ levels. Three lipophylic antioxidants (α-tocopherol, CoQ_9 and CoQ_{10}) were measured in heart mitochondrial, and the results shown that ageing led to higher concentrations at 24 months, compared with 6 months. Comparing the three antioxidants, it found no differences at 6 months between groups for α-tocopherol and CoQ_9; however the sunflower plus CoQ_{10} group had the higher values of CoQ_{10}. This evidences that the supplementation of sunflower-oil diet with CoQ_{10} increases the mitochondrial level of this antioxidant in heart. Another stress-oxidative marker measured was lipid peroxidation (lipidic hydroperoxides), where no differences were discovered at 6 months between groups. At 24 months, lower levels were found for the sunflower plus CoQ group. Ageing led to higher concentrations at 24 months for the virgin-olive-oil and sunflower-oil group while no affects to sunflower plus CoQ group. Lipid-peroxidation values, as the level of mitochondrial hydroperoxides showed a common profile characterized by higher concentrations in all groups of aged rats. In opposition to other experiments performed previously by the same group (Ochoa et al., 2003), animals fed on the MUFA-rich diet did not reach lower values for lipid-peroxidation markers than those fed on the sunflower-rich diet. On this occasion, lipid-peroxidation results did not reflect the differences found in the above-mentioned mitochondrial-lipid profile. On the other hand, animals fed on the sunflower-rich diet and supplemented throughout life with CoQ_{10} showed lower lipid-peroxidation values during ageing than in the rest of the groups. CoQ supplementation could be the responsible for the higher protection in this group against lipid peroxidation.

Protein oxidation is an important aspect of age-related oxidative stress. Several papers indicate that protein oxidation augments with ageing (Yasuda et al., 2006). Oxidative alterations to proteins include especially sensitive amino-acid residues in proteins, such as tyrosine, methionine, arginine, proline, and lysine, among others (Amici et al., 1989). Quiles et al. investigated probes of oxidation of amino acids in protein, in particular carbonyl products of metal-catalyzed oxidation of proteins (Pamplona et al., 2005). For the parameters used, ageing led to higher values at 24 months compared with the same groups at 6 months. Overall, those data suggest that MUFA can partially protect mitochondria from age-related changes and that CoQ supplementation to n-6 PUFA partially resembles some of the positive results found after the lifelong feeding of MUFA-based diet. Moreover, lipid-derived oxidative damage appears to be more important than the pure protein-derived oxidative damage during ageing.

7.5. Studies on Mitochondrial DNA Deletions, Oxidative Stress, and Ultrastructural Alterations in Brain

Mitochondria-related oxidative damage is a primary event in ageing and age-related neurodegenerative disorders (Su et al., 2010). Gilmer et al. recently reviewed that history of brain mitochondrial studies on ageing (Gilmer et al., 2010), examining many studies that have reported significant age-related decline in mitochondrial enzymatic activity and amount in various complexes isolated from whole brains or specific brain regions of mice, rats and primates. In these studies several groups report declines in enzymatic activities of certain ETC complexes with age, it is unclear whether these enzymatic changes translate into a functional decline in respiration or even a decline in ATP production (Van Remmen and Richardson, 2001). In the past few years it has been demonstrated that some antioxidants, as well as, interventions in relations to dietary fat, may be used as dietary antiageing therapies (Quiles et al., 2006c). Already seen how n-6 PUFA-rich diet lead to higher levels of lipid peroxidation and mtDNA damage in rat blood compared with MUFA-based diet (Quiles et al., 2006c; 2010); furthermore, it has been demonstrated that n-6 PUFA diet supplemented with CoQ_{10} lengthens life span, decrease lipid-peroxidation levels and enhance antioxidant capacity (Quiles et al., 2010; Ochoa et al., 2007). The next step taken by Quiles and his group was to evaluate the effect of dietary fat type and coenzyme Q_{10} on age-related changes is brain mitochondrial DNA deletion and oxidative stress (Ochoa et al., 2011). Studies of dietary fat (mainly n-3 PUFA family) effects on neurobiology and neurodegeneration have a long history (Innis, 2000). The brain is one of the less adaptable organs concerning dietary fat other than n-3 PUFAs. Only a few studies have analyzed the effects of dietary sunflower or virgin olive oil on the fatty acid profile in this organ (Yaqoob, 1995; Barzanti, 1994). On the other hand, studies using fish oil or any other n-3 PUFA source, shown an important incorporation of these fatty acid into the brain fatty acid profile (Engström et al. 2009), suggestion that the brain has a very strong preference for the incorporation of n-3 PUFA fatty acids into its membranes. Ochoa et al. analyzed the fatty-acid profile of brain mitochondrial membranes. When oleic acid was observed, no difference between the two dietary fat types were to be seen, however animals fed sunflower oil shown higher percentages of this fatty acid, with the exception of animals fed virgin olive oil at 24 months. The ratio between oleic and linoleic acids is higher in all groups fed virgin olive oil for both periods, which may suggest a good adaptation, although poorer than observed for these animals in other tissues (Quiles et al., 2002b; 2010). Respecting CoQ, animals supplemented with CoQ presented higher concentrations at 6 and 24 months than did the same groups without supplementation, so low dosages of CoQ for long time periods raise tissue CoQ levels. The fact that the animal membranes adapted well to dietary fat and CoQ_{10} supplementation is an interesting finding, because the benefits (if any) from being fed either of the two fat types and CoQ_{10} might persist throughout life, thus representing an opportunity for nutritional therapy during ageing.

Although all groups presented higher levels of hydroperoxides at 24 months than at 6 months, animals fed diets rich in n-6 PUFAs shown higher levels of lipid peroxidation than animals fed virgin olive oil. Even under ageing, it has been shown that lipid peroxidation is lower in animals fed virgin olive oil (Ochoa et al., 2003; Quiles et al., 2010). With these results, the protective action of virgin olive oil in brain of rats is demonstrated by means of lipid peroxidation markers. Furthermore, CoQ_{10} led to lower lipid-peroxidation values at all ages in the animals given the sunflower oil diet. There are various ways in which CoQ10 could induce these differences:

- Changes in the mitochondrial fatty-acid profile, thus affecting its susceptibility to lipid peroxidation.
- Increases in antioxidant defenses
- Effects on the production of free radicals.

Antioxidant defenses do not fall with physiological ageing; indeed, increases with age have been described (Halliwell and Gutteridge, 1999). It has been postulated that a compensatory antioxidant defense system exists to counteract the oxidative stress associated with ageing, and therefore some antioxidants would be expected to accumulate, such as α-tocopherol (Armeni et al., 2003; Van der Loo et al., 2002). In this study, Ochoa et al. found higher activities of antioxidant enzymes in older animals, irrespective of diet, which correlates with the increased oxidative stress found in older animals. Although CoQ_{10} increases α-tocopherol levels in the two diets, higher α-tocopherol amount were found in virgin olive oil group supplemented with CoQ_{10}, both 6 and 24 months.

Ageing has been associated with decay in the mitochondrial respiratory chain activity (Miró et al., 2000). The involvement of mtDNA in the ageing process is mainly from its location, close to the mitochondrial respiratory chain, which is the main source of ROS generation. The accumulation of somatic mtDNA mutations might play an important role in the ageing process by producing cells with a decreased oxidative capacity (Harman, 1972). Ochoa et al. studied a particular deletion from a region coding for complex I proteins, which is probably among the complexes most affected by ageing (Pamplona et al., 2002). They found that the deletion frequency differed depending on the dietary fat, CoQ_{10} supplementation and ageing, being lower in animals supplemented with CoQ_{10}. Ageing led to higher values with both dietary treatments, but they were higher for the animals fed the n-6 PUFA-rich diet, what had previously been shown to liver and heart of rats (Quiles et al, 2006c; 2010). The MUFA diet prevents the age-related increase in levels of mitochondrial DNA deletions in the brain mitochondria from aged animals. In addition, a positive effect of CoQ10 supplementation is reported. These results demonstrate that the ager-related rise in mtDNA deletions can be attenuated. Only caloric restriction has previously been shown to have such a capacity in attenuating the age-related increase in mtDNA deletion frequency (Kang et al., 1998).

SUMMARY AND CONCLUSION

The impact of the diet and dietary components on ageing and age-associated degenerative diseases has been widely recognized in recent years (Finkel and Holbrook, 2000; Meydani, 2001). Therefore, prevention through the introduction of lifestyle and proper nutrition habits ("functional foods") is now considered a primary strategy for what we call healthy ageing (Santos-González, 2011). Nutritional modulation has a major impact on mitochondria and therefore holds considerable promise as a therapeutic intervention (Schiff, 2011). Oxidative stress associated with age is closely related at the mitochondrial level to other features typical of the ageing phenotype, such as mtETC and mtDNA alterations.

The type of dietary fat will condition the mitochondrial functionality and structure, as well as it susceptibility to be oxidatively attacked. In this way, if we could build "customized" biological membranes according to a particular type of dietary fat, it would be possible to modify in a positive way the manner in which different organs age. This working hypothesis represents a new approach to the study of ageing from the viewpoint of nutrition, and it could have important implications for the study of the ageing phenomenon. Moreover, it could help us to understand the differences observed on ageing between populations with similar socioeconomic level but very different on diet (Mataix, 2008). So, it been demonstrated that populations with a Mediterranean diet, which have a distinct fat intake (sometimes even higher) to north of Europe or United States present lower level of certain age-related pathologies, like cancer or cardiovascular diseases (Roman et al., 2008; Mataix, 2001). There are another factors apart from source of dietary fat involved in these differences, but the role of fat is enough important to be taken into account from a point of view of cellular and molecular mechanisms to try to explain several age-related alterations.

With respect to dietary fat, mitochondrial oxidative stress and ageing, one of the most important findings is that is possible to modulate mitochondrial membranes through dietary fatty-acid changes and that these changes are maintained lifelong if the diet is not changed. As a consequence of such manipulation, changes in mitochondrial oxidative stress, mtDNA deletions, mitochondrial ultrastructural alterations and mitochondrial electron-transport function take place, reducing some of the deleterious effects of ageing in the mitochondria. In this sense, virgin olive oil confers greater protection to mitochondria. The antioxidant constituents of virgin olive oil, as well as its high content in monounsaturated lipids appear to be essential for the beneficial effect of this food. Virgin olive oil-rich diet extends the human lifespan improving reactive-oxygen production by reducing the unsaturation of the mitochondrial membranes.

In summary, virgin olive oil consumption leads to the preservation of mitochondrial function and its electron transport chain, with a lower level of free radical production, a blood more capable to fight against free radicals and with a DNA more protected against oxidation. Despite its many benefits, virgin olive oil has high energy content so the recommendation is not supplement the usual diet with this food, but rather to substitute olive oil for other lipids, choosing virgin olive oil as principal dietary fat, always keeping a balance between energy intake and expenditure. So, the intake throughout life of virgin olive oil like fat dietary provides a healthier ageing.

References

[1] Amici, A., Levine, R.L., Tsai, L. and Stadtman, E.R. (1989). Conversion of amino acid residues in proteins and amino acid homopolymers to carbonyl derivates by metal-catalyzed oxidation reactions, *J. Biol. Chem. 365*: 3341-3346.

[2] Anantharaju, A., Feller, A. and Chedid, A. (2002). Aging liver, *Gerontology. 48*: 343-353.

[3] Angermüller, S., Islinger, M. and Völkl, A. (2009). Peroxisomes and reactive oxygen species, a lasting challenge, Histochem. Cell. Biol. 131: 459-463.

[4] Armeni, T., Principato, G., Quiles, J.L., Pieri, C., Bompadre, S. and Battino, M. (2003). Mitochondrial dysfunctions during aging: vitamin E deficiency or caloric restriction – two different ways of modulating stress, *J. Bioenerg. Biomembr. 35*: 181-191.

[5] Barja, G. (2002). Rate of generation of oxidative stress-related damage and animal longevity, *Free Radic. Biol. Med. 33*: 1167-1172.

[6] Barja, G. and Herrero, A. (2000). Oxidative damage to mitochondrial DNA is inversely related to maximum life span in the heart and brain of mammals, *FASEBJ. 14*: 312-318.

[7] Barzanti, V., Battino, M., Baracca, A., Cavazzoni, M., Cocchi, M., Noble, R, Maranesi, M., Turchetto, E. and Lenaz, G. (1994). The effect of dietary lipid changes on the fatty acid composition and fuction of liver, heart and brain mitochondria in the rat at different ages, *Br. J. Nutr. 71*: 193-202.

[8] Battino, M., Ferreiro, M.S., Littarru, G., Quiles, J.L., Ramírez-Tortosa, M.C., Huertas, J.R., Mataix, J., Villa, R.F. and Gorini, A. (2002a). Structural damages induced by peroxidation could account for functional impairment of heavy synaptic mitochondria, *Free Rad. Res. 36*: 479-484

[9] Battino, M., Quiles, J.L., Huertas, J.R., Ramírez-Tortosa, M.C., Cassinello, M., Mañas M., López-Frías, M. and Mataix, J. (2002b). Feeding fried oil changes antioxidant and fatty acid pattern of rat and affects rat liver mitochondrial respiratory chain components, *J. Bioenerg. Biomembr. 34*: 127-134.

[10] Beckman, K.B. and Ames, B.N. (1998). The free radical theory of aging matures, *Physiol. Rev. 78*: 547-581.

[11] Bello, R.I., Gómez-Díaz, C., Buron, M.I., Navas, P. and Villalba, J.M. (2006). Differential regulation of hepatic apoptotic pathways by dietary olive and sunflower oils in the aging rat. *Exp. Gerontol. 41*: 1174-1184.

[12] Bevilacqua, L., Ramsey, J.J., Hagopian, K., Weindruch, R. and Harper, M.E. (2004). Effects of short- and medium-term calorie resctriction on muscle mitochondrial proton leak and reactive oxygen species productions, *Am. J. Physiol. Endocrinol. Metab. 286*: 852-861.

[13] Bogani, P., Galli, C., Villa, M. and Visioli, F. (2007). Postprandial anti-inflammatory and antioxidant effects of extra virgin olive oil, *Atherosclerosis. 190*: 181-186.

[14] Bohr, V.A. and Anson, R.M. (1999). Mitochondrial DNA repair pathways, *J. Bioenerg. Biomembr. 31*: 391-398.

[15] Brown-Borg, H.M. and Rakoczy, S.G. (2000). Catalase expression in delayed and premature aging mouse models, *Exp. Gerontol. 35*: 199-212.

[16] Bullon, P., Quiles, J.L., Morillo, J.M., Rubini, C., Goteri, G., Granados-Principal, S., Battino, M. and Ramírez-Tortosa, M.C. (2009). Gingival vascular damage in atherosclerotic rabbits: hydroxytyrosol and squalene benefits, *Food Chem. Toxicol. 47*: 2327-2331.

[17] Cadenas, E., and Davies, K.J.A. (2000). Mitochondrial free radical generation, oxidative stress and aging, *Free Radic. Biol. Med. 29*: 222-230

[18] Cadenas, E., Boveris, A., Ragan, C.I. and Stoppani, A.O.M. (1977). Production of superoxide radicals and hydrogen peroxide by NADH-ubiquinone reductase and ubiquinol-cytochrome c reductase from beef-heart mitochondria, *Arch. Biochem. Biophys. 180*: 248-257.

[19] Camougrand, N., Rigoulet, M. (2001). Aging and oxidative stress: studies of some genes involved both in aging and in response to oxidative stress, *Resp. Physiol. 128*: 393-401.

[20] Capri, M., Salvioli, S., Monti, D., Caruso, C., Candore, G., Vasto, S., Olivieri, F., Marchegiani, F., Sansoni, P., Baggio, G., Mari, D., Passarino, G., De Benedictis, G. and Franceschi, C. (2007). Human longevity within an evolutionary perspective: The peculiar paradigm of a post-reproductive genetics, *Exp. Gerontol. 43*: 53-60.

[21] Carrie, I., Guesnet, P., Bourre, J.M. and Frances, H. (2000). Diets containing long-chain n-3 polyunsaturated fatty acids affect behavior differently during development than ageing in mice, *British J. Nutr. 83*: 439-447.

[22] Chevanne, M., Caldini, R., Tombaccini, D., Mocali, A., Gori, G. and Paoletti, F. (2003). Comparative levels of DNA breaks and sensitivity to oxidative stress in aged and senescent human fibroblast: a distinctive pattern for centenarians, *Biogerontology. 4*: 97-104.

[23] Covas, M.I., Nyyssonen, K., Poulsen, H.E., Kaikkonen, J., Zunft, H.J, Kiesewetter, H., Gaddi, A., de la Torre, R., Mursu, J., Bäumler, H., Nascetti, S., Salonen, J.T., Fitó, M., Virtanen, J. and Marrugat, J. EUROLIVE Study Group (2006). The effect of polyphenols in olive oil on heart disease risk factors: a randomized trial, *Ann. Intern. Med. 145*: 333-341.

[24] Cross, A.R. and Jones, O.T. (1991). Enzymic mechanisms of superoxide production, *Biochim. Biophys. Acta. 1057*: 281-298.

[25] De Benedictis, G., Carrieri, G., Varcasia, O., Bonafè, M. and Franceschi, C. (2000). Inherited variability of the mitocondrial genome and successful aging in humans, *Ann. N.Y. Acad. Sci. 908*: 208-218.

[26] De Benedictis, G., Qihua, T., Jeune, B., Christensen, K., Ukraintseva, S.V., Bonafê, M., Franceschi, C., Vaupel, J.W., and Yashin, A.I. (2001). Recent advances in human gene-longevity association studies, *Mech. Ageing Develop. 122*: 909-920.

[27] De Souza-Pinto, N.C., Wilson, D.M., Stevnsner, T.V. and Bohr, V.A. (2008). DNA Repair, *Amst. 7*: 1098-1109.

[28] Engler, M.M., Engler, M.B. and Nguyen, H. (1998). Age-related changes in plasma and tissue fatty acid composition in fischer 344 rats, *Biochem. Mol. Biol. Int. 46*: 1117-1126.

[29] Engström, K., Saldeen, A.S., Yang, B., Mehta, J.L. and Saldeen, T. (2009). Effect of fish oils containing different amounts of EPA, DHA, and antioxidants on plasma and brain fatty acids and brain nitric oxide synthase activity in rats, *Ups. J. Med. Sci. 114*: 206-213.

[30] Esterbauer, H., Schaur, R.J. and Zollner, H. (1991). Chemistry and biochemistry of 4-hydroxynonenal, malondialdehyde and related aldehydes, *Free Radic. Biol. Med. 11*: 81-128.

[31] Everitt, A.V., Rattan, S.I., Le Couteur, D.G. and de Cabo, R. eds (2010). Calorie Restriction, Aging and Longevity; *New York: Springer Press*.

[32] Finch, C.E., and Ruvkun, G. (2001). The genetics of aging, *Annu. Rev. Genomics Human Genet. 2*: 435-462.

[33] Finkel, T. and Holbrook, N.J. (2000). Oxidants, oxidative stress and biology of ageing, *Nature. 408*: 239-247.

[34] Forsmark-Andree, P., Lee, C.P., Dallner, G. and Ernster, L. (1997). Lipid peroxidation and changes in the ubiquinone content and the respiratory chain enzymes of submitochondrial particles, *Free Radic. Biol. Med. 22*: 391-400.

[35] Fraga, M.F. (2009). Genetic and epigenetic regulation of aging, *Curr. Opin. Immunol. 21*: 446-453.

[36] Furukawa, T., Meydani, S.N. and Blumberg, J.B. (1987). Reversal of age-associated decline in immune responsiveness by dietary glutathione supplementation in mice, *Mech. Ageing Develop. 38*: 107-117.

[37] Fusco, D., Colloca, G., Lo Monaco, M.R. and Cesari, M. (2007). Effects of antioxidant supplementation on the aging process, *Clin. Interv. Aging. 2*: 377-387.

[38] Gilmer, L.K., Ansari, M.A., Roberts, K.N. and Scheff, S.W. (2010). Age-related changes in mitochondrial respiration and oxidative damage in the cerebral cortex of the Fischer 344 rat, *Mech. Ageing Dev. 131:* 133-143.

[39] Granados-Principal, S., Quiles, J.L., Ramírez-Tortosa, C.L., Camacho-Coherencia, P., Sáncherz-Rovira, P., Vera-Ramírez L. and Ramírez-Tortosa, M.C. (2011). Hydroxytyrosol inhibits growth and cell proliferation and promotes high expression of sfrp4 in rat mammary tumours, *Mol. Nutr. Food Res. 55*: 117-126.

[40] Granados-Principal, S., Quiles, J.L., Ramírez-Tortosa, C.L., Sánchez-Rovira, P. and Ramírez-Tortosa, M.C. (2010). Hydroxytyrosol: from laboratory investigations to future clinical trials, *Nutrition Reviews. 68*: 191-206.

[41] Gredilla, R., Bohr, V.A. and Stevnsner, T. (2010). Mitochondrial DNA repair and association with aging – an update, *Exp. Gerontol. 45*: 478-488.

[42] Gutiérrez-Mariscal, F.M., Pérez-Martínez, P., Delgado-Lista, J., Yubero-Serrano, E.M., Camargo, A., Delgado-Casado, N., Cruz-Teno, C., Santos-González, M., Rodríguez-Cantalejo, F., Castaño, J.P., Villalba-Montoro, J.M., Fuentes, F., Pérez-Jiménez, F. and

López-Miranda, J. (2011). Mediterranean diet supplemented with coenzyme Q10 induces postprandial changes in p53 in response to oxidative DNA damage in elderly subjects, *Age. Mar 15.*

[43] Hagopian, K., Harper, M.E., Ram, J.J., Humble, S.J., Weindruch, R. and Ramsey, J.J. (2005). Long-term calorie restriction reduces proton leak and hydrogen peroxide production in liver mitochondria, *Am. J. Physiol. Endocrinol. Metab. 288*: 674-684.

[44] Halliwell, B. and Gutteridge, J.M.C. Eds (1999) Free radicals in biology and medicine. *Third edition, Oxford University Press, Oxford, UK.*

[45] Harman, D. (1956). Aging: a theory based on free radical and radiation chemistry, *J. Gerontol. 11*: 298-300.

[46] Harman, D. (1962). Role of free radicals in mutations, cancer, aging and maintenance of life, *Radiat. Res. 16*: 752-763.

[47] Harman, D. (1972). The biologic clock: the mitochondria, *J. Am. Geriatr. Soc. 20*: 145-147.

[48] Harman, D. (2006). Free radical theory of aging: an update, *Ann. N.Y. Acad. Sci. 1067*: 10-21.

[49] Hauptmann, N., Grimsby, J., Shih, J.C. and Cadenas, E. (1996). The metabolism of tyramine by monoamine oxidase A/B causes oxidative damage to mitochondrial DNA, *Arch. Biochem. Biophys. 335*: 295-304

[50] Hayflick, L. and Moorehead, P.S. (1961). The cultivation of human diploid cell strains, *Exp. Cell. Res. 25*: 585-621.

[51] Herrero, A., Portero-Otin, M., Bellmunt, M.J., Pamplona, R. and Barja, G. (2001). Effect of the degree of fatty acid unsaturation of rat heart mitocondria on their rates of H2O2 production and lipid and protein oxidative damage, *Mech. Ageing Dev. 122*: 427-443.

[52] Huertas, J.R., Battino, M., Lenaz, G., and Mataix, F.J. (1991a). Changes in mitocondrial and microsomal rat liver coenzyme Q9 and Q10 content induced by dietary fat and endogenous lipid peroxidation, *FEBS Lett. 287*: 89-92.

[53] Huertas, J.R., Battino, M., Mataix, F.J. and Lenaz, G. (1991b). Cytochrome oxidase induction after oxidative stress induced by adriamycin in liver of rats fed with dietary olive oil, *Biochem. Biophys. Res. Commu. 181*: 375-382.

[54] Huertas, J.R., Martínez-Velasco, E., Ibáñez, S., López-Frías, M., Ochoa, J.J., Quiles, J.L., Parenti-Castelli, G., Mataix, J. and Lenaz, G. (1999). Virgin olive oil protects heart mitocondria from peroxidative damage during aging, *BioFactors. 9*: 337-343.

[55] Imre, S., Firbas, J.H. and Noble, R.C. (2000). Reduced lipid peroxidation capacity and desaturation as biochemical markers of aging, *Arch. Gerontol. Geriatry. 31*: 5-12.

[56] Ingram, D.K., Anson, R.M., deCabo, R., Mamczarz, J., Zhu, M., Mattison, J., Lane, M.A. and Roth, G.S. (2004). Development of calorie restriction mimetics as a prolongevity strategy, *Ann. N. Y. Acad. Sci. 1019*: 412-423.

[57] Ingram, D.K., Zhu, M., Mamczarz, J., Zou, S., Lane, M.A., Roth, G.S. and deCabo, R. (2006). Calorie restriction mimetics: an emerging research field, *Aging Cell. 5*: 97-108.

[58] Innis, S.M. (2000). Essential fatty acids in infant nutrition: lessons and limitations from animal studies in relation to studies on infant fatty acid requirements, *Am. J. Clin. Nutr. 71*: 238-244.

[59] Judge, S. and Leeuwenburgh, C. (2007). Cardiac mitochondrial bioenergetics, oxidative stress and aging, *Am. J. Physiol. Cell Physiol. 292*: 1983-1992.

[60] Kajstura, J., Cheng, W., Sarangarajan, R., Li, P., Li, B., Nitahara, J.A., Chapnick, S., Reiss, K., Olivetti, G. and Anversa P. (1996). Necrotic and apoptotic myocyte cell death in the aging heart of Fischer 344 rats, *Am. J. Physiol. 271*: 1215-1228.

[61] Kang, C.M., Kristal, B.S. and Yu, B.P. (1998). Age-related mitochondrial DNA deletions: effect of dietary restriction, *Free Radic. Biol. Med. 24*: 233-238.

[62] Kipling, D. (2001).Telomeres, replicative senescence and human ageing, *Maturitas. 38*: 25-37.

[63] Kirkwood, T.B., and Austrad, S.N. (2000). Why do we age? *Nature. 408*: 233-238

[64] Kirkwood, T.B., and Rose, M.R. (1991). Evolution of senescence: late survival sacrificed for reproduction. *Philos. Trans. R. Soc. London. B332*: 15-24.

[65] Ksenzenko, M., Konstantinov, A.A., Khomutov, G.B., Tikhnov, A.N. and Ruuge, E.K. (1983). Effect of electron transfer inhibitors on superoxide generation in the cytochrome bc1 site of the mitochondrial respiratory chain, *FEBS Lett. 155*: 19-24.

[66] Lai, W.F. and Chan, Z.C. (2011). Beyond sole longevity: a social perspective on healthspan extension, *Rejuvenation Res. 14*:83-88.

[67] Lambert, A.J., Boysen, H.M., Buckingham, J.A., Yang, T., Podlutsky, A., Austad, S.N., Kunz, T.H., Buffenstein, R. and Brand, M.D. (2007). Low rates of hydrogen peroxide production by isolated heart mitochondria associate with long maximum lifespan in vertebrate homeotherms, *Aging Cell. 6*: 607-618.

[68] Lambert, A.J. and Brand, M.D. (2009). Reactive oxygen species production by mitochondrial, *Methods. Mol. Biol. 554*: 165-181.

[69] Le Couteur, D.G., McLachlan, A.J., Quinn, R.J., Simpson, S.J. and deCabo, R. (2011). Aging biology and novel tarjets for drug discovery, *J. Gerontol. A. Biol. Sci. Med. Sci. Jun 21.*

[70] Lee, C.M., Weindruch, R. and Aiken, J.M. (1997). Age-associated alterations of the mitochondrial genome, *Free Radic. Biol. Med. 22*: 1259-1269.

[71] Lenaz, G. (1998). Role of mitochondria in oxidative stress and ageing, *Biochim. Biophys. Acta. 1366*: 53-67

[72] Lippe, G., Comelli, M., Mazzilis, D., Sala, F.D. and Mavelli, L. (1991). The inactivation of mitochondrial F1 ATPase by H2O2 is mediated by iron ions not tightly bound in the protein, *Biochem. Biophys. Res. Commun. 181*: 764-770.

[73] Lithgow, G.J. and Kirkwood, T.B. (1996). Mechanism and evolution of aging. *Science. 273 (5271)*: 80.

[74] Masoro, E.J. (2000). Caloric restriction and aging: an update, *Exp. Gerontol. 35*: 299-305.

[75] Mataix, J. (2001). Aceite de olive virgin: nuestro patrimonio alimentario. *Granada: Universidad de Granada and PULEVA Food.*

[76] Mataix, J., Battino, M., Ramírez-Tortosa, M.C., Bertoli, E., Quiles, J.L. (2008). Virgin olive oil: a key healthy component of the Mediterranean diet, *Mediterr. J. Nutr. Metab. 1*: 69-75.

[77] Mataix, J., Ochoa, J.J. and Quiles, J.L. (2004). Olive oil, dietary fat and ageing, a mitochondrial approach, *Grasas y aceites. 55*: 84-91.

[78] Mataix, J., Ochoa, J.J. and Quiles, J.L. (2006). Olive oil and mitochondrial oxidative stress, *Int. J. Vit. Nutr. Res. 76*: 178-183

[79] Mataix, J., Quiles, J.L., Huertas, J.R., Battino, M., and Mañas, M. (1998). Tissue specific interactions of exercise, dietary fatty acids, and vitamin E in lipid peroxidation, *Free Radic. Biol. Med. 24*: 511-521.

[80] Maxwell, S.R.J. (1995). Prospects for the use of antioxidant therapies, *Drugs. 49*: 345-361.

[81] Maynard, S., de Souza-Pinto, N.C., Scheibye-Knudsen, M. and Bohr, V.A. (2010). Mitochondrial base excision repair assays, *Methods. 51*: 416-425.

[82] McCay, C.M., Crowell, M.F. and Maynard, L.A. (1989). The effect of retarded growth upon the length of life spam and upon the ultimate body size. 1935, *Nutrition. 5*: 155-171

[83] McKeown, R.E. (2009). The epimediologic transition: changing patterns of mortality and population dynamics, *Am. J. Lifestyle Med. 3*: 19-26.

[84] Medvedev, Z. (1990). An attempt at a rational classification of theories of aging, *Biol. Rev. 65*: 375-398.

[85] Meydani, M. (2001). Nutrition interventions in aging and age-associated disease, *Ann N.Y. Acad. Sci. 928*: 226-235.

[86] Michikawa, Y., Mazzucchelli, F., Bresolin, N, Scarlato, G. and Attardi, G. (1999). Aging-dependent large accumulation of point mutations in the human mtDNA control region for replication, *Science. 286*: 774-779.

[87] Mikhelson, V.M. (2001). Replicative mosaicism might explain the seeming contradictions in the telomere theory of aging, *Mech. Ageing Dev. 33*: 1361-1365.

[88] Minor, R.K., Allard, J.S., Younts, C.M., Ward, T.M. and deCabo, R. (2010). Dietary interventions to extend lifespan and healthspan based on calorie restriction, *J. Gerontol. 65*: 695-703.

[89] Miquel, J. and Economos, A.C. (1979). Favorable effects of the antioxidants sodium and magnesium thiazolidine carboxylate on the vitality and the life span of Drosophila and mice, *Exp. Gerontol. 14*: 279-285.

[90] Miquel, J., Economos, A.C., Fleming, J.E., and Johnson, J.E. (1980). Mitochondrial role in cell aging, *Exp. Gerontol. 15*: 579-591.

[91] Miró, O., Casademont, J., Casals, E., Perea, M., Urbano-Márquez, A., Rustin, P. and Cardellach, F. (2000). Aging is associated with increased lipid peroxidation in human hearts, but not with mitocondrial respiratory chain enzymes defect, *Cardiovasc. Res. 47*: 624-631.

[92] Molina, H. and García, M. (1997). Enzymatic defenses of the rat heart against lipid peroxidation, *Mech. Ageing Dev. 97*: 1-7.

[93] Montine, T.J., Neely, M.D., Quinn, J.F. Beal, F., Markesbery, W.R., Roberts, L.J. and Morrow, J.D. (2002). Lipid peroxidation in aging brain and alzheimer's disease, *Free Radic. Biol. Med. 33*: 620-626.

[94] Niki, E., Noguchi, N., Tsuchihashi, H. and Gotoh, N. (1995). Interaction among vitamin C, vitamin E, and beta-carotene, *Am. J. Clin. Nutr. 62*: 1332-1326.

[95] Ochoa, J.J., Pamplona, R., Ramírez-Tortosa, M.C., Granados-Principal, S., Pérez-López, P., Naudí, A., Portero-Otín, M., López-Frías, M., Battino, M. and Quiles, J.L. (2011). Age-related changes in brain mitocondrial DNA deletion and oxidative stress are differentially modulated by dieарty fat type and coenzyme Q10, *Free Radic. Biol. Med. 50*: 1053-1064.

[96] Ochoa, J.J., Quiles, J.L., Ibáñez, S., Martínez, E., López-Frías, M., Huertas, J.R. and Mataix, J. (2003). Aging-related oxidative stress depends on dietary lipid source in rat postmitotic tissues, *J. Bioenerg. Biomemb. 35*: 267-275.

[97] Ochoa, J.J., Quiles, J.L., López-Frías, M., Huertas, J.R. and Mataix, J. (2007). Effect of lifelong coenzyme Q10 supplementation on age-related oxidative stress and mitochondrial function in liver and skeletal muscle of rats fed on a polyunsaturated fatty acid (PUFA)-rich diet, *J. Gerontol. A Biol. Sci. Med. Sci. 62*: 1211-1218.

[98] Ochoa, J.J., Quiles, J.L., Ramírez-Tortosa, M.C., Mataix, J. and Huertas, J.R. (2002). Dietary oils high in oleica cid but with different unsaponifiable fraction contens have different effects in lipid profile and peroxidation in rabbit-LDL, *Nutrition. 18*: 60-65.

[99] Ochoa-Herrera, J.J., Huertas, J.R., Quiles, J.L., and Mataix, J. (2001). Dietary oils high in oleic acid, but with different non-glyceride contents, have different effects on lipid profiles and peroxidation in rabbit hepatic mitochondria, *J. Nutr. Biochem. 12*: 357-364.

[100] Olovnikov, A.M. (1973). A theory of marginotomy. The incomplete copying of template margin in enzymic synthesis of polynucleotides and biological significance of the phernomenon, *J. Theor. Biol. 41*:181-190.

[101] Page, M.M., Robb, E.L., Salway, K.D. and Stuart, J.A. (2010). Mitochondrial redox metabolism: Aging, longevity and dietary effects, *Mech. Ageing Develop. 131*: 242-252.

[102] Pamplona, R., Barja, G. and Portero-Otin, M. (2002). Membrane fatty acid unsaturation, protection against oxidative stress, and máximum life span: a homeoviscous-longevity adaptation? *Annu. N.Y. Acad. Sci. 959*: 475-490.

[103] Pamplona, R., Dalfo, E., Ayala, V., Bellmunt, M.J., Prat, J., Ferrer, I. and Portero-Otin, M. (2005). Proteins in humans brain cortex are modified by oxidation, glycoxidation and lipoxidation, *J. Biol. Chem. 280*: 21522-21530.

[104] Pamplona, R., Portero-Otin, M., Requena, J.R., Thorpe, S.R., Herrero, A. and Barja, G. (1999). A low degree of fatty acid unsaturation leads to lower lipid peroxidation and lipoxidation-derived protein modification in heart mitocondria of the longevous pigeon than in the short-lived rat, *Mech. Ageing Dev. 106*: 283-296.

[105] Pamplona, R., Portero-Otin, M., Requena, J.R., Thorpe, S.R., Lopez-Torres, M. and Barja, G. (2000b). Low fatty acid unsaturation: a mechanism for lowered lipoperoxidative modification of tissue proteins in mammalian species with long life spans, *J. Gerontol. A Biol. Sci. Med. Sci. 55*: 286-291.

[106] Pamplona, R., Portero-Otin, M., Riba, D., Ruiz, C., Prat, J., Bellmunt, M.J. and Barja, G. (1998). Mitochondrial membrane peroxidizability index is inversely related to maximum life span in mammals, *J. Lipid Res. 39*: 1989-1994.

[107] Pamplona, R., Portero-Otin, M., Ruiz, C., Gredilla, R., Herrero, A. and Barja, G. (2000a). Double bond content of phospholipids and lipid peroxidation negatively correlate with maximum longevity in the heart of mammals, *Mech. Ageing Dev. 112*: 169-183.

[108] Pamplona, R., Portero-Otin, M., Sanz, A., Requena, J. and Barja, G. (2004). Modification of the longevity-related degree of fatty acid unsaturation modulates oxidative damage to proteins and mitocondrial DNA in liver and brain, *Exp. Gerontol. 39*: 725-733.

[109] Partridge, L., and Gems, D. (2002). A lethal side-effect, *Nature. 418*: 921.

[110] Pearl, R. (1928). The rate of living. *Knopf, London.*

[111] Ploszaj, T., Robaszkiewicz, A. and Witas, H. (2010). Oxidative damage of mitochondrial DNA: the result or consequence of enhanced generation of reactive oxygen species, *Postepy Biochem. 56*: 139-146.

[112] Quiles, J.L, Ochoa, J.J., Ramírez-Tortosa, M.C., Battino, M., Huertas, J.R., Martín, Y. and Mataix J. (2004b) Dietary fat type (virgin oil versus sunflower oil) affects age-related changes in DNA double-strands-breaks, antioxidant capacity and blood lipid, *Exp. Gerontol. 39*: 1189-1198.

[113] Quiles, J.L. (1995). *Comparative study of virgin olive and sunflower oils on lipid peroxidation in rats under physical exercise.* PhD Thesis. University of Granada. Granada. Spain

[114] Quiles, J.L., Barja, G., Battino, M., Mataix, J. and Solfrizzi, V. (2006a). Role of olive oil and monounsaturated fatty acids in mitochondrial oxidative stress and aging, *Nutr. Rev. 64*: 31-39.

[115] Quiles, J.L., Huertas, J.R., Battino, M., Mataix, J. and Ramírez-Tortosa, M.C. (2002a). Antioxidant nutrients and adriamycin toxicity, *Toxicology. 180*: 79-95.

[116] Quiles, J.L., Huertas, J.R., Battino, M., Ramírez-Tortosa, M.C., Cassinello, M., Mataix, J., López-Frías, M. and Mañas, M. (2002c). The intake of fried virgin olive or sunflower oils differentially induces oxidative stress in rat liver microsomes, *British J. Nutr. 88*: 57-65.

[117] Quiles, J.L., Huertas, J.R., Mañas, M., Battino, M., and Mataix, J. (1999a). Physical exercise affects the lipid profile of mitocondrial membranes in rats fed with virgin olive oil or sunflower oil, *British J. Nutr. 81*: 21-24.

[118] Quiles, J.L., Huertas, J.R., Mañas, M., Ochoa, J.J., Battino, M. and Mataix, J. (1999b). Oxidative stress induced by exercise and dietary fat modules the coenzyme Q and vitamin A balance between plasma and mitochondria, *Int. J. Vit. Nutr. Res. 69*: 243-249.

[119] Quiles, J.L., Huertas, J.R., Mañas, M., Ochoa, J.J., Battino, M. and Mataix, J. (2001). Dietary fat type and regular exercise affect mitochondrial composition and function depending on specific tissue in rat, *J. Bioenerg. Biomembr. 33*: 127-143.

[120] Quiles, J.L., Martínez, E., Ibáñez, S., Ochoa, J.J., Martin, Y., López-Frías, M., Huertas, J.R. and Mataix, J. (2002b). Ageing-related tissue-specific alterations in mitochondrial composition and function are modulated by dietary fat type in the rat, *J. Bioenerg. Biomembr. 34*: 517-524

[121] Quiles, J.L., Ochoa J.J., Huertas, J.R. and Mataix J. (2004a) Coenzyme Q supplementation protects from age-related DNA double-strands breaks and increases life span in rats fed on a pufa-rich diet. *Exp. Gerontol. 39*:189-194.

[122] Quiles, J.L., Ochoa, J.J., Ramírez-Tortosa, M.C., Huertas, J.R. and Mataix, J. (2006c). Age-related mitocondrial DNA deletion in rat liver depends on dietary fat unsaturation, *J. Gerontol. A Biol. Sci. Med. Sci. 61*: 107-114.

[123] Quiles, J.L., Pamplona, R., Ramírez-Tortosa, M.C., Naudí, A., Portero-Otin, M., Araujo-Nepomuceno, E., López-Frías, M., Battino, M. and Ochoa, J.J. (2010). Coenzyme Q addition to an n-6 PUFA-rich diet resembles benefits on age-related mitochondrial DNA detection and oxidative stress of a MUFA-rich diet in rat heart, *Mech. Ageing Develop. 131*: 38-47.

[124] Quiles, J.L., Ramírez-Tortosa, M.C., Yaqoob, P. Eds. (2006b). Olive oil and Health. *CABI Publishing group, Wallingford, UK.*

[125] Ramírez-Tortosa, M.C., López-Pedrosa, J.M., Suárez, A., Ros, E., Mataix, J. and Gil, A. (1999b). Olive oil and fish oil enriched diets modify plasma lipids and susceptibility of low density lipoprotein to oxidative modification in free-living male patiens with peripheral vascular disease: the Spanish Nutrition Study, *British J. Nutr. 82*: 31-39.

[126] Ramírez-Tortosa, M.C., Suárez, A., Gómez, M.C., Mir, A., Ros, E., Mataix, J. and Gil, A. (1999a). Effect of extra-virgin olive oil and fish-oil supplementation on plasma lipids and susceptibility of low-density lipoprotein to oxidative alteration in free-living Spanish male patients with peripheral vascular disease, *Clin Nutr. 18*: 167-174.

[127] Reaven, P.D. and Witztum, J.L. (1996). Oxidized low density lipoproteins in atherogenesis: role of dietary modification, *Annu. Rev. Nutr. 16*: 51-71.

[128] Richter, C., Park, J.W. and Ames, B.N. (1988). Normal oxidative damage to mitochondrial and nuclear DNA is extensive, *Proc. Natl. Acad. Sci. USA. 85*: 6465-6467.

[129] Roman, B., Carla, L., Martínez-González, M.A. and Serra-Majem, L. (2008). Effectiveness of the Mediterranean Diet in the elderly, *Clin. Interv. Aging. 3*: 97-109.

[130] Rosamond, W., Flegal, K., Furie, K., Go, A., Greenlund, K., Hasse, N., Hailpern, S.M., Ho, M., Howard, V., Kissela, B., Kittner, S., Lloyd-Jones, D., McDermott, M., Meigs, J., Wilson, M., Hong, Y,. American Heart Association Statistics Committee and Stroke Statistics Subcommitee (2008). Heart disease and stroke statistics-2008 update: a report from the American Heart Association Statistics Committee and Stroke Statistics Subcommittee, *Circulation. 117*: 25-146.

[131] Roth, G.S., Ingram, D.K. and Lane, M.A. (1999). Caloric restriction in primates: will it work and how will we know? *J. Am. Geriatr. Soc. 47*: 896-903.

[132] Sacher, G.A. (1980). Theory in gerontology. Part 1. *Annu. Rev. Gerontal. Geriatr. 1*: 3-25

[133] Salvioli, S., Bonafè, M., Capri, M., Monti, D. and Franceschi, C. (2001). Mitochondria, aging and longevity – a new perspective, *FEBS Lett., 492*: 9-13.

[134] Santos-González, M., López-Miranda, J., Pérez-Jiménez, F., Navas, P. and Villalba, J.M. (2011). Dietary oil modifies the plasma proteome during aging in the rat, *Age. April 7.*

[135] Sanz, A., Caro, P. Sánchez, J.G. and Barja, G. (2006c). Effect of lipid restriction on mitocondrial free radical production and oxidative DNA damage, *Ann. N.Y. Acad. Sci. 1067*: 200-209.

[136] Sanz, A., Caro, P., Ibáñez, J., Gómerz, J., Gredilla R. and Barja, G. (2005). Dietary restriction at old age lowers mitocondrial oxygen radical production and leak at complex I and oxidative DNA damage in rat brain, J. Bioenerg. Biomembr. 37: 83-90.

[137] Sanz, A., Gómez, J. Caro, P. and Barja, G. (2006b). Carbohydrate restriction does not change mitocondrial free radical generation and oxidative DNA damage, J. Bioenerg. Biomembr. 38: 327-333.

[138] Sanz, A., Pamplona, R., and Barja, G. (2006a). Is the mitochondrial free radical theory of aging intact? *Antioxid. Redox Signal. 8*: 582-599

[139] Sastre, J., Pallardo, F.V., De La Asuncion, G.J. and Viña, J. (2000). Mitochondria, Oxidative Stress and Aging, *Free Radic. Biol. Med. 32*: 189-198.

[140] Sauvain, J.J., Setyan, A., Wild, P., Tacchini, P., Lagger, G., Storti, F., Deslarzes, S., Guillemin, M., Rossi, M.J. and Riediker, M. (2011). Biomarkers of oxidative stress and

its association with the urinary reducing capacity in bus maintenance workers, *J. Occup. Med. Toxic. 6*: 18.

[141] Schiff, M., Bénit, P., Coulibaly, A., Loublier, S., El-Khoury, R. and Rustin, P. (2011). Mitochondrial response to controlled nutrition in health and disease, *Nutrition Reviews. 69*: 65-75.

[142] Selivanov, V.A., Zeak, J.A., Roca, J., Cascante, M., Trucco, M. and Votyakova, T.V. (2008). The role of external and matrix pH in mitocondrial reactive oxygen species generation, *J. Biol. Chem. 283*: 29292-29300.

[143] Shimomura, Y., Nishikimi, M. and Ozawa, T. (1985). Novel purification of cytochrome c1 from mitochondrial complex III. Reconstitution of antimycin-insesitive electron transfer with the iron-sulfur protein and cytochrome c1, *J.Biol. Chem. 260*: 15075-15080.

[144] Sohal, RS., Mockett, RJ., and Orr, WC. (2002). Mechanisms of aging: an appraisal of the oxidative stress hypothesis, *Free Radic. Biol. Med. 16*: 621-626.

[145] Souza-Pinto, N., Croteau, D.L., Hudson, E.K., Heansford, E.G. and Bohr, V.A. (1999). Age-associated increase in 8-oxo-deoxyguanosine glycosylase/AP lyase activity in rat mitochondria, *Nucl. Acids Res. 27*: 1935-1942.

[146] Su, Y., Sun, H., Fang, J., Hu, G. and Xiao, M. (2010). Brain mitochondrial dysfunction in ovariectomized mice injected with D-galactose, *Neurochem. Res. 35*: 399-404.

[147] Tanaka, M., Gong, J., Zhang, J., Yamada, Y., Borgeld, H. and Yagi, K. (1998). Mitochondrial genotype associated with longevity, *Lancet. 351*: 185-186.

[148] Thomas, R.P., Guigneaux, M., Wood, T. and Evers, M.B. (2002). Age-associated changes in gene expression patterns in the liver, *J. Gastrointest. Surg. 6*: 445-454.

[149] Tzagoloff, A. (1982). Mitochondria, *New York: Plenum Press.*

[150] Ulmann, L., Blond, J.P., Maniongui, C., Poisson, J.P., Duran, G., Bezard, J. and Pascal, G. (1991). Effects of age and dietary fatty acids on desaturase activities and on fatty acid composition of liver microsomal phospholipids of adult rats, *Lipids.26*: 127-133.

[151] Upritchard, J.E., Schuurman, C.R., Wiersma, A., Tijburg, L.B., Coolen, S.A., Rijken, P.J. and Wiseman, S.A. (2003). Spread supplemented with moderate doses of vitamin E and carotenoids reduces lipid peroxidation in healthy, nonsmoking adults, *Am. J. Clin. Nutr. 78*: 985-992.

[152] Van der Loo, B., Labugger, R., Aebischer, C.P., Skepper, J.N., Bachnschmid, M., Spitzer, V., Kilo, J., Altwegg, L., Ullrich, V. and Lüscher, T.F. (2002). Cardiovascular aging is associated with vitamin E increase, *Circulation. 105*: 1635-1638.

[153] Van Remmen, H. and Richardson, A. (2001). Oxidative damage to mitochondria and aging, *Exp. Gerontol. 36*: 957-968.

[154] Vendelbo, M.H. and Nair, K.S. (2011). Mitochondrial longevity pathways, *Biochim. Biophys. Acta. 1813*: 634-644.

[155] Vijg, J. and Suh, Y. (2005). Genetics of longevity and aging, *Annu. Rev. Med. 56*: 193-212.

[156] Walford, R.L. (1969). The immunologic theory of aging. *Munksgaard. Copenhagen, Denmark.*

[157] Watson, W.H., Cai, J. and Jones, D.P. (2000). Diet and apoptosis, *Annu. Rev. Nutr. 20*: 485-505.

[158] Weinert, B.T., and Timiras, P.S. (2003). Invited review: Theories of aging, *J. Appl. Physiol. 95*: 1706-1716.

[159] Wessells, R.J. and Bodmer, R. (2007). Cardiac aging. *Semin. Cell Dev. Biol. 18*: 111-116.

[160] Yaqoob, P., Sherrington, E.J., Jeffery, N.M., Sanderson, P., Harvey, D.J., Newsholme, E.A. and Calder, P.C. (1995). Comparison of the effects of a range of dietary lipids upon serum and tissue lipid composition in the rat, *J. Biochem. Cell. Biol. 27*: 297-310.

[161] Yasuda, K., Ishii, T., Suda, H., Akatsuka, A., Hartman, P.S., Goto, S., Miyazawa, M. and Ishii, N. (2006). Age-related changes of mitochondrial structure and function in Caenorhabditis elegans, *Mech. Ageing. Dev. 127*: 763-770.

[162] Yin, D. and Chen, K. (2005). The essential mechanisms of aging: irreparable damage accumulation of biochemical side-reactions, *Exp. Gerontol. 40*: 455-465.

[163] Yoneda, M., Katsumata, K., Hayakawa, M., Tanaka, M. and Ozawa, T. (1995). Oxygen stress induces an apoptotic cell death associated with fragmentation of mitochondrial genome, *Biochem. Biophys. Res. Commun. 209*: 723-729.

[164] Yu, B.P. and Yang, R. (1996). Critical evaluation of the free radical theory of aging: a proposal of oxidative stress hypothesis, *Ann. NY Acad Sci. 786*: 1-11.

In: Olive Consumption and Health
Editors: C. A. Savalas and S. M. Nicolau
ISBN: 978-1-62100-774-6

Chapter 3

VIRGIN OLIVE OIL ANTIOXIDANTS

Maria Tasioula-Margari*

Department of Chemistry, Section of Industrial and Food Chemistry,
University of Ioannina, Ioannina, Greece

ABSTRACT

The Mediterranean diet is associated with reduced risk of atherosclerosis, cardiovascular disease, and certain types of cancer and this has partially been explained by the consumption of virgin olive oil (VOO). Historically, the healthful properties of VOO were attributed to a high proportion of monounsaturated fatty acids, namely oleic acid, which represents 60–80% of the fatty acids present in virgin olive oil. In addition, virgin olive oil contains minor, yet significant phenolic components that other seed oils lack. Hydrophilic phenols are the most abundant natural antioxidants of VOO, in which, however, tocopherols and carotenes are also present. The prevalent classes of hydrophilic phenols found in VOO are complex phenols such as ligstroside aglycon and the dialdehydic form of elenolic acid linked to tyrosol, oleuropein aglycon and the dialdehydic form of elenolic acid linked to hydroxytyrosol. Simple phenols such as phenolic alcohols, (hydroxytyrosol, tyrosol) phenolic acids, (vanillic, caffeic, p-coumaric and ferullic acid) flavonoids, (luteolin, apigenin) and lignans, (pinoresinol, 1-acetoxypinoresinol) are present in olive oil at lower concentrations. The qualitative and quantitative composition of VOO phenols is strongly affected by the agronomic and technological conditions of production such as olive cultivar, degree of ripeness olive fruit, processing and storage conditions of the oil. A median of total phenols content of 300 ppm (as gallic acid) is reported, although the above individual phenols ranged widely (100-400 ppm). Those compounds are important for the sensory quality and storage life of VOO. Specifically 'sweet', 'fruity' and 'bitter' taste correlated with low, moderate and high amounts of phenolic compounds respectively. Bitterness is a common and desirable attribute of virgin olive oil flavour when present at low to moderate intensity. The stability of VOO is influenced by their concentration and type of phenols. Tocopherols are the major group of hydrophobic antioxidants occurring in VOO. Nearly 95% of the

* Assistant Proffessor, Department of Chemistry, Section of Industrial and Food Chemistry, University of Ioannina, Ioannina 45110, Greece, Tel.: 0030 2651008345, fax: 0030 2651008795, e-mail: mtasioul@cc.uoi.gr.

total tocopherols content is α-tocopherol, which exhibits the highest biological activity. The antioxidant activity is dependent on both concentration and lipid system factors, such as hydroperoxides concentration, metals presence, temperature, and singlet oxygen presence e.g. Natural concentration of α–tocopherol, varies between 100-400 ppm. These compounds are included in the designation of vitamin E and correlated with preventive action against reactive oxygen species (ROS) in biological systems such as plasma, membranes, and tissues.

1. Introduction

Currently, the olive oil produced in the European Union EU/27countries accounted for close to 75% of world production. The breakdown of this percentage between its chief producing countries shows shares of 46% for Spain, 15% for Italy, 11% for Greece and 2% for Portugal (International Olive Oil Council, IOOC).More than 95% of the world's olive trees grow in the Mediterranean Basin. About 84% of total olive production comes from the European Community (Spain, Italy, Greece, Portugal, and France) with the Near East (Turkey, Syria, Lebanon, Israel, Jordan, and Iran) contributing 5.5% and North Africa (Tunisia, Algeria, Morocco, Libya, and Egypt) supplying about 8.5%. The remaining 2% is of American origin, chiefly from Argentina, and Mexico, the United States, Chile, Peru, and Uruguay (Emmons, 1996).

In the last couple of years the number of reports describing the beneficial properties of olive oil has dramatically increased. It has been postulated that the lower incidence of coronary heart disease and prostate and colon cancers in Greece, Italy and Spain is due to the Mediterranean diet. The Mediterranean diet is largely vegetarian in nature and the consumption of olive oil is the principal source of fat. Olive oil has been generally considered to be nutritionally desirable for its health properties and oxidative stability not only because of its relatively high content of oleic acid but also due to the abundance of its natural phenolic antioxidants. Oxidative stability is an important parameter in evaluating the quality of oils and fats, as it gives a good estimation of their susceptibility to oxidative degeneration, the main cause of their alteration. Lipid oxidation is a degradative, free radical mediated process responsible for the development of objectionable odors and flavors in oils, fats, and foods containing them. Moreover, oxidation of the polyunsaturated fatty acids (PUFA) of the biomembranes causes functional abnormalities and pathological changes. Oleic acid is less prone to lipid peroxidation than linoleic acid and is incorporated as a major long-chain fatty acid in cellular membranes, when consumption is high. The mechanisms responsible for lipid oxidation have been extensively studied and documented in many books and excellent reviews (Chan, 1987, Halliwell, 1989, Frankel, 1991, Aruoma, 1998).

It is well-known that linoleate hydroperoxides decompose faster than oleate ones. The oleate/linoleate/linolenate oxidation ratio has been reported to be of the order of 1/12/25, based on peroxide formation (Lea, 1952). At the same time, any reaction preventing the propagation of peroxidation, or removing free radicals, plays an important role in the oxidation mechanism. Chain breaking antioxidants, such as phenolic compounds, react with lipid radicals to form nonreactive radicals, stopping the propagation chain (Simic, 1981). In fact, these compounds are able to donate a hydrogen atom to the lipid radical formed during the propagation phase of lipid oxidation (Shahidi, 1992). Findings from studies (human, animal, in vivo and in vitro) have demonstrated that olive oil phenolics have positive effects on certain physiological parameters, possibly reducing the risk of chronic disease development. Increased ROS and decreased plasma antioxidant capacity have been suggested to be involved in the development of a number of chronic diseases including, atherosclerosis, cardiovascular diseases, certain cancers, and Alzheimer's disease. Thus, the Mediterranean diet, with its favourable fatty acid composition and relatively high levels of polyphenolic antioxidants, provides greater resistance to oxidative stress, which is regarded to be a major etiologic factor for many cancers and heart diseases (Simic, 1992, Bartsch, 1999, Owen, 2000a, Bartsch, 2002, Fito, 2005, Ebaid, 2005, Ruano, 2005, Tripoli, 2005, Bogani, 2007, Covas, 2007, Cicerale, 2010).

2. Olive Oil Components, Description and Quality Factors

Standard applies to olive oils and olive-pomace oils by commercial partners for human consumption described in ***CODEX STAN 33-1981***:

- ***Olive oil*** is the oil obtained solely from the fruit of the olive tree (*Olea europaea* L.), to the exclusion of oils obtained using solvents or re-esterification processes and of any mixture with oils of other kinds.
- ***Virgin olive oil***s are the oils obtained from the fruit of the olive tree solely by mechanical or other physical means under conditions, particularly thermal conditions, that do not lead to alterations in the oil, and which have not undergone any treatment other than washing, decanting, centrifuging and filtration.
- ***Olive-pomace oil*** is the oil obtained by treating olive pomace with solvents or other physical treatments, to the exclusion of oils obtained by re-esterification processes and of any mixture with oils of other kinds.

The free fatty acid content is used to distinguish the various classes of virgin olive oil (VOO), from extra virgin to lampante (EC 1991, amendment 1989/2003). Product may only be sold direct to the consumer are those with the following characteristics:

- ***Extra virgin olive oil***: virgin olive oil with a free acidity, expressed as oleic acid, of not more than 0.8 grams per 100 grams and whose other characteristics correspond to those laid down for this category.
- ***Virgin olive oil***: virgin olive oil with a free acidity, expressed as oleic acid, of not more than 2.0 grams per 100 grams and whose other characteristics correspond to those laid down for this category.
- ***Ordinary virgin olive oil***: virgin olive oil with a free acidity, expressed as oleic acid, of not more than 3.3 grams per 100 grams and whose other characteristics correspond to those laid down for this category. This product may only be sold direct to the consumer if permitted in the country of retail sale.
- ***Refined olive oil***: olive oil obtained from virgin olive oils by refining methods which do not lead to alterations in the initial glyceridic structure. It has a free acidity,

expressed as oleic acid, of not more than 0.3 grams per 100 grams and its other characteristics correspond to those laid down for this category.

- ***Olive oil:*** oil consisting of a blend of refined olive oil and virgin olive oils suitable for human consumption. It has a free acidity, expressed as oleic acid, of not more than 1 gram per 100 grams and its other characteristics correspond to those laid down for this category. The country of retail sale may require a more specific designation.

The organoleptic characteristics (odour and taste) of virgin olive oils used to distinguish the first three classes of virgin olive oil are shown in Table 1:

Table 1. Organoleptic characteristics of virgin olive oils

	Median of the defect	Median of the fruity attribute
Extra virgin olive oil	Me = 0	Me > 0
Virgin olive oil	0 < Me ≤ 2.5	Me > 0
Ordinary virgin olive oil	2.5 < Me ≤ 6.0 *	

* or when the median of the defect is less than or equal to 2.5 and the median of the fruity attribute is equal to 0.

The composition of olive oil is primarily triacylglycerols with fatty acid composition rich in oleic acid (55-83%) and linoleic acid (3.5-21%), as shown in **Table 1** (CODEX STAN 33-1981).

Table 2. Fatty acid composition as determined by gas chromatography (%)

Fatty acid	Virgin olive oils	Olive-pomace oil Refined olive-pomace oil
C14:0	0.0 - 0.05	0.0 - 0.05
C16:0	7.5 – 20.0	7.5 - 20.0
C16:1	0.3 - 3.5	0.3 - 3.5
C17:0	0.0 - 0.3	0.0 - 0.3
C17:1	0.0 - 0.3	0.0 - 0.3
C18:0	0.5 - 5.0	0.5 - 5.0
C18:1	55.0 - 83.0	55.0 - 83.0
C18:2	3.5 – 21.0	3.5 - 21.0
C18:3*	<1	<1
C20:0	0.0 - 0.6	0.0 - 0.6
C20:1	0.0 - 0.4	0.0 - 0.4
C22:0	0.0 - 0.2	0.0 - 0.3
C24:0	0.0 - 0.2	0.0 - 0.2
Trans fatty acids		
C18:1 T	0.0 - 0.05	0.0 - 0.40
C18:2 T + C18:3 T	0.0 - 0.05	0.0 - 0.35

*Pending the results of IOOC survey and further consideration by the Committee on Fats and Oils, national limits may remain in place.

Minor components, amounting to about 2% of the total oil weight, include more than 230 chemical compounds, e.g., aliphatic and triterpenic alcohols, sterols, hydrocarbons, volatile compounds, pigments, tocopherols, phenols and related compounds (Servili, 2002).

2.1. Methodology Used for Phenolic Compounds Determination

The literature reviewed on olive oil antioxidants is extensive and often difficult to interpret. Several potential problems become apparent from literature published in the past several decades on different kinds of olive oils and a wide variation in test methods used to evaluate phenolic antioxidants (Pirisi, 2000). The source of this discrepancy could be due to inaccuracy and variability of the methods commonly used to determine phenolic content. A colorimetric analysis based on the Folin-Ciocalteau reagent for total phenols (which is not specific for individual phenols) was the first recognised methodology employed (Gutfinger, 1981). However, it is known that responses of single phenols to the Folin-Ciocalteau reagent are significantly different from each other, thus making this method unsuitable for the exact measurement of phenolic content.

Very interesting systematic studies of the individual classes of hydrophilic phenols in VOO have been developed up to now, and it is possible to say that the composition of VOO is today largely elucidated by high performance liquid chromatography (HPLC) coupling with several detection systems, (which is limited by the extraction procedure and the complexity of the phenolic fraction). Apart from UV diode array detection, the use of fluorimetric detection (Selvaggini, 2006) to analyse phenolic acids in VOO compared with electrochemical and UV detectors (Brenes, 2000a) concluding that fluorescence detectors present clear advantages in terms of sensitivity and selectivity being specially promising for characterization of lignans. Its main limitation is that not all phenolic compounds of VOO are able to fluoresce. The limited application of gas chromatography (GC-MS) methods for analysis of phenolic compounds is that a silylation step is required, in order to increase volatility and thermostability of the analytes. In addition, derivatization often produces mixtures of partially derivatized phenolic compounds or hydrolysis of complex phenols, thus decreasing sensitivity and involving errors. Nevertheless, Angerosa et al. (1996) have shown GC-MS to be an effective tool for phenol identification after extraction from olive oil and derivatization with bis(trimethylsilyl)trifluoracetamide. Improvement in the identification of compounds was obtained with sophisticated analytical techniques such as Liquid Chromatography with Postcolumn Solid-Phase Extraction to Nuclear Magnetic Resonance Spectroscopy (LC-SPE-NMR) (Christophoridou, 2005), or analyte collection using preparative-scale HPLC and off-line identification by GC-MS (Tasioula-Margari, 2001a). In many instances, LC-MS with pneumatically assisted electrospray ionisation (LC-ESI-MS) (Rovellini, 1997, Ryan, 1999, De la Torre-Carbot, 2005, Obied, 2007) or atmospheric pressure ionization (LC-API-MS) (Bianco, 2003) was able to elucidate several structures of phenols. Strong correlations between methodologies based on 31P NMR spectroscopy and high performance liquid chromatography for the main phenolic compounds have also been reported (Dais, 2007). Recently, high resolution 1H NMR spectroscopy has been employed for the development of a versatile and rapid method for identification and quantitation of various classes of phenolic compounds such as simple phenols, flavonols, lignans and some secoiridoids (Christophoridou, 2009) as well as, gas chromatography–atmospheric pressure chemical ionization-time of flight mass spectrometry (GC-APCI-TOF-MS) has been used for screening, structural assignment and quantitative determination of phenolic compounds from virgin olive oils (Garcia-Villalba, 2011).

2.2. Identification of Phenolic Compounds

VOO contains different classes of phenolic compounds such as phenolic acids, phenolic alcohols, flavonoids, hydroxy-isocromans, secoiridoids, and lignans as shown in Figure 1. Phenolic acids with the basic chemical structure of C6-C1 (benzoic acids) and C6-C3 (cinnamic acids), such as caffeic, vanillic, syringic, p-coumaric, o-coumaric, protocatechuic, sinapic, and p-hydroxybenzoic acid, were the first group of phenols observed in VOO. Several authors confirmed the occurrence of phenolic acids (Montedoro, 1992, Caponio, 1999, Owen, 2000b, Pancorbo, 2004) and flavonoids (Rovellini, 1997, Mateos, 2001) as minor components in VOO.

The prevalent phenols of VOO, however, are the secoiridoids of olive fruits, such as oleuropein, demethyloleuropein, and ligstroside. Breakdown products of two major phenolic constituents of the olive fruit, oleuropein and ligstroside, due to the activity of endogenous b-glucosidases, form the majority of the phenolic fraction known as secoiridoids. The most abundant secoiridoids of VOO are the dialdehydic form of elenolic acid linked to hydroxytyrosol or tyrosol (3,4-DHPEA-EDA or p-HPEA-EDA respectively) and oleuropein aglycone (3,4-DHPEA-EA). These complex phenolic compounds were characterized by Montedoro et al. (1992), who also assigned their chemical structure by NMR (Montedoro, 1993,). Angerosa et al. (1996), using GC-MS for phenol identification after derivatization with bis(trimethylsilyl)trifluoracetamide, have shown that peaks in the mass spectra at *m/z* 192 or *m/z* 280, related only to tyrosol and hydroxytyrosol, were attributed to a McLafferty rearrangement of linked phenols. Later these structures were confirmed by other authors (Servili, 1999, Caponio, 1999, Brenes, 1999, Tasioula-Margari, 2001a) in many cultivars from Spain, Italy and Greece.

Hydroxytyrosol (3,4-dihydroxyphenyl-ethanol) and tyrosol (p-hydroxyphenyl-ethanol) are the main phenolic alcohols in VOO. It has also been reported the occurrence in VOO of hydroxytyrosol acetate (Brenes, 1999), tyrosol acetate (Mateos, 2001), and a glucosidic form of hydroxytyrosol (Bianco, 1998), as minor components.

Lignans are also found as prevalent phenolic compounds in VOO. Owen et al. (2000b) and Brenes et al. (2000b) have isolated and characterized (+)-1-acetoxypinoresinol, (+)-pinoresinol, and (+)-1-hydroxypinoresinol as the most frequent lignans in VOO. The lignan syringaresinol has also been detected in VOO (Christophoridou, 2005).

Finally some oxidation products of phenolic compounds have been demonstrated to occur only in traces. Specifically, a new class of phenolic compounds, hydroxy-isochromans, was found in different samples of extra-VOO. In particular, the presence of 1-phenyl-6,7-dihydroxy-isochroman and 1-(3′-methoxy-4′-hydroxy)phenyl-6,7-dihydroxy-isochroman. They are formed during oil extraction by reaction between hydroxytyrosol and benzaldehyde or vanillin (Bianco, 2001). Moreover, two oxidized phenolic compounds (tyrosol and OH-tyrosol oxidized products) were detected in virgin olive oils, (Rovellini, 2002), in heated VOO (Rios, 2005) and in both stored and heated VOO (Daskalaki, 2009). Morello et al. (2004) reported a marked increase of structural isomers of secoiridoid derivatives such as 3,4-

DHPEA-EDA and p-HPEA-EDA in stored oils. Finally, eleven unknown oxidized phenolic compounds were detected in oil samples subjected to accelerated oxidation (Armaforte, 2007).

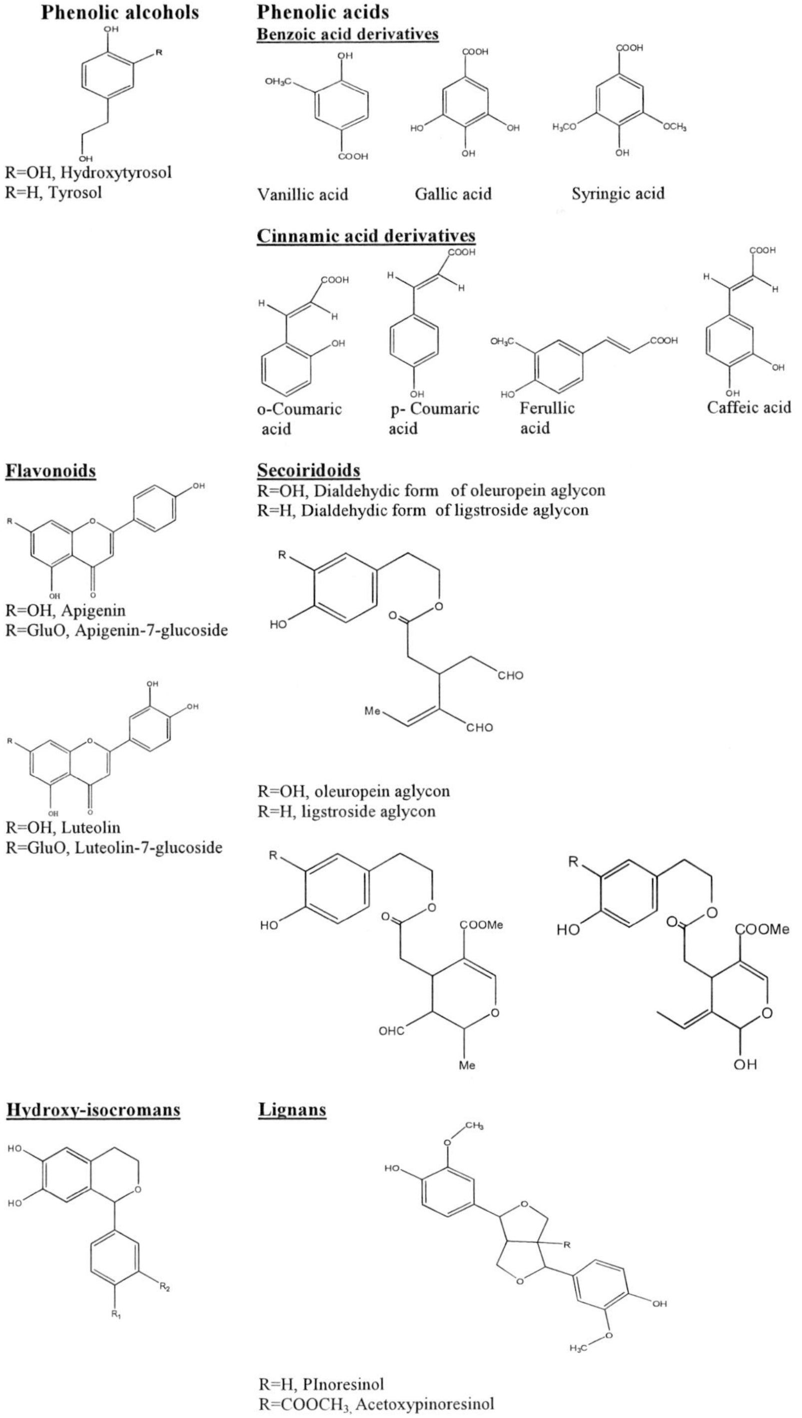

Figure 1. Strucrures of virgin olive oil phenolic compounds.

2.3. Quantitation of Phenolic Compounds

Many analytical procedures for the determination of the complete phenolic profile have been proposed. However, the variety of extraction techniques, chromatographic conditions, and methods of quantification existed, have contributed to differences in reported levels of virgin olive oil phenolics. In general, an analytical procedure for the determination of individual phenolic compounds in VOO involves three basic steps: extraction from the oil sample, analytical separation, and quantification.

Extraction of Phenolic Compounds from the Oil Sample

Traditionally, the phenolic fraction of olive oil has been isolated by extraction of an oil solution in a lipophilic solvent (liquid-liquid extraction, LLE) with several portions of methanol or methanol/ water (with different levels of methanol that range between 60, 80 and 100%, followed by solvent evaporation of the aqueous extract and a cleanup of the residue by solvent partition (Montedoro, 1992, Angerosa, 1996). Hexane has been the most commonly used solvent. Montedoro et al. (1992) reported a mixture of CH_3OH/H_2O (80:20, v/v) as the most efficient extraction solvent for simple and hydrolysable phenolic compounds, whereas, Angerosa et al. (1996) proposed the use of pure methanol. In another study, VOO samples subjected to extraction using both aqueous methanol after dissolution in hexane, and a solvent system consisting of methanol and an isopropanol-methanol mixture in order to be evaluated the effectiveness of the extraction procedure (Tasioula-Margari, 2001b). Results obtained, suggest that simple phenols were better extracted with 60% aqueous methanol while complex phenols were better extracted with methanol and isopropanol/ methanol (20:80, v/v) mixture. It should also be noted that with the exclusion of water from the extraction solvents, the formation of an emulsion between oil and water-methanol layer, which can adversely affect recovery yield, is prevented. However, using pure methanol for extraction, additional steps are needed, as the combined methanol extracts are brought to dryness and the residue is taken up to acetonitrile, following by washing with hexane. Consequently, it could be concluded that the concentration of phenols in extracts were dependent on extraction solvents and the class of phenolic compounds present in olive oil.

Extraction with N,N-dimethylformamide, followed by HPLC analysis, seemed to show interesting results in terms of recovery efficiency and sample manipulation (Brenes, 2000b).

Promising results were obtained by Mateos et al. (2001), who worked with diol-bond phase SPE cartridges (solid phase extraction, SPE) and found high recovery (>90%) of all major olive phenolic compounds. On the contrary, the results obtained in a study carried out by Hrncirik and Fritsche (2004) showed that LLE using 60:40 methanol–water v/v as extraction solvent, led to higher extraction efficiencies of total phenolics (93%) than SPE-diol (68%) and SPE-C18 (38%). From these examples, it can be deduced that a wide variation in extraction methods and the diversity of protocols used for different olive oil phenolic content can justify differences between the results obtained by different research groups.

Spectrophotometric Determination of Total Phenols

One method that is widely used for the quantitative determination of total phenols in VOO is colorimetric assay, based on the reaction of Folin-Ciocalteu reagent with the functional hydroxy groups of phenolic compounds (Gutfinger, 1881). Folin-Ciocalteu phenol reagent consists of a mixture of the heteropoly acids, phosphomolybdic and phosphotungstic acids, in which the molybdenum and tungsten are in the 6+ state. On reduction with certain reducing agents, so-called molybdenum blue and tungsten blue are formed, in which the mean oxidation state of the metals is between 5 and 6. As the reduced Folin-Ciocalteu reagent is blue, it is possible to carry out the detection with a spectrophotometer in the range of 500 to 750 nm. The method consists of calibration with a pure phenolic compound, extraction of phenols from the sample, and the measurement of absorbance after the colour reaction. The calibration curve is usually constructed by different researchers, using different standard solutions such as gallic acid, caffeic acid or tyrosol, consequently results obtained can't be compared. The popularity of this assay can mainly be attributed to its simplicity and speed of analysis. The major disadvantage of the colorimetric assay is its low specificity, as the color reaction can occur with any oxidizable phenolic hydroxy group. Furthermore, the method does not distinguish between individual compounds differing in molar mass thus, samples with comparable total phenolic content, but widely varying phenolic composition, will give a different response in the colorimetric method (Carrasco-Pancobro, 2005).

Chromatographic Determination of the Phenolic Profile of Virgin Olive Oils

The limited volatility of many phenols has restricted the use of GC for their separation, so HPLC currently represents the most popular and reliable technique for analysis of phenols. The most common mode of separation exploits reversed-phase systems typically with C18 columns and various mobile phases. Detection is routinely achieved by ultraviolet absorption often involving a photodiode array detector (UV-DAD).

Numerous mobile phases have been employed, but binary systems comprising an aqueous component and a less polar organic solvent such as acetonitrile or methanol remain common. Acid (acetic, formic, or phosphoric acid) is usually added to both components to maintain a constant acid concentration during gradient runs. There are significant differences in absorption maximal and molar absorptivities of even the major phenols identified in olive oil, creating problems in quantification (Obied, 2007). Dual wavelength detection has been applied for routine detection, 280 nm which represents a suitable compromise for phenolic compounds, and 340 nm for flavonoids. **Figure 2** shows a representative HPLC chromatogram of the phenolic compounds from Koroneiki variety.

The limited availability of suitable standards is a problem for quantitation of phenolic compounds identified in olive oil. Response factors for the main phenolic compounds (relationship between peak area and concentration) for quantitation of the dialdehydic form of decarboxymethyl oleuropein aglycon, pinoresinol, 1-acetoxypinoresinol, and the aldehydic forms of oleuropein aglycon and ligstroside aglycon has been suggested by Mateos et al. (Mateos, 2001). The limited availability of suitable standards for quantitation can be overcome, in part, by using the most relevant available compounds such as "Tyrosol" for tyrosol derivatives quantification, multiplied by their molecular weight ratio (304:138 and 362:138 for p-HPEA-EDA and p-HPEA-EA respectively), "Oleuropein" for hydroxytyrosol derivatives quantification, multiplied by their molecular weight ratio (154:540, 320:540 and 378:540 for hydroxytyrosol, 3,4-DHPEA-EDA or 3,4-DHPEA-EA respectively) and "Pinoresinol" for 1-acetoxypinoresinol quantification, multiplied by their molecular weight ratio 358:416 (Oliveras-Lopez, 2007, Daskalaki, 2009).

Unfortunately, the HPLC chromatograms showed incomplete separation of many phenolic components analyzed. The existence of co-eluted compounds in each of the three fractions corresponding to a) 3,4-DHPEA-EDA), b) p-HPEA-EDA+lignans and c) 3,4-DHPEA-EA, indicated the presence of significantly larger number of components in these fractions (Tasioula-Margari, 2001a). It must be noted that an oxidation product (with m/z 335) has the same retention time with pinoresinol in HPLC columns used for the phenolic compounds separation, **Figure 2**, (Daskalaki, 2009).

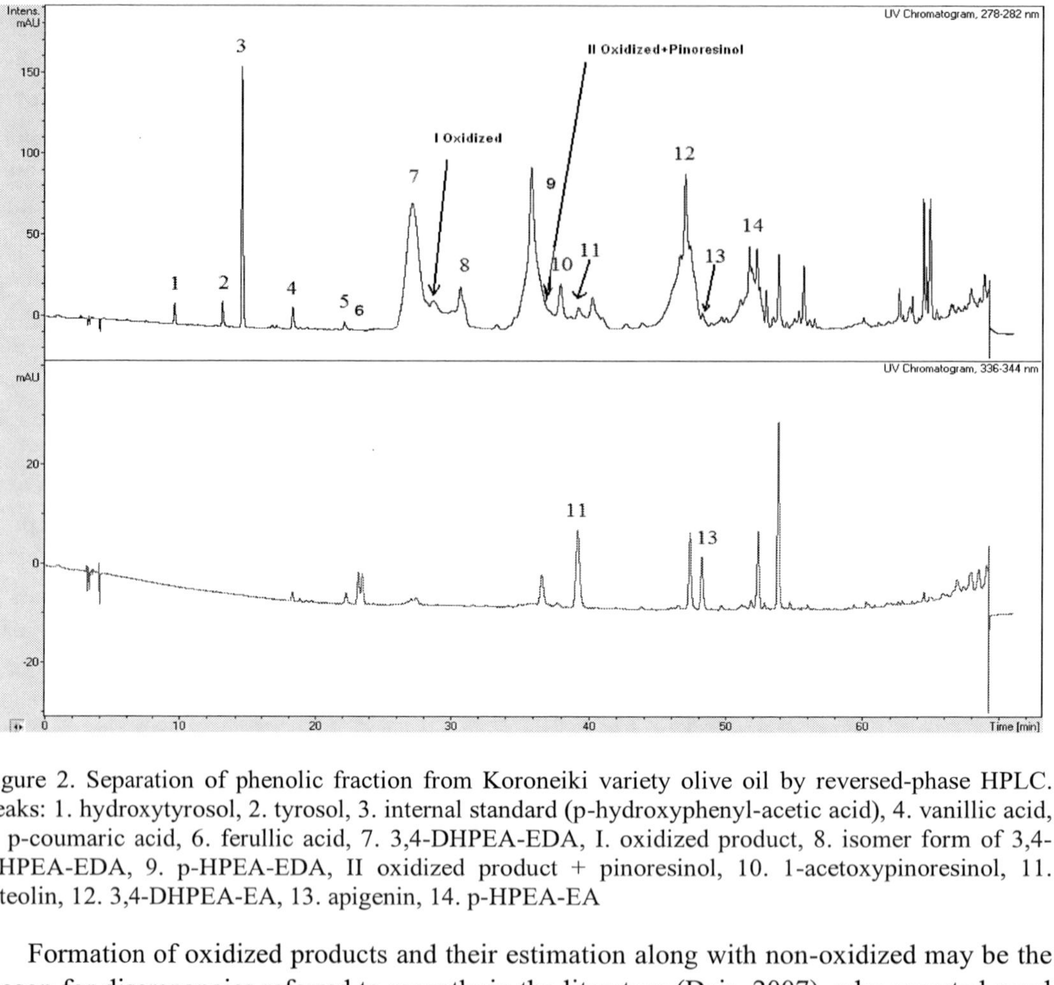

Figure 2. Separation of phenolic fraction from Koroneiki variety olive oil by reversed-phase HPLC. Peaks: 1. hydroxytyrosol, 2. tyrosol, 3. internal standard (p-hydroxyphenyl-acetic acid), 4. vanillic acid, 5. p-coumaric acid, 6. ferullic acid, 7. 3,4-DHPEA-EDA, I. oxidized product, 8. isomer form of 3,4-DHPEA-EDA, 9. p-HPEA-EDA, II oxidized product + pinoresinol, 10. 1-acetoxypinoresinol, 11. luteolin, 12. 3,4-DHPEA-EA, 13. apigenin, 14. p-HPEA-EA

Formation of oxidized products and their estimation along with non-oxidized may be the reason for discrepancies referred to recently in the literature (Dais, 2007), who reported good correlations between methodologies based on 31P NMR spectroscopy and high performance liquid chromatography for the main phenolic compounds in VOO, except for pinorecinol. Nevertheless, amounts of oxidized products are low, values recorded ranged from 0-11 $mg.kg^{-1}$ for 15 months storage in the dark, (Daskalaki, 2009).

Tyrosol acetate is coeluted with 3,4-DHPEA-EDA cinnamic acid with acetoxypinoresinol (Gutierrez-Rosales, 2003) an oxidation product (with m/z 335) has the same retention time with pinoresinol (Daskalaki, 2009), stereoisomers of 3,4-DHPEA-EDA along with p-HPEA-EDA (De la Torre-Carbot, 2005, Christophoridou, 2005). Fortunately, compounds coeluted with the main phenolic compounds of VOO occur only in traces.Consequently, better efficiency and quantitation were obtained for phenyl alcohols and 3,4-DHPEA-EA, (**Figure 2**, Peaks: **1**. hydroxytyrosol, **2**. tyrosol, **12**. 3,4-DHPEA-EA) but lower efficiency and quantitation were found for 3,4-DHPEA-EDA, p-HPEA-EDA and lignans (Peaks:**7** 3,4-DHPEA-EDA, I. oxidized product, **9**. p-HPEA-EDA, II oxidized product and pinoresinol, **14**. p-HPEA-EA and isomers). Therefore, concentrations of olive phenols reported in the literature greatly differ depending on the wide variety of analytical procedures used for extraction, separation or detection and drastically influenced by the standard selected and/or by the expression of the results in different formats.

3. TOCOPHEROLS, STRUCTURE, ANTIOXIDANT ACTIVITY AND QUANTITATION

Vitamin E compounds (tocopherols and tocotrienols) are well recognized for their effective inhibition of lipid oxidation in foods and biological systems. Since vitamin E is only synthesized by plants, it is a very important dietary nutrient for humans and animals.

While studying the influence of nutrition on rat reproduction, Evans and Bishop, (1922) discovered vitamin E (at that time α-tocopherol) as a factor essential for reproduction. The name tocopherol, then, came from 'toketos' (childbirth) and 'phero' (to bring forth) and the suffix '-ol' was added to indicate the phenolic nature. Now the term 'vitamin E' is a generic name for all tocopherol and tocotrienol derivatives qualitatively exhibiting the biological activity of α-tocopherol. Structurally, the tocopherols and tocotrienols can be viewed as consisting of a chroman head (with two rings: one phenolic and one heterocyclic) and a phytyl tail (**Figure 3**). The four tocopherols have saturated tails and vary only in the number of methyl substituents and the patterns of substitution in the phenolic ring. The four tocotrienols have chroman heads similar to those in their corresponding tocopherols but contain three isolated double bonds in their phytyl tails.

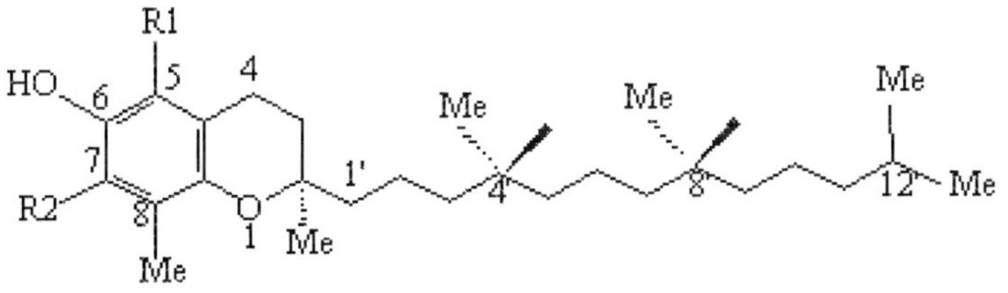

Tocopherols	R1	R2	Trivial names
α-Tocopherol	Me	Me	5,7,8-Trimethyltocol
β- Tocopherol	Me	H	5,8-Dimethyltocol
γ- Tocopherol	H	Me	7,8-Dimethyltocol
δ- Tocopherol	H	H	8-Monomethyltocol

Figure 3. The Structures and Chemical Names of Tocopherols.

3.1. Antioxidant Activity of Tocopherols

The antioxidant activity of the tocopherols and tocotrienols (grouped as chromanols) is mainly due to their ability to donate their phenolic hydrogens to lipid free-radicals. The tocopherols not only inhibit free radical-induced lipid autoxidation, but they also inhibit the oxidations induced by the electronically excited singlet oxygen (O_2 $1\Delta g$), both in vivo and in vitro. The efficiency of the tocopherols as singlet oxygen quenchers (in the light) was mentioned to have a direct correlation with their concentrations.

Nagaoka et al. (1992) offered a probable explanation for the mechanism of antioxidant action of the tocopherols (TOH). Initially, the tocopherol molecule and the peroxy radicals (susceptible to donating and accepting an electron, respectively) approach each other and their electron clouds begin to overlap. Thus, a transition state which has the property of the charge transfer species (LOO^{-}---TOH^{+}) will be reached. When the tocopherol molecule and the peroxy radical approach each other to an appreciable extent ($LOO^{\delta-}$---$TOH^{\delta+}$), proton tunneling will take place where the chromanol molecule will lose a hydrogen atom to a lipid peroxy radical forming the chromanoxyl radical (Eq. 1).

$$LOO^{\bullet} + TOH \xrightarrow{Ka} LOOH + TO^{\bullet} \tag{1}$$

The chromanoxyl radical ($TO^{\bullet}$) may undergo radical-radical coupling with other radicals forming adducts (Eq. 2). The chromanoxyl radicals react differently with carbon-centered and oxygen-centered oxidized lipid radicals.

$$(n-1)(LOO^{\bullet}) + TO^{\bullet} \rightarrow adducts \tag{2}$$

In the absence of antioxidants, the rate of the lipid oxidation reaction is given by:

$$-d[O_2] / dt = Ri \bullet Kp[RH] \tag{3}$$

and the inhibitory effect of an antioxidant on lipid oxidation reactions can be represented as follows:

$$-d[O_2] / dt = (Ri \bullet Kp[RH]) / (n \bullet Ka[TOH]) \tag{4}$$

where: Ri, Kp, and Ka are the rate constants for the initiation, propagation, and antioxidation reactions, respectively. Thus, the antioxidant effect of the tocopherols and tocotrienols is dependent on their stoichiometric factors (n), the rate constants of their reactions with peroxy radicals (Ka), and their concentrations (TOH).

Since each tocopherol molecule can neutralize two peroxy radicals by reactions (Eqs. 1 and 2), the stoichiometric factor (n) for the four tocopherol isomers is theoretically considered to be equal to 2.0. Values of n = 1.3-1.6 were reported for α-tocopherol in the autoxidation of polyunsaturated fatty acids (PUFA) within the microsomal membranes. The stoichiometric factors (n) for β-, γ-, and δ-tocopherols were reported as 2.04, 1.89, and 1.78 relative to a standard value of 2.00 for α-tocopherol. Values of Ka for the four tocopherol isomers were measured for the inhibition of styrene oxidation initiated by 2,2′-bis(isobutyronitrile) at tocopherol concentrations of 2×10^{-4}-7×10^{-2} M at 30 °C. The Ka values were 23.5, 16.6, 15.9, and 6.5×10^{5} $M^{-1}s^{-1}$ for α-, β-, γ-, and δ-tocopherols, respectively, suggesting a relative antioxidant potency of the order α > β ≈ γ > δ. The magnitude of Ka for α-tocopherol was also measured at room temperature in a number of substrates and values reported ranged from as low as 2×10^{5} $M^{-1}s^{-1}$ for $C_6H_5.CMe_2.OO^{\bullet}$ at 60 °C to as high as 5×10^{8} $M^{-1}s^{-1}$ for $Cl_3OO^{\bullet}$. The value of Ka is, thus, not only dependent on the tocopherol isomer but also on the substrate and reaction conditions. Since lipid peroxy radicals react with the tocopherols several orders of magnitude faster than their reactions with acyl lipids, one tocopherol molecule can protect about 10^{3}-10^{8} PUFA molecules at low peroxide levels.

The tocopherols also can react with alkoxy radicals (LO•), formed in the propagation step (Eq. 5), or undergo self-coupling to form dimers and/or trimers (Eq. 6).

$$LO^{\bullet} + TOH \rightarrow TO^{\bullet} + LOH \tag{5}$$

$$TO^{\bullet} + TO^{\bullet} \rightarrow TO - TO \tag{6}$$

In very special cases, when oxygen is present in trace amounts and hydroperoxides are present in negligible concentrations, the tocopherols can react directly with alkyl radicals (L•):

$$TOH + L^{\bullet} \rightarrow TO^{\bullet} + LH \tag{7}$$

The oxidation of α-tocopherol by the reactive oxygen species, hydroxyl ($^{\bullet}OH$), perhydroxy ($^{\bullet}OOH$), and superoxide ($O_2^{\bullet-}$) radicals, was studied in micelles and liposomes. The hydroxy radicals were efficient oxidants of α-tocopherol through an indirect reaction, due to their low diffusivity. The $HO^{\bullet}$ first react with the solvent (ethanol, membrane lipids, etc.) molecules in their vicinity compared to the tocopherol molecules (Eq. 8) and the solvent radicals will afterward oxidize the tocopherol molecules (Eq. 9):

$$OH^{\bullet} + SH \rightarrow H_2O + S^{\bullet} \tag{8}$$

$$S^{\bullet} + TOH \rightarrow SH + TO^{\bullet} \tag{9}$$

The $HO_2^{\bullet}$ and $O_2^{\bullet-}$ radicals are always present in equilibrium (Lewis acid and base) in protonated solvents:

$$O_2^{\bullet-} + H^{+} \leftrightarrow HO_2^{\bullet} \tag{10}$$

The oxidizing ability of the three radicals was in the order $OH^{\bullet} > HO_2^{\bullet} > O_2^{\bullet-}$. Although $HO_2^{\bullet}$ is reactive enough to attack lipids, the concentration ratio $O_2^{\bullet-}$ / $HO_2^{\bullet}$ in protonated solvents and at neutral pH is 400. Under these conditions, the oxidation is very slow and it has also to compete with the dismutation (Eq. 11):

$$2HO_2^{\bullet} \xrightarrow{H^+} H_2O_2 + O_2 \qquad (11)$$

The tocopherols not only inhibit free radical-induced lipid autoxidation, but they also inhibit the oxidations induced by the electronically excited singlet oxygen ($O_2\ ^1\Delta_g$) both *in vivo* and *in vitro*. Tocopherols react with singlet oxygen either by physical quenching or by chemical reactions. The balance of these processes depends on the properties of an initially formed exciplex to which three options were offered: reversion to reactants, collapse to ground state *via* intersystem crossing, and evolution to products. As a rule, physical quenching predominates but chemical quenching is by no means a negligible process, at least in polar solvents. In physical quenching, excited state singlet oxygen ($O_2\ ^1\Delta_g$) is deactivated to ground state triplet oxygen ($O_2\ ^3\Sigma_g$) through a charge transfer mechanism. The charge transfer mechanism involves donation of an electron by the tocopherol to the electron-deficient singlet oxygen forming a charge transfer exciplex. The exciplex then undergoes intersystem crossing and then dissociates into a tocopherol molecule and a molecule of triplet oxygen (Eq. 12):

$$TOH + {}^1O_2 \xrightarrow{Kq} \left[TOH^{\delta+} --{}^1O_2^{\delta-}\right] \rightarrow \left[TOH^{\delta+} --{}^3O_2^{\delta-}\right] \rightarrow TOH + {}^3O_2 \qquad (12)$$

Furthermore, the tocopherols also react chemically with singlet oxygen and are destroyed after the reaction. The rate of physical quenching (Kq) of singlet oxygen by the tocopherols is several orders of magnitude higher than the rates of chemical reactions. The chemical reaction proceeds through an intermediate hydroperoxide which will decompose to form the secondary products.

Effective antioxidants should generally yield radicals that are unreactive toward stable molecules (mainly molecular oxygen, lipid molecules, and lipid hydroperoxides) and that are limiting their reactions only to donation of hydrogen(s) to radicals and to radical-radical coupling. This goal is not ideally achieved since the antioxidants and/or their radicals often undergo other side reactions, which may be classified as prooxidative. The degree of such reactions is determined by different factors, mainly the antioxidant structure, concentration, temperature, etc. The optimum concentration varies from one substance to another, and the natural amounts of tocopherols in natural systems are close to their optimal values (Kamal-Eldin, 1996).

3.2. Quantitation of Tocopherols

Quantitative determination of tocopherols is commonly performed by normal or reversed phase HPLC (Wahyuni, 1988). Normal phase chromatography is advantageous for resolving β -and γ-tocopherols which cannot be resolved by RP-HPLC. However, separation of α-, β-, γ-, and δ-tocopherols has been achieved with an octadecyl polyvinyl alcohol column. (Abidi, 1997). HPLC detectors used to measure tocopherols include ultraviolet, fluorescence and amperometric (Carpenter, 1979; Dionisi, 1995; IUPAC, 1987). Fluorescence detection is more sensitive and selective than UV detection (Hoehler, 1998). However, it is not suitable for detecting the ester form of α-tocopherol which fluoresce to a much lesser extent than free α-tocopherol. A saponification step is therefore needed to convert α-tocopherol esters to their free alcohol form with the risk of partial loss of tocopherols. Reports on simultaneous analysis of phenolic substances and tocopherols by HPLC dealt with phenolic antioxidants and tocopherols either directly in VOO samples (Andrikopoulos, 1991) or after their co-extraction from VOO (Tasioula-Margari, 2001b). With direct injection, most compounds of lower concentrations and extinction coefficients cannot be detected whereas after their co-extraction, α-tocopherol and phenolic compounds can be sufficiently concentrated and therefore analysed simultaneously by reversed phase HPLC. However, extraction was not complete; recovery achieved reached up to 70% and 80% for simple phenols and for α-tocopherol respectively.

4. Factors Affecting Antioxidant Content of Virgin Olive Oil

4.1. Agronomic Factors

There is much variation in the composition and concentration of phenolic compounds among virgin olive oils. Several agronomic parameters can modify the phenolic concentration of VOO. The most studied aspects reviewed by Servili el al. (2004), include cultivar, fruit ripening, geographic region, pedo-climatic conditions of production and some agronomic techniques such as the irrigation. Phenolic compounds decreased as the level of irrigation water increased and maturation of the olive fruit at harvest increased (Tovar, 2001). In contrast to this observation, using the same variety, a clear increase of the total amount of phenolic compounds associated with the increase in irrigation has recently been reported (Dabbou, 2010, Gómez-Rico, 2007). Such discrepancies may be due to other macro-climatic conditions of production as reported by Tura et al., (2007), who reported that antioxidants were influenced by area with diverse climates and soil characteristics. In addition, different fertilization treatments can affect VOO phenolic content. Recently, a decline has been reported in total phenol concentration in VOO when treated with a mixture of a seaweed extract plus nitrogen and boron (Chouliaras, 2009).

Maturation of the olive fruit at harvest has also been shown to affect phenolic composition and concentration in virgin olive oil. During maturation of the fruit chemical and enzymatic reactions take place, resulting in free phenols formation. Different concentrations of certain phenolics are present at differing stages of olive maturity. Hydroxytyrosol, tyrosol, and luteolin increased their concentration in oils with maturation of fruits, while glucoside aglycons diminished their concentration with maturation (Brenes 1999). In general, the total content and α-tocopherol and phenolic compounds decrease during the ripening process. Variability by crop year was due to the rainfall levels, and oils from the drier crop year showed the highest tocopherol content, however, this effect was cultivar-dependent (Beltran, 2005). α-tocopherol seems to be the least affected, although the level of antioxidants decreased throughout ripening Gutierrez, 1999). Total tocopherol content has ranged between 84 and 463 mg/kg, with α-tocopherol represented more than 95%, from thirty Spanish olive cultivars (Beltran, 2010) and between 39-425 mg/kg, from 18 Italian cultivars (Tura, 2007). It had been concluded that tocopherols in virgin olive oil have a significant genetic component.

4.2. Processing Conditions

The processing of olive fruit to oil has a substantial effect on concentrations of phenolics in virgin olive oil. Since the occurrence of hydrophilic phenols in VOO is strictly related to the activities of various endogenous enzymes of olive fruit, their concentration in the oil is strongly affected by the extraction conditions (Servili, 2004). Crushing and malaxation are the most important critical points of the oil mechanical extraction process (Caponio 1999). The system of extraction used (classical, two-phase centrifugal, three-phase centrifugal, percolation) is critical for total phenol content. Oils produced by the continuous centrifugal system generally present lower polyphenol content than oils extracted with other systems (classical, percolation). One important innovation in the olive oil industry is the use of dual-phase or ecological decanters. Virgin olive oils extracted using two-phase centrifugation have been noted to contain a significantly higher phenolic concentration in comparison to virgin olive oils obtained from three-phase centrifugation. In such systems of extraction the oily phase is separated from the paste without requiring the addition of warm water. In this way no waste water is produced and the natural water from the olives remains in the pomace. Oils produced, using two typical Italian cultivars such as Coratina and Oliarola, shown higher concentration of hydrophilic phenols in VOO extracted using two-phases decanters as compared to the traditional three-phases centrifuges (for Coratina, 673 versus 585 mg/kg and for Oliarola, 304 versus 263 mg/kg for two or three-phases respectively) (Servili, 2002). Other factors affecting the minor composition of VOO are kneading, malaxation temperature and time of olive paste. The content of phenolic compounds in virgin olive oil was affected by the malaxation temperature as fpllows: the 3,4-DHPEA-EDA content increased by 220-630 % when the temperature was increased from 20 to 40°C (Gomez-Rico, 2009). On the other hand, oxidative reactions catalysed by endogenous oxidoreductases such as polyphenoloxidase and peroxidase can promote the phenolic oxidation during processing. Oleuropein and ligstroside derivatives, such as 3,4-DHPEA-EDA, 3,4-DHPEA-EA and *p*-HPEA-EDA, were highly affected by the O_2 concentration during malaxation, whereas lignans, such as pinoresinol and acetoxypinoresinol, were less modified; in fact, they seem to be independent of the O_2 level in the malaxer (Servili, 2008). As consequence, the control of O_2 concentration in the paste during processing, temperature and time of malaxation, can be use to optimize the phenolic concentration in VOO (Servili, 2003). Neither extraction processing system (two-phase centrifugation and three-phase centrifugation) affects the levels of tocopherols, as those molecules are lipophilic compounds (Gimeno, 2002).

Apparently, the many variables involved in the entire process are responsible for differences in antioxidant content. Cultivar, fruit ripening, pedo-climatic conditions of production and some agronomic techniques can modify the antioxidant content of VOO. Small diversities in the machinery of olive crushing, the temperatures applied, the total volume of water used and the duration of contact with the water and with O_2, may cause significant changes in the total polyphenol content. In fact, for phenol-rich cultivars such as Picual and Coratina, or unripe olive fruit, a reduction in the phenolic content of the final virgin olive oil would improve the sensory properties of the product by means of a desirable decrease in its sensory bitterness, without significantly affecting its oxidative stability and shelf life. On the contrary, in the case of phenol-poor cultivars such as the Spanish Arbequina or Morisca and the Italian Leccino and Taggiasca, a further increase, during extraction processes, of their naturally occurring antioxidants is of course advisable and, therefore, a compromise should be established in each case (Gomez-Rico, 2009).

Total phenol content in olive oil, based on the Folin-Ciocalteau reagent for total phenols, has been reported to vary between 800-1000 mg/kg (Visioli, 1998), to be over 500 mg/kg (Montedoro, 1992, Servili, 2004), 320 ± 191 mg/kg expressed as tyrosol equivalent (Tasioula-Margari, 2002b).

On average, olive oils from Italian market contained 232 ±15 mg/kg (complex phenols were expressed as OH-tyrosol) in extra-virgin olive oil and 62 ± 12 mg/kg in refined olive oil as judged by HPLC analysis (Owen, 2000a). The main phenolic compounds detected in monovarietal Picual oil, representing 25% of Spanish production, were the aglycon of oleuropein followed by the other secoiridoid aglycons. Lignans' concentration in oil showed low variability with season and harvesting time, and pinoresinol in particular was present at a concentration of about 40 ppm. The total polyphenol content of this monovarietal oil ranged from 300 to 700 ppm as judged by HPLC analysis after extraction using *N,N*-dimethylformamide (Garcia, 2002). A paper on phenolic extracts from 2 French monocultivar olives and 3 Spanish monocultivar olives, reported similar phenolic compounds. French olive oils total phenol content ranged (230.85 ±30.62 and 222.38 ±30.49 mg/kg for the 2 cultivars) and in Spanish samples ranged (218.22 ±33.27, 232.72 ±43.43 and 238.29 ±69.2 mg/kg for the three cultivals) (Andjelkovic, 2008). Extraction of phenolic compounds was performed on solid phase extraction (SPE) with diol-phase cartridges and quantification by HPLC–DAD detection. Pinoresinol was detected in the highest amount in all olive oil samples ranged from 98.69 mg/kg, in the French oil "Tanche", to 123.10 mg/kg in the Spanish oil "Picual". Pinoresinol content in the Picual variety was higher than that previously reported by Garcıa et al. (2002), due to the differences in extraction and/or the origin of the samples. On the contrary, pinoresinol was found at low concentrations (2–5% of total phenols) and acetoxypinoresinol was the main compound in Taggiasca and Arbequina varieties, in a more recent study of the phenolic composition of Spanish and Italian monocultivar extra virgin olive oils (Oliveras-Lopez, 2007). Oils from cultivar Picual showed similar characteristics to those of Seggianese oils, with total amounts of secoiridoids of 498.7 and 619.2 mg/kg, respectively. The phenolic composition of Arbequina oils is close to that of the Taggiasca variety with lignans among the main compounds. Similar phenolic compounds profile has been reported for the main Greek varieties such as Koroneiki which ranged between 105-750 mg/kg and Lianolia which ranged between 80-870 mg/kg expressed as individual compounds, determined by HPLC (Daskalaki, 2009) or 142±85 mg/kg expressed as tyrosol equivalent (Okogeri, 2002). Although the concentrations of the above phenols ranged widely between different samples, the main phenolic compounds in both varieties were tyrosol and hydroxytyrosol derivatives. The Koroneiki variety contained a higher amount of lignans, consisting mainly from 1-acetoxypinoresinol, compared to Lianolia, whereas both varieties contained low amounts of simple phenols.

In conclusion, total phenolic content in olive oil of good quality, based on the Folin-Ciocalteau reagent and reported so far, ranged 300 ±200 mg/kg expressed as gallic acid or tyrosol. Those values correspond to 300 to 700 ppm of phenolic compounds in different ratios, as judged by HPLC analysis and expressed at corresponding class of compounds. Total tocopherol content has ranged between 84 and 463 mg/kg, with α-tocopherol represented more than 95%, from thirty Spanish olive cultivars (Beltran, 2010), between 39-425 mg/kg, from 18 Italian cultivars (Tura, 2007), and between 98-370 mg/kg from ninety Greek virgin olive oils (Psomiadou, 2000).

5. Changes Occurring in Olive Oil Antioxidants During Storage and Cooking

5.1. Effect of Phenolic Compounds on Virgin Olive Oil Flavor

A large increase in demand for high/quality olive oil during the past few years can be attributed not only to its potential health benefits (Visioli, 1998), but also to reports of its fragrant flavor. Hence, virgin olive oil commands a high price in the market, and a comprehensive knowledge of the chemical compounds responsible for its flavor is therefore desirable. The delicate, fragrant aroma of virgin olive oils is the sum of sensations perceived when several chemicals, transported by the air streams during inhalation and expiration actions, reach and stimulate the odor receptors located in neurons if the olfactory epithelium. A specific vocabulary has been developed to describe flavors of virgin olive oils. Generally descriptions of the fragrant and delicate aroma of virgin olive oils fall into two main groups: (a) *olive fruity*, the sensation that recalls olive fruit, and (b) *green notes*, which are reminiscent of leaves or green fruits. Volatiles compounds are mainly responsible for virgin olive oil aroma, whereas phenolic compounds are considered to be related to virgin olive oil taste. The presence of phenolic compounds gives rise to the special flavor of virgin olive oil and is responsible for the sensory attributes of VOO (e.g. bitter, astringent, pungent, throat-catching). When occur at low to medium concentrations, phenolic compounds provide the oil with its delicate and unique flavour highly appreciated by consumers (Garcıa-Gonzalez, 2008). In fact, recent studies showed that the sensory intensity of the bitterness attribute in VOO is associated mainly to secoiridoid derivatives of hydroxytyrosol, particularly 3,4-DHPEA-EDA and 3,4-DHPEA-EA (Gutierrez-Rosales, 2003). The sensory qualities of the isolated polyphenols, using reversed phase HPLC, were evaluated, and almost all fractions containing polyphenols were described as bitter and astringent. However, the fraction containing deacetoxy-ligstroside aglycon produced a strong burning pungent sensation at the back of the throat. In contrast, the fraction containing the analogous deacetoxy-oleuropein aglycon, at an equivalent concentration, produced only a slight burning/numbing sensation, which was perceived more on the tongue. No other polyphenol fractions from the analyzed oils produced the intense burning sensation; thus, deacetoxy-ligstroside aglycon is the polyphenol responsible for the majority of the burning pungent sensation found in pungent extra virgin olive oils (Andrewes, 2003).

5.2. Changes Occurring in Virgin Olive Oil Antioxidants During Storage

The characteristic resistance to oxidation of virgin olive oil is related to its unique fatty acid composition, relatively high oleic acid content, in addition to minor components such as phenolic compounds and tocopherols having a catechol group, which degrade to a certain degree (Zhang, 1999). Although olive oils are generally stable to oxidation, they are still susceptible to oxidation due to their PUFAs (5-15%) and minor constituents including chlorophylls, carotenoids, and metal impurities such as Fe, Cu. The in vitro activities of antioxidants are not only dependent on their absolute chemical reactivity toward hydroperoxy and other free radicals, but also on many other factors such as concentrations, temperature, light, type of substrate, solvent, and other chemical species acting as prooxidants and synergists in the system (Moure, 2001). The antioxidants and/or their radicals often undergo other side reactions, which may be classified as prooxidative. The degree of such reactions is determined by different factors, mainly the antioxidant structure, concentration, temperature, etc. These factors affect the absolute and relative potency of antioxidants and may explain the inconsistency in the reported relative activities of the different tocopherols *in vivo* and *in vitro*. The prooxidant effect of α-tocopherol was related to its tocopheroxyl radicals (α-TO$^•$). This was based on the assumption that when TO$^•$ is present at high concentration, there is more possibility for a number of undesirable side reactions, which may initiate a reaction chain or enhance the rate of peroxidation (Kamal-Eldin, 1996). When more than a single component (antioxidant) is present in an oxidizing lipid system, their net antioxidant effect is frequently more than the sum of their individual effects (a phenomenon known as synergism). We can recognize at least three mechanisms by which synergism to the tocopherols can be explained. The first mechanism, which involves some sort of tocopherol 'sparing', occurs when the tocopherol is present with another real antioxidant working by the same or by a different mechanism (i.e., a radical scavenger). OH-containing benzoic acids (VOO phenolic compounds) were mentioned to function as peroxy radical scavengers and, thereby, can have a sparing effect on the tocopherols. The second mechanism operates when the tocopherol is present together with other substance(s) which is/are capable of 'regenerating' it from its radicals or oxidation products (e.g., vitamin C). The third mechanism by which many synergists work is through 'trace metal chelation'. Tocopherols showed synergistic effects with dihydroxy-phenols, which are mainly due to the metal-chelating properties of the latter. Thus, the mode in which the phenols and α-tocopherol react is significantly affected by the interplay of all the chemical and physical parameters of the system.

Several studies on factors that influence the oxidative processes of olive oil have been reported. The predominant phenolic compounds of virgin olive oil have an antioxidant effect, which increases in the order: hydroxytyrosol > oleuropein > tyrosol (Chimi, 1991). Commercial olive oil samples were evaluated to determine the factors influencing their oxidative stability (Satue, 1995). Phenolic compounds extracted from VOOs increased the oxidative stability when added to the control refined, bleached and deodorized (RBD) olive oil. The phenolic extract had the best antioxidant activity at 50 ppm gallic acid equivalents (GAE) on the basis of peroxide value, but better antioxidant activity was observed at 100 and 200 ppm GAE on the basis of hexanal formation measured by static headspace GC. α-tocopherol behaved as a prooxidant at high concentrations (>250 ppm GAE) based on peroxide value for hydroperoxide formation, but was more effective than the other phenolic antioxidants in inhibiting hexanal formation in RBD olive oil. Baldioli et al. (1996) reported that, the oxidative stability of virgin olive oils correlates mainly with the concentration of hydrophilic phenols and, in particular with the oleosidic forms of hydroxytyrosol. The concentration of α-tocopherol, which is quantitatively the most important tocopherol in the oil, shows synergistic activity in mixtures with hydroxytyrosol and its oleosodic forms in purified olive oil. In another study, in the presence of strong antioxidants, such as orthodiphenols, α-tocopherol did not show any significant additional antioxidant effect during the period of low peroxide accumulation. α-tocopherol acted as antioxidant added at levels of 100, 500 and 1000 ppm in purified olive oil kept in the dark at 40°C, although the antioxidant effect was greater at 100 ppm than at higher concentrations. In the initial stage of autoxidation a slightly pro-oxidant effect was observed (Blekas, 1995). With regard to olive oil stability and individual phenolic substances changes, during accelerating oxidation at moderate temperatures of 60°C and 100°C, it has been reported (Nissiotis, 2002) that hydroxytyrosol derivatives are the first compounds to be oxidized, providing therefore oxidative stability to the oil, wherhas α-tocopherol seems to be oxidized after a significant decrease on hydroxytyrosol derivatives content. Tyrosol derivatives are the antioxidants that decrease with the lowest rate, providing the oil with the less antioxidant activity. With regard to the biological value of virgin olive oil (peroxide value lower than 20 meq/kg) hydroxytyrosol derivatives is destroyed first and it is possibly absent even in fine virgin olive oil or in olive oils after unsuitable storage conditions. Tyrosol derivatives and α-tocopherol are quite stable up to a peroxide value of 20 meq/kg. Similar results reported for the radical scavenging and antioxidant activities of phenolic compounds from olive pulp and olive oils, which were due mainly to 3,4- dihydroxymoiety linked to an aromatic ring (Morello, 2005). Glucosides and complex phenolics were more active antioxidants in liposomes and aglycons in bulk lipids. The antioxidant activity of VOO was mainly due to the dialdehyde of elenolic acid linked to hydroxytyrosol (3,4- DHPEA-EDA). In addition, it has been concluded that o-diphenols prevent oxidation of α-tocopherol (Nissiotis, 2002; Mateos, 2003).

The effect of storage conditions on olive oil phenolic content has also been reported in a number of studies. Several factors can influence the oxidative processes that extend or shorten the self-life and phenolic content of olive oil. Among them, the oxygen availability in the bottle headspace, storage temperature and the ratio of oleic acid/linoleic acid content, are the most important. The effects of changes in the concentrations of α-tocopherol, total phenols, and complex phenols were studied during storage of VOO of Lianolia variety, with bottles' headspace 3% (Okogeri, 2002). α-tocopherol was decomposed by 79% and total phenols by 45%, after 4 months of storage under diffused light. After storage in the dark, α-tocopherol was decomposed by 39-45% and total phenols by 50-62% after 12 months. When the olive oil reached a PV of 20 meq/kg, the remaining levels of tphenolic compounds ranged between 50 and 73% under diffused light and between 40 and 62% in the dark. In another study during storage of VOO of Lianolia and Koroneiki varieties for 15 months in the dark with bottles' headspace <1.5%, the peroxide value did not exceed the upper limit of 20 meq/kg set by the European Community Regulation. Changes occurring in phenolic compounds are dependent on the peroxide value and approximately 70% of hydroxytyrosol derivatives, 90% tyrosol derivatives and 100% lignans remained in the oil. Lianolia is more susceptible to oxidative degradation than Koroneiki due to its higher linoleic acid content (9% versus 5%). Higher degradation rate in phenolic compounds observed in the first work is owed to the higher bottles' headspace 3%, compared to 1.5% in the second work.

The changes of phenolic compounds and tocopherols content in oils stored for 2 years in amber glass bottles in the dark and for 6 months in the light have also been recorded in Picual olive oils (Garcia, 2002). In both cases, a decrease in polyphenols with storage time was observed, though this effect was more pronounced at the beginning of the storage period. The decrease in polyphenols in VOOs stored for two years was less than 30% and tocopherol loss was less than 20%. This monovarietal olive oil is very stable due to its high content of oleic acid. Similarly, when Cornicabra oil from Spain, having high oleic acid 80% percentage, was stored at 4°C in darkness without headspace, the oils did not exceed the upper limit of 20 meq/kg during the storage period of 21 months. The reduction of total phenolic compounds ranged in that work from 43% to 73% (Gómez-Alonso, 2007). In another study, using olive oil from Arbequina variety with low oleic acid, 65%, a noticeable decrease was observed in hydroxytyrosol derivatives after 12 months of storage (Morello, 2004).

Finally, in a stability study of bottled VOOs, changes were reported in minor polar compounds after storage for 18 months at 18°C in the dark (Romani, 2007). Concentrations of tyrosol and OH-hydroxytyrosol were relatively stable for the first 12 months and then rapidly decreased between 12 and 18 months of storage. Similarly, the secoiridoids and diacetoxy-oleuropein aglycone were depleted by 34-55 and 38-61%, respectively, after the same storage period. These reactions lead to a decrease in bitterness and pungent intensity; positive attributes that are characteristic of a fresh VOO (Bendini 2009).

It must be stressed that the decrease in polyphenols in the most representative Greek olive oil, Koroneiki variety stored for 15 months was less than 30% (Daskalaki, 2009), which is in agreement with data reported previously on the most representative Spanish olive oil, Picual (Garcia 2002). Therefore, it could be said that most of the antioxidants in virgin olive oils remained in the oil after 18 months of storage, which is the maximum storage time for olive oil, under ideal commercial conditions. Those conditions are low oxygen head space in the bottles <1% and low storage temperature <15°C in the dark, especially, for the olive oils having a low oleic/inoleic acid ratio.

5.3. Changes Occurring in Olive Oil Antioxidants During Cooking

At room or moderate temperatures, autoxidation reactions taking place through chain reactions of free radicals are relatively slow; the hydroperoxides are the major products formed and their concentration increases until advanced stages of oxidation. However, oxidation at the high temperatures of food processes like frying or boiling is far more complex because both oxidative and thermal reactions are simultaneously involved. The hydroperoxides decompose rapidly and are practically absent above 150°C, indicating that the decomposition of hydroperoxides becomes faster than their formation. These processes can affect the phenolic compounds content of oils to a certain degree, depending on each one treatment. Chemical degradation of antioxidants seems to be the major pathway for antioxidant loss at high temperatures although volatilization and steam distillation due to both the high temperature and the large amount of steam water escaping from the food have also been postulated. In a work studing the changes of phenolic compounds at heat treatment, simulating common domestic cooking processing, such as boiling and frying conducted by Daskalaki et al. (2009), thermal oxidation of oils at 180°C (frying) caused a significant decrease in hydroxytyrosol derivatives (60% reduction after 30 min and 90% reduction after 60 min) and, to a lower degree, in tyrosol derivatives. No changes were observed in the content of lignans. On the other hand, thermal oxidation of oils at 100°C (boiling) for 2 h caused a decrease of less than 20% in all classes of phenolic compounds. Similar trends for the reduction of the main groups of phenolic compounds (hydroxytyrosol derivatives consumed after 2 h whereas tyrosol derivatives and lignans were more stable) were reported for an Italian extra virgin olive oil (Bertolli oil) subjected to thermal treatment in an oven at 180°C (Carrasco-Pancobro, 2007). They reported that after heating at 180°C for 30 min the levels of hydroxytyrosol (61.5%), elenolic acid (56%), decarboxymethyl oleuropein aglycon (28.3%), and oleuropein aglycon (25.3%) were rapidly depleted, but tyrosol (19.9%), hydroxytyrosol acetate (5%), and the lignan aglycon (3%) were more thermally resistant. On the contrary, findings reported in the literature for Arbequina and Picual oil, which are the most popular varieties in Spain, resulted in a minor loss of polyphenols (Brenes, 2002). In this case, total loss of orthodiphenols was achieved in a longer period of time 5–15 h. in this work a different quantity of olive oil (different surface/volume ratio) was subjected to treatment in a Rancimat apparatus at 180°C. However, heating olive oils without foods at frying temperatures is known to cause excessive thermal damage without the tempering influence of steam produced by the moisture in foods, which means that losses in VOO phenols may be even lower at usual culinary practices.

In conclusion, during frying at 180°C, the content of phenolic compounds in VOO was remarkably reduced, especially hydroxytyrosol derivatives. During boiling at 100°C, all phenolic compounds remained stable, only 20% were decomposed. When virgin olive oil is stored under environmental conditions in the dark, the reduction of phenolic compounds depends on olive oil unsaturation, headspace oxygen availability and temperature. Under diffused light, α-tocopherol was almost totally depleted in 4 months storage time. The decrease in polyphenols in VOOs stored for 18 months is less than 30% and tocopherol loss is less than 20%, under ideal commercial conditions. Those conditions are low oxygen head space in the bottles (<1%) and low storage temperature (<18°C) in the dark. In addition, it has been concluded that o-diphenols prevent oxidation of α-tocopherol in the dark.

References

Abidi S. L., & Mounts T. L. Reversed-phase high-performance liquid chromatographic separation of tocopherols. *J. Chromatogr. A* 1997, 782, 25–32.

Andjelkovic M., Van Camp J., Pedra M., Renders K., Socaciu C., Verhe′ R. Correlations of the phenolic compounds and the phenolic content in some Spanish and French olive oils. *J. Agric. Food Chem.* 2008, 56, 5181–5187.

Andrewes P., Busch J., De Joode T., Groenewegen A., Alexandre H. Sensory properties of virgin olive oil polyphenols: Identification of deacetoxy-ligstroside aglycone as a key contributor to pungency. *J. Agric. Food Chem.* 2003, 51, 1415-1420.

Andrikopoulos N. K., Brueschweller H., Felber H., & Taeschler C. HPLC analysis of phenolic antioxidants, tocopherols and triglycerides. *J. Am. Oil Chem. Soc* 1991, 68, 359–364.

Angerosa F., D'Alessandro N., Konstantinou P., Corana F., Mellerio G. Characterization of phenolic and secoiridoid aglycons present in virgin olive oil by gas chromatography-chemical-ionization mass spectrometry. *J. Chromatogr.* 1996, 736, 195-203.

Armaforte E, Mancebo-Campos V, Bendini A, Salvasor MA, Fregapane G, Carretani L. Retention effects of oxidized polyphenols during analytical extraction of phenolic compounds of virgin olive oil. *J. Sep. Sci.* 2007, 30, 2401-2406

Aruoma O.I. Free radicals, Oxidative stress, and Antioxidants in human health and disease. *J. Am. Oil Chem. Soc.* 1998, 75, 199-212.

Baldioli M., Servili M., Perretti G., & Montedoro G. F. Antioxidant activity of tocopherols and phenolic compounds of virgin olive oil. *J. Am. Oil Chem. Soc.* 1996, 73, 1589–1593.

Bartsch H., Nair J., Owen R.W. Dietary PUFA's and cancer of the breast and colorectum: compelling evidence for their role as risk modifiers. *Carcinogenesis* 1999, 20, 2209-2218.

Bartsch H., Nair J., Owen R.W. Exocyclic DNA adducts as oxidative stress markers in colon carcinogenesis: potential role of lipid peroxidation, dietary fat and antioxidants. *Biology and Chemistry* 2002, 383, 915-921.

Beltran G., Aguilera M.P., Del Rio C., Sanchez S., Martinez L. Influence of fruit ripening process on the natural antioxidant content of Hojiblanca virgin olive oils. *Food Chem.* 2005, 89, 207-215

Beltran G., Jimenez A., Del Rio C., Sanchez S., Martinez L., Uceda M., & Aguilera M. P. Variability of vitamin E in virgin olive oil by agronomical and genetic factors, *Journal of Food Composition and Analysis* 2010, 23, 633–639.

Bendini A., Cerretani L., Salvador M.D., Fregapane G., Lercker G. Stability of the sensory quality of virgin olive oil during storage: An overview. *Ital. J. Food Sci.* 2009, 21, 389-406.

Bianco A., Coccioli F., Guiso M., Marra C. The occurrence in olive oil of a new class of phenolic compounds: hydroxy-isochromans. *Food Chem.* 2001, 77, 405-411.

Bianco A.,Buiarelli F.,Cartoni G.,Coccioli F.,Jasionowska R.,Margherita M. Analysis by liquid chromatography–tandem mass spectrometry of biophenolic compounds in virgin olive oil, Part II. *J. Sep. Sci.* 2003, 26, 417–424.

Bianco A.D, Mazzei R.A., Melchioni C., Romeo G., Scarpati M.L., Soriero A., Uccella N. Microcomponents of olive oil-III. Glucosides of 2(3,4-dihydroxy-phenyl)ethanol. *Food Chem.* 1998, 63, 461-464.

Blekas,G., Tsimidou M. & Boskou D. Contribution of α -tocopherol to olive oil stability. *Food Chem..* 1995, 52 289-294.

Bogani P., Galli C., Villa M., Visioli F. Postpradial anti-flammatory and antioxidant effects of extra virgin olive oil. *Atherosclerosis* 2007, 190, 181-186.

Brenes M., Garcia A., Dobarganes M. C., Velasco J., Romero C. Influence of thermal treatment simulating cooking processes on the polyphenol content in virgin olive oil. *J. Agric. Food Chem.* 2002, *50*, 5962–5967.

Brenes M., Garcıa A., Garcıa P, Rios J.J., Garrido A. Phenolic compounds in Spanish olive oils. *J. Agric. Food Chem.* 1999, 47, 3535-3540.

Brenes M., Garcıa A., Garcıa P., Garrido A. Rapid and complete extraction of phenols from olive oil and determination by means of a coulometric electrode array system. *J. Agric. Food Chem.* 2000a, 48, 5178-5183.

Brenes M., Hidalgo F.J., Garcia A., Rios J.J., Garcia P., Zamora R., Garrido A. Pinoresinol and 1-Acetoxypinoresinol, Two New Phenolic Compounds Identified in Olive Oil. *J. Am. Oil Chem. Soc.* 2000b, 77, 715-720.

Caponio F., Alloggio V., Gomes T. Phenolic compounds of virgin olive oil: influence of paste preparation techniques. *Food Chem.* 1999, 64, 203-209.

Carpenter A. P. J. Determination of tocopherols in vegetable oils. *J. Am. Oil Chem. Soc.* 1979, 5, 668–671

Carrasco-Pancobro A., Cerretani L., Bendini A., Segura-Carretero A., Lercker G., Fernández-Gutiérrez A. Evaluation of the influence of thermal oxidation on the phenolic composition and on the andioxidant activity of extra-virgin olive oil. *J. Agric. Food Chem.* 2007, *55*, 4771–4780.

Carrasco-Pancorbo A., Cerretani L., Bendini A., Segura-Carretero A., Gallina-Toschi T., Fernandez-Gutierrez A. Analytical determination of polyphenols in olive oils. *J. Sep. Sci.* 2005, 28, 837–858.

Chan H. W.S. The Mechanism of Autoxidation, in Autoxidation of Unsaturated Lipids, Chan, H.W.S., Academic Press, London, 1987, p. 1.

Chimi H., Cillard J., Cillard P., Rahmani M. Peroxyl and Hydroxyl Radical Scavenging Activity of Some Natural Phenolic Antioxidants. *J. Am. Oil Chem. Soc.* 1991, 68, p. 307.

Chouliaras V., Tasioula-Margari M., Chatzissavvidis C., Therios I., Tsabolatidou E. The effects of a seaweed extract in addition to nitrogen and boron fertilization on productivity, fruit maturation, leaf nutritional status and oil quality of the olive (*Olea europaea* L.) cultivar Koroneiki. *J. Sci. Food Agric.* 2009, 89, 984-988.

Christophoridou S., Dais P. Detection and quantification of phenolic compounds in olive oil by high resolution 1H nuclear magnetic resonance spectroscopy. *Anal. Chim. Acta* 2009, 633, 283–292.

Christophoridou S., Dais P., Tseng L.I.-H., Spraul M. Separation and identification of phenolic compounds in olive oil by coupling high-performance Liquid Chromatography with Postcolumn Solid-Phase Extraction to Nuclear Magnetic Resonance Spectroscopy (LC-SPE-NMR). *J. Agric. Food Chem.* 2005, 53, 4667-4679.

Cicerale S., Lucas L., Keast R. Biological Activities of Phenolic Compounds Present in Virgin Olive Oil. *Int. J. Mol. Sci.* 2010, 11, 458-479.

CODEX STAN 33-1981 Standard for Olive Oils and Olive Pomace Oils *http://www.codexalimentarius.net/web/standard_list.jsp*

Covas M. I. Olive oil and Cardiovascular system. *Pharm. Res.* 2007, 55, 175-186.

Dabbou S., Cheha, H., Faten B., Dabbou S., Esposto S., Selvaggini R., Taticchi A., Servili M., Montedoro G.F., Hammami M. Effect of three irrigation regimes on Arbequina olive oil produced under Tunisian growing conditions. *Agricultural Water Management* 2010, 97, 763–768.

Dais P., Spyros A., Christophoridou S., Hatzakis M., Fragaki G., Agiomyrgianaki A., Salivaras E., Siragakis G., Daskalaki D., Tasioula-Margari M., Brenes M. Comparison of analytical methodologies based on 1H and 31P NMR spectroscopy with conventional methods for the determination of some olive oil constituents. *J. Agric. Food Chem.* 2007, 55, 577-584.

Daskalaki D., Kefi G., Kotsiou K., Tasioula-Margari M. Evaluation of phenolic compounds degradation in virgin olive oil during storage and heating. *J. Food and Nutr. Research* 2009, 48, 31-41.

De la Torre-Carbot K., Jauregui O., Gimeno E., Castellote I.A., Lamuela-Raventoäs M.R., Loäpez-Sabater M.C. Characterization and quantification of phenolic compounds in olive oils by solid-phase extraction. HPLC-DAD and HPLC-MS/MS. *J. Agric. Food Chem.* 2005, 53, 4331-4340.

Dionisi F., Prodolliet J., & Tagliaferri, E. Assessment of olive oil adulteration by reversed-phase high-performance liquid chromatography/amperometric determination of tocopherols and tocotrienols. *J. Am. Oil Chem. Soc.* 1995, 72, 1505–1511.

Ebaid G.M.X., Seiva F.R.F., Rocha K. KHR, Souza G. A. and Novelli E. L.B. Effects of olive oil and its minor phenolic constituents on obesity-induced cardiac metabolic changes. *Eur. J. Nutr.* 2005, 44, 121-127.

EC. Commission Regulation No. 2568/91 of 11 July 1991 on the characteristics of olive oil and olive-residue oil and on the relevant methods of analysis. Official Journal, L 248:1–83 and later amendments 1989/2003, L 295.

Emmons E.W., Fedeli E., Firestone D. Olive Oil, in Bailey's Industrial Oil and Fat Products, Fifth Edition, Volume 2, Edible Oil and Fat Products: Oils and Oil Seeds, Ed. Y.H. Hui, John Wiley and Sons, Inc., New York, 1996, p.90.

Evans H.M., Bishop K.S. On the Existence of a Hitherto Unrecognized Dietary Factor Essential for Reproduction. *Science* 1922, 56, 650-651.

Fito M., Cladellas M., De la Torre R. Marti J., Alcantara M., Pujadas-Bastardes M., Marrugat J., Bruguera J., Lopez-Sabater M.C., Vila J, Covas M.I. Antioxidant of virgin olive oil in patients with stable coronary heart dease: rarandomezed, crossover,controlled clinical trial. *Atherosclerosis* 2005,181, 149-158.

Frankel E.N. Recent Advances in Lipid Oxidation. *J. Sci. Food Agric.* 1991, S4, 495-511.

García A., Brenes M., Romero C., García P., Garrido A. Study of phenolic compounds in virgin olive oils of the Picual variety. *Eur Food Res. Technol.* 2002, 215, 407–412

Garcia-Gonzalez D., Aparicio-Ruiz R., Aparicio R. Virgin olive oil-chemical implications on quality and health. *Eur. J. Lipid Sci. Technol.* 2008, 110, 602–607.

Garcia-Villalba R., Pacchiarotta T., Carrasco-Pancorbo A., Segura-Carretero A., Fernαndez-Gutiιrrez A., Deelder A.M., Mayboroda O.A., Gas chromatography–atmospheric pressure chemical ionization-time of flight mass spectrometry for profiling of phenolic compounds in extra virgin olive oil. *J. Chromatogr. A* 2011, 1218, 959–971.

Gimeno E., Castellote A.I., Lamuela-Raventós R.M., De la Torre M.C., López-Sabater M.C. The effects of harvest and extraction methods on the antioxidant content (phenolics, α-tocopherol, and β-carotene) in virgin olive oil. *Food chemistry* 2002, 78, 207-211

Gómez-Alonso S., Mancebo-Campos V., Desamparados-Salvador M., Fregapane, G. Evolution of major and minor components and oxidation indices of virgin olive oil during 21 months storage at room temperature. *Food Chem.* 2007, 100, 36–42.

Gomez-Rico A., Inarejos-Garcia A.M. Salvador M.D., and Fregapane G. Effect of Malaxation Conditions on Phenol and Volatile Profiles in Olive Paste and the Corresponding Virgin Olive Oils (Olea europaea L. Cv. Cornicabra) *J. Agric. Food Chem.* 2009, 57, 3587–3595.

Gómez-Rico A., Salvador M.D., Moriana A., Pérez D., Olmedilla N., Ribas F., Fregapane, G. Influence of different irrigation strategies in a traditional Cornicabra cv. olive orchard on virgin olive oil composition and quality. *Food Chem.* 2007, 100, 568-578.

Gutfinger T., Polyphenols in olive oils. *J. Am. Oil Chem. Soc.* 1981, 58, 966–968.

Gutierrez F., Jimenez B., Ruιz A., & Albi M.A. Effect of olive ripeness on the oxidative stability of virgin olive oil extracted from the varieties Picual and Hojiblanca and on the different components involved. *J. Agric. Food Chem.* 1999, 44, 121–127.

Gutierrez-Rosales F., Rios J.J., Gomez-Rey M.L. Main polyphenols in the bitter taste of virgin olive oil. Structural confirmation by on-line high-performance liquid chromatography electrospray ionization mass spectrometry. *J. Agric. Food Chem.* 2003, 51, 6021–6025.

Halliwell B., Gutteridge J.M.C. Free Radicals in Biology and Medicine. Oxford University Press, Oxford, 1989, p. 84.

Hoehler D., Frohlich A. A., Marquardt R. R., & Stelsovsky H. Extraction of tocopherol from serum prior to reversed-phaseliquid chromatography. *J. Agric. Food Chem.* 1998, 46, 973–978.

Hrncirik K., Fritsche S. Comparability and reliability of different techniques for the determination of phenolic compounds in virgin olive oil. *Eur. J. Lipid Sci. Technol.* 2004, 106, 540–549.

International Olive Oil Council (IOOC*) http://www.internationaloliveoil.org/store/view/49-olivae-115-english*

IUPAC. Standard methods for the analysis of oils, fats and derivatives. Method 2.411 (7th ed.), International Union of Pure and Applied Chemistry, London: Blackwell Scientific Publication, 1987.

Kamal-Eldin A., and Appelquist L.A. The Chemistry and Antioxidant Properties of Tocopherols and Tocotrienols, *Lipids,* 1996, 31, 671-701.

Lea C.H., Methods for determining peroxide in lipids. *J. Sci. Food Agric.*1952, 3, 586-594.

Mateos R., Dominguez M., Espartero J.L., Cert A. Antioxidant effect of phenolic compounds, α-tocopherol, and other minor components in virgin olive oil. *J. Agric. Food Chem* 2003, 51, 7170–7175.

Mateos R., Espartero J. L., Trujillo M., Rıos J.J., Leon-Camacho M., Alcudia F., Cert A. Determination of Phenols, Flavones, and Lignans in Virgin Olive Oils by Solid-Phase Extraction and High-Performance Liquid Chromatography with Diode Array Ultraviolet Detection. *J. Agric.Food Chem.* 2001, 49, 2185-2192.

Montedoro G., Servili L.M., Baldioli M., Selvaggini R., Miniati E., Macchionii A. Simple and Hydrolyzable Compounds in Virgin Olive Oil. 3. Spectroscopic Characterizations of the Secoiridoid Derivatives. *J. Agric. Food Chem.* 1993, 41, 2228-2234.

Montedoro G., Servili N., Baldioli M., Miniati E. Simple and hydrolysable phenolic compounds in virgin olive oil: their extraction, separation, and quantification and semiquantitative evaluation by HPLC. *J. Agric. Food Chem.* 1992, 40, 1571-1576.

Morello J.R., Motilva M.J., Tovar M.J., Romero M.P. Changes in commercial virgin olive oil (cv Arbequina) during storage, with special emphasis on the phenolic fraction. *Food Chem.* 2004, 85, 357-364.

Morello J.R., Vuorela S., Romero M.P., Motilva M.J., Heinonen M. Antioxidant activity of olive pulp and olive oil phenolic compounds of the Arbequina cultivar. *J. Agric. Food Chem.* 2005, 53, 2002–2008.

Moure A., Cruz J. M., Franco D., Dominguez J. M., Sineiro J., Dominguez H., Nunez M. J., Parajo J. C. Natural antioxidants from residual sources. *Food Chem.* 2001, *72*, 145-171.

Nagaoka S., Sawada K., Fukumoto Y., Nagashima U., Katasumata S., and Mukai,K. Mechanism of Antioxidant Reaction of Vitamin E: Kinetic, Spectroscopic and ab initio Study of Proton-Transfer Reactions. *J. Phys. Chem.* 1992, 96, 6663-6668.

Nissiotis M., Tasioula-Margari M. Changes in antioxidant concentration of virgin olive oil during thermal oxidation. *Food Chem.* 2002, 77, 371-376.

Obied H. K., Bedgood Jr D. R,. Prenzler P.D,, Robards K. Chemical screening of olive biophenol extracts by hyphenated liquid chromatography. *Anal. Chim. Acta* 2007, 603 176–189.

Okogeri O., Tasioula-Margari M. Changes occuring in phenolic compounds and α-tocopherol during storage of virgin olive oil. *J. Agric. Food Chem.* 2002, 50 (5), 1077-1080.

Oliveras-Lopez M.J., Innocenti M., Giaccherini C., Ieri F., Romani A., Mulinacci N. Study of the phenolic composition of spanish and italian monocultivar extra virgin olive oils: Distribution of lignans, secoiridoidic, simple phenols and flavonoids, *Talanta* 2007, 73, 726-732.

Owen R.W., Giacosa A., Hull W.E., Haubner R., Spiegelhalder B., Bartsh H. The antioxidant/anticancer potential of phenolic compounds isolated from olive oil. *Europ. J. Cancer* 2000a, 36, 1235-1247.

Owen R.W., Mier W., Giacosa A., Hull W.E., Spiegelhalder B., Bartsch H. Phenolic compounds and squalene in olive oils: The concentration and antioxidant potential of total phenols, simple phenols, secoiridoids, lignans and squalene. *Food Chem. Toxicol.* 2000b, 38, 647-659.

Pancorbo A.C., Cruces-Blanco C., Segura-Carretero A., Gutierrez A. Sensitive determination of phenolic acids in extra-VOO by Capillary Zone Electrophoresis. *J. Agric. Food Chem.* 2004, 52, 6687-6693.

Pirisi F.M., Cabras P., Cao C.F., Magliorini M., Suggelli M. Phenolic compounds in virgin olive oil. 2. Reappraisal of the extraction, HPLC separation, and quantification procedures. *J. Agric. Food Chem.* 2000, 48, 1191-1196.

Psomiadou E., Tsimidou, M., and Boskou D. α-Tocopherol content of Greek virgin olive oils. *J. Agric. Food Chem.* 2000, *48,* 1770-1775.

Rios J.J., Gil M.J., Gutierrez-Rosales F., Solid phase extraction gas chromatography – ion trap – mass spectrometry qualitative method for evaluation of phenolic compounds in virgin olive oil and structural confirmation of oleuropein and ligstroside aglycons and their oxidation products. *J. Chromatogr. A* 2005, 1093, 167-176.

Romani A., Lapucci C., Cantini C., Ieri F., Mulinacci N., Visioli F. Evolution of minor polar compounds and antioxidant capacity during storage of bottled extra virgin olive oil. *J. Agric. Food Chem.* 2007, 55, 1315–1320.

Rovellini P., Cortesi N., Fedeli E., Analysis of flavonoids from Olea europaea by HPLC-UV and HPLC-Electrospray- MS. *Riv. Ital. Sost. Grasse* 1997, 74, 273–279.

Rovellini P., Cortesi N., Liquid chromatography – mass spectrometry in the study of oleuropein and ligstroside aglycons in virgin olive oil: Aldehydic forms and their oxidized products. *Riv. Ital. Sost. Grasse,* 2002, 77, 1-14.

Ruano J., Lopez-Miranda J., Fuentes F., Moreno J. A., Bellido C., Perez-Martinez P., Lozano A., Gomez P., Jimenez Y., Perez J. F. Phenolic content of virgin olive oil improves ischemic reactive hyperemia in hypercholesterolemic patients. *J. Am. Coll. Cardiol.* 2005, 46, 1864-1868

Ryan D, Robards K, Prenzler P, Jardine D, Herlt T, Antolovich M. Liquid chromatography with electrospray ionisation mass spectrometric detection of phenolic compounds from Olea europaea. *J Chromatogr A.* 1999; 855: 529–537.

Satue M. T., Huang S.W., Frankel E. N. Effect of natural antioxidants in virgin olive oil on oxidative stability of refined, bleached, and deodorized olive oil. *J. Am. Oil Chem. Soc.* 1995, 72, 1131–1137.

Selvaggini R., Servili M., Urbani S., Esposto S., Taticchi A., Montedoro G.F. Evaluation of phenolic compounds in virgin olive oil by direct injection in high-performance liquid chromatography with fluorometric detection. *J. Agric. Food Chem.* 2006, 54, 2832–2838.

Servili M., Baldioli M., Selvaggini R., Macchioni A., Montedoro G.F. Phenolic compounds of olive fruit: one- and two dimensional nuclear magnetic resonance characterization of nuzhenide and its distribution in the constitutive parts of fruit. *J. Agric. Food Chem.* 1999, 47, 12–18.

Servili M., Montedoro G. Contribution of phenolic compounds to virgin olive oil quality. *Eur. J. Lipid Sci. Technol.* 2002, 104, 602–613.

Servili M., Selvaggini R., Esposto S., Taticchi A., Montedoro G.F., Morozzi G. Health and sensory properties of virgin olive oil hydrophilic phenols: agronomic and technological aspects of production that affect their occurrence in the oil. *J. Chromatogr.* A 2004, 1054, 113–127.

Servili M., Selvaggini R., Taticchi A., Esposto S., Montedoro G.F., Volatile compounds and phenolic composition of virgin olive oil: optimization of temperature and time of exposure of olive pastes to air contact during the mechanical extraction process. *J. Agric. Food Chem.* 2003, 51, 7980–7988.

Servili M., Taticchi A, Esposto S, Urbani,S.,Selvaggini R.and Montedoro GF, Influence of the Decrease in Oxygen during Malaxation of Olive Paste on the Composition of Volatiles and Phenolic Compounds in Virgin Olive Oil *J. Agric. Food Chem.* 2008, *56,* 10048–10055.

Shahidi F., Pegg R.B. Nutrite-free meat curing systems; Update and review. Food Chem., 1992, 43, 185-191.

Simic M.G. Urinary biomarkers and the rate of DNA damage in carcinogenesis and anticarcinogenesis. *Mutation Research/Fundamental and Molecular Mechanisms of Mutagenesis* 1992, 267, 277-290.

Simic, M.G. Free Radical Mechanisms in Autoxidation Processes. *J. Chem. Educ.* 1981, 58, p. 125-131.

Tasioula-Margari M., Okogeri O. Isolation and Characterization of Virgin Olive Oil Phenolic Compounds by HPLC/UV and GC-MS. *J. Food Sci.* 2001a, 66, 530-534.

Tasioula-Margari M., Okogeri O. Simultaneous determination of phenolic compounds and tocopherols in virgin olive oil using HPLC and UV detection. *Food Chem.* 2001b, 74, 369-375.

Tovar M. J., Motilva M. J., and Romero M. P. Changes in the Phenolic Composition of Virgin Olive Oil from Young Trees (Olea europaea L. cv. Arbequina) Grown under Linear Irrigation Strategies. *J. Agric. Food Chem.* 2001, 49, 5502-5508.

Tripoli E., Giammanco M,. Tabacchi G, Di Majo D., Giammanco S. and. La Guardia M. The phenolic compounds of olive oil: Structure, biologigical activity and beneficial effect on human health. *Nutr. Research Reviews.* 2005, 18, 98-112.

Tura D., Gigliotti C., Pedó S., Failla O., Bassi D., Serraiocco A. Influence of cultivar and site of cultivation on levels of lipophilic and hydrophilic antioxidants in virgin olive oils (Olea Europea L.) and correlations with oxidative stability. *Scientia Horticulturae* 2007, 112, 108-119.

Visioli F., Galli C. Olive oil phenols and their potential effects on human health. *J. Agric. Food Chem.* 1998, 46, 4292–4296.

Wahyuni W. T. & Jinno K. Separation of tocopherols on various chemically bonded phase in microcolumn liquid chromatography. *J. Chromatogr.* 1988, 448, 398–403.

Zhang H. Y. Theoretical methods used in elucidating activity differences of phenolic antioxidants. *J. Am. Oil Chem. Soc.* 1999, *76*, 745-748.

In: Olive Consumption and Health
Editors: C. A. Savalas and S. M. Nicolau

ISBN: 978-1-62100-774-6

Chapter 4

OLIVE OIL AND POSTPRANDIAL LIPEMIA

Javier S. Perona*
Instituto de la Grasa (IG-CSIC), Av. Padre García Tejero Nº4,
41012, Seville, Spain

ABSTRACT

The postprandial lipid period takes place after the intake of food, involves the metabolic processes that occur following the ingestion of a meal containing fat, and it is characterized by a considerable increase in plasma triglyceride levels. An impaired metabolism of postprandial triglyceride-rich lipoproteins (TRL), comprising chylomicrons, very-low-density lipoproteins (VLDL) and their remnants, is believed to contribute to the onset and development of atherosclerosis. Recent research has pointed out that these particles are highly atherogenic because, in contrast to low-density lipoproteins, can penetrate into the intima and be taken up by macrophages without need for prior oxidation, leading to the initiation of atherogenesis. The atherogenicity of TRL depends on their lipid composition, which is, in turn, influenced by the composition of dietary fats.

The intake of oleic-acid rich oils, like olive oil, have been shown to modulate the production of postprandial TRL and their subsequent metabolism and it is likely that both the fatty acid and minor component compositions of the oil may have a role. The postprandial triglyceride response seems to be dependent mainly upon the triglyceride molecular species composition and not on the minor components. However, the unsaponifiable components of virgin olive oil and pomace olive oil can have important effects on the uptake of postprandial TRL by macrophages and other cells involved in the processes related to the development of atherosclerosis.

Keywords: Triglyceride-rich lipoproteins, chylomicron, olive oil, triglyceride, minor components, fatty acid, atherosclerosis

* Corresponding author: Instituto de la Grasa (CSIC). Av. Padre Garcia Tejero, 4. 41012 Seville. Spain. E-mail: perona@ig.csic.es. Tel.: +34954611550. Fax: +34954616790.

Abbreviations

MUFA	Monounsaturated Fatty Acids
PUFA	Polyunsaturated Fatty Acids
SFA	Saturated Fatty Acids
CM	Chylomicrons
TRL	Triglyceride-rich lipoproteins
VLDL	Very low-density lipoproteins
VOO	Virgin olive oil
FA	Fatty acid
LPL	Lipoprotein lipase
SR	Scavenger receptor.

Introduction

After decades of epidemiological, clinical and experimental research, consumption of specific foods and, particularly, dietary patterns, have a profound influence on health outcomes, including coronary heart disease. In this regard, the Mediterranean Diet has been ascribed as the dietary pattern that best fulfills the need for nourishment, health and pleasure, with olive oil as its characteristic culinary fat (Hu, 2003).

There is now sufficient scientific evidence to support that increasing adherence to the Mediterranean diet is associated with a reduction of overall, cardiovascular and cancer mortality (Trichopoulou et al., 2003; Psaltopoulou et al., 2004; Trichopoulou et al., 2005a; Trichopoulou et al., 2005b; Panagiotakos et al., 2008; Sofi et al., 2008). Although it is difficult to elucidate the effect solely due to olive oil, from that of the other components of the Mediterranean Diet, olive oil has been proposed as a key factor for the health benefits associated with the Mediterranean Diet (Hu, 2003; Perez-Jimenez et al., 2005).

The beneficial effects of olive oil on cardiovascular risk have been attributed to its high monounsaturated fatty acid (MUFA) content, but new evidences are now suggesting that minor though highly bioactive components of olive oil have also an important role (Table 1).

A significant number of the new outcomes of the beneficial effects of olive oil and its major and minor components, are related to its effect postprandially. Recently, it was shown that the triglyceride concentration of triglyceride-rich lipoproteins (TRL) and their particle size were higher and the number of TRL particles was lower after virgin olive oil consumption, with a high content of non-polar constituents, than after refined olive oil (Cabello-Moruno et al., 2007a). Furthermore, intake of high-oleic sunflower oil (HOSO) was associated with higher postprandial triglyceride increases compared with virgin olive oil or virgin olive oil enriched with non-polar components. Moreover, incubation of postprandial TRL formed after ingestion of virgin olive oil with endothelial cells was associated with a greater reduction in eicosanoid production (Perona et al., 2004). During the postprandial state, diets rich in saturated fatty acids (SFA) impair vascular reactivity, while consumption of virgin olive oil preserves endothelial function (Fuentes et al., 2008).

The present article summarizes the current knowledge of the effects of olive oil consumption during the postprandial state and its implications in cardiovascular disease, with emphasis in the first events occurring in the development of the atherosclerotic plaque. The article will also focus on the possible mechanisms by which olive oil components, like oleic acid (18:1, n-9), but more importantly minor components, contribute to its beneficial effect as part of the Mediterranean diet.

Table 1. Beneficial effects of dietary olive oil intake and its active components

Effect	Active components	References
Lower cardiovascular mortality	MUFA phenolic compounds	Covas et al., 2009 Lairon, 2007
Improved blood lipid profile	MUFA	Covas et al., 2009 Huang and Sumpio, 2008 Covas, 2007 Cabello-Moruno et al., 2007
Reduced blood pressure	MUFA phenolic compounds	Covas, 2007 Perez-Jiminez et al., 2007
Lower inflammation	MUFA phenolic compounds oleuropein oleocanthal α-tocopherol β-sitosterol oleanolic acid	Covas et al., 2009 Covas, 2007 Perez-Jiminez et al., 2007 Perona et al., 2006
Reduced oxidative damage	MUFA phenolic compounds α-tocopherol	Bester et al., 2010 Raederstorff, 2010 Fito et al., 2007
Reduced cancer risk	MUFA squalene	Bosetti et al., 2009 Waterman and Lockwood, 2007 Escrich et al., 2007
Increased life span		Perez-Lopez et al., 2009 Perez-Jimenez et al., 2005 Trichopoulou et al., 2005a

ATHEROSCLEROSIS AS A POSTPRANDIAL DISEASE

Postprandial lipemia refers to the transient increase in blood lipids, that takes place after a meal containing fat and it is characterized by a considerable increase in plasma triglyceride levels (Perez-Martinez et al., 2008). In Western societies, in which 3-4 four meals are usually consumed during the day, individuals may spend most of the wakefulness period in this state and only very few hours are in the fasting phase (Sharrett et al., 2001). The role of postprandial lipemia in atherogenesis was first proposed by Zilversmit (1979) more than thirty years ago, and it is currently supported by a great deal of evidence from epidemiological, clinical and experimental studies (Goldberg et al., 2000; Hyson et al., 2003; O'Keefe et al., 2007; Alipour et al., 2008).

Together with elevated plasma triglyceride, an impaired metabolism of postprandial triglyceride-rich lipoproteins (TRL) is believed to contribute to the onset and development of atherosclerosis (Ginsberg, 2002). TRL comprise a very heterogeneous group of nascent and metabolically modified lipoproteins, including chylomicrons, very-low-density lipoproteins

(VLDL) and their remnants. Chylomicrons are assembled in the intestine and contain mainly dietary lipids, while VLDL include lipids from endogenous origin. In recent years, there is accumulating evidence showing that postprandial TRL are strongly atherogenic (Mamo, 1995; Yu and Cooper, 2001; Wilheim and Cooper 2003; Alipour et al. 2008). CM remnants have been shown to penetrate the artery wall and to interact with vascular cells (Mamo, 1995; Proctor et al., 2002). A delay in their clearance from the circulation has been found to correlate with the development of atherosclerotic lesions (Patsch et al., 1992; Benlian et al., 1996) and has been linked with atherosclerosis progression in two recent large scale prospective trials, independently of other risk factors (Bansal et al., 2007; Nordestgaard et al., 2007).

Current evidence suggests that postprandial lipoproteins may be involved in promoting atherosclerosis both directly, via an influence on events in the vasculature, and indirectly, by causing a more atherogenic lipoprotein profile when their levels are abnormally raised (Hyson et al., 2003; Wilheim and Cooper 2003; Alipour et al., 2008). TRL become remnant particles after partial depletion of their triglyceride content by means of lipoprotein lipase (LPL) activity. In the postprandial phase, the resulting fatty acids are incorporated into extrahepatic tissues, mainly adipose tissue (Fielding and Frayn, 1998). The remaining triglycerides and the other dietary lipids are retained in the remnant particle and delivered to the liver in order to obtain energy or for the synthesis of complex lipids such as phospholipids (Redgrave, 1983; Yu and Cooper, 2001). Fatty acids in the liver may be re-synthesized into triglycerides, returned to the blood in the form of VLDL (Nguyen et al., 2008). During their transport to the liver, remnant particles may enter the artery wall and are retained in the sub-endothelial space, where they have the opportunity to influence atherosclerosis development by interacting directly with cells in the tissue (Proctor et al., 2002).

Atherosclerosis is initiated by dysfunction of the vascular endothelium followed by the formation of macrophage foam cells, generated by lipid uptake from plasma lipoproteins. Accumulation of foam cells and the proliferation of smooth muscle cells causes the appearance of fatty streaks, the first visible lesions in the vessel wall (Kadar and Glasz, 2001). In contrast to low-density lipoproteins, TRL can penetrate into the intima and be taken up by macrophages without need for prior oxidation, leading to foam cell formation (Cohn et al., 1999; Napolitano et al., 2003). Other pro-inflammatory and potentially atherogenic effects of postprandial lipoproteins include activation of leukocytes, promoting adhesion to the endothelium and invasion of the artery wall (Alipour et al., 2008; Bentley et al., 2008).

Postprandial Triglyceride Response to Diet

Postprandial lipemia is modulated by many lifestyle factors, including diet, and postprandial hyperlipidemia is a feature of diseases linked to the Western lifestyle, including obesity, insulin resistance and diabetes (Lopez-Miranda et al., 2007). Western dietary habits, involve the intake of several meals throughout the day, thus the plasma triglyceride concentration is continuously elevated except for a few hours.

Lipids from the diet, including macronutrients, such as triglycerides, and micronutrients, such as lipid soluble antioxidants, are absorbed in the intestine and are incorporated into the bloodstream, via the lymphatic system, as part of large chylomicrons. These TRL, synthesized in the enterocyte, transport exogenous dietary lipids within the circulation, causing an increase in plasma triglyceride concentrations in the postprandial state. Chylomicrons contain apolipoprotein B-48 (apo B-48) as structural protein, and are very large but heterogeneous in size, which depends on the rate of fat absorption, type and amount of fat absorbed (Table 2).

Table 2. Key features of postprandial triglyceride-rich lipoproteins

Origin	Heterogeneous group of nascent and metabolically modified lipoproteins, including chylomicrons, very-low-density lipoproteins and their remnants.
Structure	TRL contain a single molecule of apolipoprotein B per particle and it is not exchanged with other lipoproteins.
Composition	The fatty acid composition of TRL partially reflects the composition of the diet, affecting their metabolism and rate of clearance.
Metabolism	Chylomicrons and very-low-density lipoproteins compete for the same clearance mechanisms.
Atherogenicity	TRL can penetrate into the arterial intima and induce foam cell formation, one of the first steps in atherogenesis, without need of prior oxidation.

The process of chylomicron formation in enterocytes involves the synthesis of apo B-48, and other apolipoproteins, transport of lipids to the site of CM assembly, association of lipids with the formed apolipoproteins and incorporation of the lipid mass into the lipoprotein (Hussain, 2000). Triglycerides are absorbed after hydrolysis by pancreatic lipase in the intestinal lumen, as free fatty acids and 2-monoglycerides. By what mechanism these molecules travel to the endoplasmic reticulum is not clear and although two fatty acid binding proteins have been identified, the intestinal and the liver fatty acid binding protein, their role in the intracellular trafficking of fatty acid remains unclear (Storch and Thumser, 2000). 2-monoglycerides and fatty acids are reconstituted to form triglycerides by the action of acyl-coenzyme A: monoacylglycerol acyltransferase (MGAT) first, and then by acyl-coenzyme A: diacylglycerol acyltransferase (DGAT) in the cytoplasmic surface of the endoplasmic reticulum (Kuksis and Manganaro, 1986). Since triglycerides have a low solubility in phospholipid bilayers, it has been postulated that triglyceride molecules saturate the membrane rapidly, splitting the bilayer and forming a small lens (Kindel et al. 2010). Addition of preformed phospholipids and a small amount of triglycerides leads to the formation of the so-called primordial particle. This primordial particle is filled with triglycerides by the action of the microsomal triglyceride transfer protein (MTP) and the fusion of the particle with stable lipid droplets within the enterocyte. Early (30-90 min) secreted chylomicrons have been reported to be small dense particles that would represent mainly primordial particles. However, as absorption progresses, the amount of less dense particles increases (Silva et al., 2001).

Whereas VLDL secretion by the liver is under strict regulation via insulin control (Karpe, 1999), chylomicron synthesis and secretion are much more dependent on the dietary lipid composition. The size of the nascent chylomicron particles that are secreted to the lymph would be partially determined by the size of the triglyceride droplets they fuse with. Likewise, the size and composition of the these droplets depends on the triglyceride composition of the diets. Fat meals containing > 30g fat have been shown to cause postprandial lipemia, with dose dependence up to about 80g (Dubois et al., 1998; Lopez-Miranda et al., 2007, Lairon, 2008). It should be taken into account that the average fat content of a Western-style meal has been estimated in 20-40g 3-4 times a day (Sharrett et al., 2001).

The fatty acid composition of the triglyceride present in nascent chylomicrons reflects the composition of dietary fat, although not completely faithfully (Hussain, 2000). It has been suggested that incorporation of MUFA or polyunsaturated fatty acids (PUFA) into enterocytes could lead to the formation of more stable lipid droplets that would enhance the recruitment of primordial particles into the active secretory pathway (Williams et al., 2004). Therefore, the fatty acid composition of the diet determine the size and composition of mature chylomicrons. In addition, dietary fatty acids may regulate key proteins involved in chylomicron assembly, like MTP (Van Greevenbroek et al., 1998). These authors suggested that oleic acid-rich triglycerides may activate MTP to a greater extent than linoleic (18:2, n-6) or palmitic (16:0) acid-containing triglycerides.

Despite dietary fatty acid composition are relatively conserved in postprandial TRL, some authors have described significant differences in the absorption of certain fatty acids. Hunter et al. (2001) found that after the intake of an experimental meal enriched with oleic acid, there was an increase in the percentage of palmitic and linoleic acid in chylomicrons when compared with the fatty acid composition of the meal. It is well-known for years, that in animal models, infusion of palmitic acid stimulated output of VLDL and CM-sized lipoproteins, whereas linoleic acid led to the formation of larger CM-sized particles (Tso et al., 1984). In addition, we found significant differences between the composition of dietary oils and postprandial TRL when molecular species of triglycerides were studied (Abia et al., 2001). A subsequent publication provided evidence that meal fatty acids result in significant compositional differences in postprandial TRL of exogenous dietary origin, which could determine differences in their metabolism, as well as their interaction with other potentially atherogenic lipoproteins (Silva et al., 2003).

Fatty acids stimulate differently the secretion of triglycerides and apo B-48 from enterocytes, as observed in experiments carried out in the human epithelial colorectal adenocarcinoma cells (Caco-2) cell line. When unsaturated fatty acids are applied to polarized Caco-2 cells, all secreted lipoproteins have the size of chylomicrons or VLDL (d<1.006 g/mL Sf>400). However, when the cells are incubated with saturated fatty acids the size of most of the secreted lipoproteins is in the LDL/HDL range (1.009-1.068 g/mL) (Field et al., 1988). In addition, van Greevenbroek et al. (1996, 2000) proposed that triglyceride molecular species that are synthesized in these intestine cells after incubation with unsaturated fatty acids may be more efficiently incorporated into chylomicrons, whereas SFA would suppress *de novo* synthesis of triglycerides. Cartwright and Higgins (1999) found that the rates of triglycerides and apo B-48 synthesis by primary enterocytes from rabbits were higher after the animals received diets rich in sunflower oil, compared to a Western diet, with fish oil producing the lowest effect on lipoprotein secretion by these cells.

Diets enriched in unsaturated fatty acids promote the synthesis of large chylomicron from enterocytes in either model investigated. The mechanism underlying this effect is related to both a greater triglyceride synthesis and accumulation in the form of big intracellular triglyceride droplets but also a more efficient assembly of the lipoproteins by regulation of the function of the proteins involved. Van Greevenbroek et al. (2000) suggested that after the intake of a meal enriched in MUFA, larger chylomicrons are secreted from the enterocyte to the circulation. In contrast, when saturated fatty acids are absorbed, smaller particles, containing mainly saturated fatty acids, are secreted.

The effects of the consumption of different types of fat in the longer term on postprandial lipemia is currently being assessed. A number of studies have shown that n-3 PUFA also reduce postprandial hypertriglyceridemia, both when chronically present in the diet and when given as a supplement for periods from 4 weeks to 6 months, in normal and hyperlipidemic subjects (Harris and Muzio, 1993; Westphal et al., 2000; Kelley et al., 2007; Rein et al., 2009). Other types of fatty acids tend to have less marked effects on postprandial lipemia than n-3 PUFA, but, in general, diets containing or supplemented with MUFA and n-6 PUFA as compared to SFA (from plant oils) have been found to cause a reduced response (Lopez-Miranda et al., 2007; Lairon, 2008).

Once they form part of chylomicrons, the degree of saturation and chain length of fatty acids are also suggested to affect LPL activity (Martins et al., 1996). A more efficient contact with LPL lowers the residence time of chylomicrons in plasma and, thus, their atherogenicity. In the postprandial period, both chylomicrons and VLDL compete for a common lipolytic pathway (Björkegren et al., 1996) however, this competence is unbalanced: since LPL shows a preference for large chylomicrons, an accumulation of VLDL occurs (Cohn et al., 1988; Schneeman et al., 1993; Karpe et al., 1993; Björkegren et al., 1996). The size and fatty acid composition of the particles are determinant in such preference. It has been shown that chylomicrons enriched in n-6 PUFA were processed by LPL faster than chylomicrons enriched in SFA, MUFA or n-3 PUFA, which may contribute to their increased rate of removal from circulation (Botham et al., 1997). However, Sato et al. (1999) prepared TRL enriched in palmitic, oleic, linoleic or α-linolenic acids (18:3, n-3), formed from rats fed palm, olive, safflower and linseed oils, respectively. They found that the LPL specificity for TRL enriched in oleic acid was higher than that for linoleic acid, and was correlated to a reduction in lipoprotein fluidity, suggesting that this effect might enhance the affinity of the particles for the enzyme.

The fatty acid composition of TRL also influences their uptake and lipid accumulation in macrophages, leading to foam cell formation. Dietary SFA carried in chylomicron remnants may enhance their propensity to induce macrophage foam cell formation, providing a link between TRL composition and their atherogenicity. A work by Botham and colleagues has pointed out that the fatty acid composition of chylomicron remnant-like particles (CRLPs) markedly influences their induction of macrophage foam cell formation. In these studies, they reported that CRLPs enriched in SFA are taken up more rapidly and cause greater lipid accumulation in macrophages than those enriched in n-6 or n-3 PUFA (De Pascale et al., 2006). More recently, these authors showed that chylomicron remnants suppress he transcription factor nuclear factor-κB (NF-κB) activity in macrophages, which is implicated in the inflammation processes that take place during the development of atherosclerosis, and that this effect is modulated by their fatty acid composition (De Pascale et al., 2009).

Effects of Olive Oil and its Components on Postprandial Triglyceridemia

Several studies have demonstrated that the main fatty acid in human TRL isolated after the intake of olive oil is oleic acid, reflecting the presence of the most abundant fatty acid in the oil. However, it has been observed that the relative concentration of oleic acid is lower in TRL compared to the concentration in the original oil, in contrast to other minority fatty acids, such as palmitic or linoleic acid, whose percentages usually are increased in postprandial lipoproteins (Abia et al., 2001).

Oleic acid has been regarded as the most potent fatty acid when it comes to stimulating chylomicron assembly and secretion, which may be explained by a more efficient absorption due to a higher preference of intestinal pancreatic lipase for monounsaturated fatty acids (Yang et al., 1990). A number of studies have demonstrated that oleic acid is better absorbed than SFA (Thompson, 1980; Vallot et al., 1985; Roche et al., 1998). Bergstedt et al. (1990) observed a greater efficiency in absorption and transference to lymph of triolein compared to tristearin in rats fed emulsions of these triglycerides. We compared the fatty acid and triglyceride incorporation into human postprandial TRL after the intake of two high-oleic dietary oils, such as HOSO and olive oil. In spite of a virtually equal triglyceride contribution from the diet, the triglyceride content in TRL was significantly higher after the intake of HOSO (Figure 1).

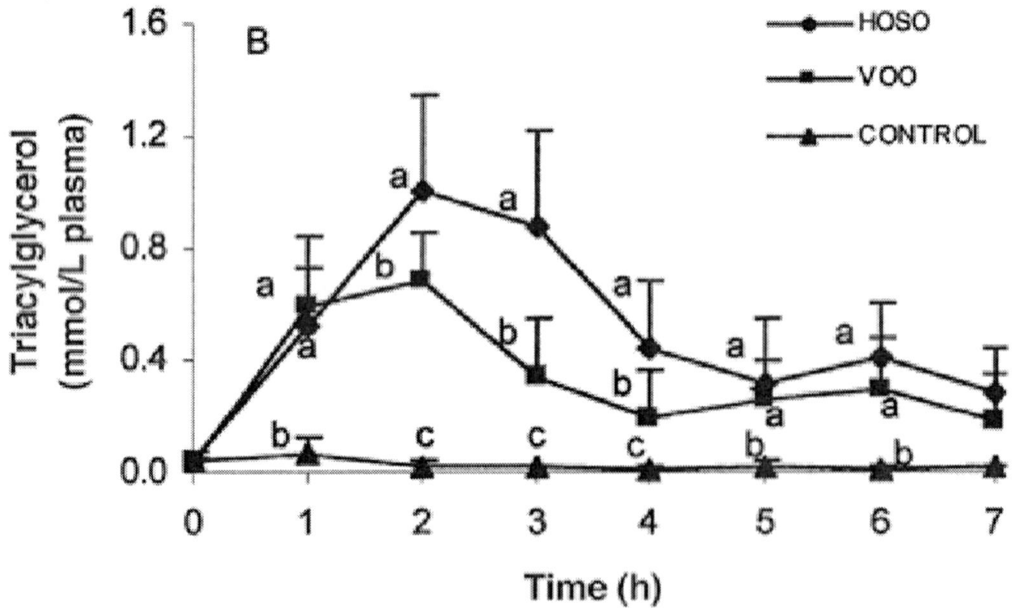

Figure 1. Mean (±SD) Triglyceride concentration during the postprandial period in the triglyceride-rich lipoprotein (TRL) fraction after virgin olive oil (VOO), high-oleic sunflower oil (HOSO) intake and control experiments. N=8. Different letters at same time point inidicate significant differences ($p<0.05$, ANOVA). Data from Abia et al. (2001).

This effect was not attributed to enhanced triglyceride absorption due to the presence of elevated amounts of oleic acid, because the concentration of this fatty acid in both oils was similar, but to the higher triolein content in HOSO (Abia et al., 2001). Actually, very slight differences were found when the fatty acid composition of TRL obtained after the intake of both high-oleic rich oils was studied. In contrast, relevant differences appear when triglyceride molecular species were analyzed: TRL formed after olive oil consumption showed a higher proportion of triglyceride species containing palmitic acid. In addition, the proportion of different triglyceride molecular species changed during the postprandial processes that lead to remnant formation and clearance, and values returned toward basal levels faster in TRL isolated after olive oil intake. Therefore, apart from the fatty acid composition of TRL, their distribution within the triglyceride molecule may be determinant when assessing the effects of dietary fat on the rates of secretion and clearance of postprandial lipoproteins.

Absorption of oleic acid-containing triglycerides is, therefore faster, leading to larger chylomicron particles. Compared with linoleic and palmitic acids, oleic acid treatment of Caco-2 cells induces a higher rate of triglyceride synthesis and secretion (Field et al., 1988). The capacity to support triglyceride secretion by addition of fatty acids was in the order oleic>linoleic>linolenic>palmitic=myristic. Later work showed that increasing the oleic acid/palmitic acid ratio caused an incremental increase in triglyceride output and increased proportion of large TRL at the expense of small denser particles. Jackson et al. (2002) examined the effect of the type of fat ingested on the density distribution of chylomicrons in the Svedberg flotation rate (Sf). Ingestion of olive oil resulted in a greater postprandial response in the Sf>400 fraction compared with palm or safflower oils, suggesting that olive oil ingestion causes the formation of a greater number of large particles. However, these authors also pointed out that the majority of particles secreted were in the Sf 60-400 fraction, rather than the Sf>400 fraction. This might explain the results of other researches who reported that ingestion of n-6 PUFA-rich dietary oils or olive oil by humans have showed comparable magnitudes of postprandial lipemia (Lichtenstein et al., 1993; Tholstrup et al., 2001; Mekki et al., 2002). In regard to SFA-rich fats or oils controversy remains: when butter was compared with olive oil the postprandial TG response was exacerbated (Thomsen et al., 1999) or considerably lower (Mekki et al., 2002). Such discrepancies have been attributed to the amount of fat, composition of test meals and the background diet of the subjects involved. Perez-Martinez et al., (2011) recently showed that consumption of an olive oil-rich meal leads to the formation of a reduced number of larger TRL particles compared with butter and walnut-based meals, after a chronic intake of diets containing the same meals. These authors suggested that chronic intake of olive oil may influence key steps involved in the formation or metabolism of TRL, like faster rates of digestion, absorption and secretion of large TRL and more efficient processing of these particles.

Olive oil has been shown to promote apo B-48 secretion by enterocytes postprandially (de Bruin et al., 1993; Higashi et al., 1997; Jackson et al., 2002), which supports the suggestion that olive oil causes a higher production of chylomicrons also in humans, perhaps through enhanced expression of apo B messenger RNA editing enzyme. However, the secretion of larger particles after oleic acid intake has also been related to a lower production of apo B-48. In this regard, Silva et al. (2003), reported that an increase in chronic MUFA intake led to a marked reduction (by 21–54%) in apo B-48 production following the test meal compared with an SFA-rich diet, leading to the formation of larger chylomicrons.

Nevertheless, despite the increase in the number of postprandial particles after MUFA intake, these particles are cleared more rapidly than those synthesized after the ingestion of SFA (Roche et al., 1998).

The lipid minor components contained in olive oil may also influence the composition of postprandial TRL. This conclusion was drawn from a study comparing the effects of two MUFA-rich oils that differ in their unsaponifable fraction content (Cabello-Moruno et al., 2007a,b), refined and pomace olive oils. The unsaponifiable fraction is comprised of all non-polar minor components of an edible oil, and thus is devoid of polar components like polyphenols. The TRL fraction isolated after the intake of test meals enriched with pomace olive oil, which is rich in unsaponifiable components, contained more triglyceride molecules than those obtained after the intake of refined olive oil. The presence of these minor components, also affected the apo B concentration in TRL. This implied a higher size of TRL particles when they were isolated after the intake of pomace olive oil, calculated as the ratio TG:apo B. Furthermore, the particle size changed rapidly during the postprandial period as a consequence of LPL activity, resulting in smaller particles after the intake of pomace olive oil. The unsaponifiable fraction was regarded as responsible for the lower apo B concentration in TRL fractions isolated after pomace olive oil intake compared with those obtained after refined olive oil consumption, showing a lower number of circulating TRL. Thus, the intake of this type of oil, rich in compounds from the unsaponifiable fraction, seemed to attenuate the postprandial apo B response. However, differences were only significant between particles were isolated 6 hours after the intake of both types of oil, which could also reflect changes in their rate of clearance.

Olive Oil and the First Events Ocurring on the Onset of Atherosclerosis

For a long time, it was suggested that the entry of lipoproteins into the arterial wall and the induction of atherogenesis was inversely related to the size of the particles, leading to the thought that TRL were not atherogenic (Stender and Zilversmit, 1981; Nordestgaard and; Ziversmit, 1988). However, subsequent studies demonstrated unequivocally that these particles are able to penetrate the artery wall and are retained within the intima (Mamo et al., 1998; Proctor et al., 2002). Proctor et al. (2002) also found that although, in terms of numbers of particles, many fewer of the larger chylomicron remnants than LDL are retained in the intima, the mass of cholesterol retained from the remnants is more than 2 fold greater. Since these authors established that the remnant particles enter the artery wall and are retained in the sub-endothelial space, it is clear that the lipids they carry have the opportunity to influence atherosclerosis development by interacting directly with cells in the tissue, including endothelial cells, smooth muscle cells and macrophages.

Endothelial Cells

Endothelial dysfunction is one of the first events occurring during the development of atherosclerosis. The endothelium is a single layer of cells lining large and small blood vessels that release a range of mediators in response to circulating or locally produced stimuli. When dysfunctional, the endothelium increases flow disturbances due to improper vasoreactivity and it initiates inflammatory responses by releasing pro-inflammatory cytokines and chemokines (Félétou and Vanhoutte, 2006). Circulating monocytes are attracted by these molecules and adhere to the endothelium, from which they transmigrate to the subendothelial space. Once within the endothelium, monocytes differentiate into macrophages, which scavenge oxidized LDL and chylomicron remnants, becoming engorged and acquiring the aspect of foam cells (Ross, 1999).

That a fatty meal induces endothelial dysfunction has been shown by most (Vogel et al., 2000; de Koning and Rabelink, 2002; Maggi et al., 2004) but not all (West, 2001; Sanderson et al., 2004) studies. Several studies have provided direct evidence for the actions of postprandial lipoproteins on endothelium (Botham, 2008) and in general they suggest detrimental effects. In fact, studies using TRL or remnant-like particles have shown reductions in acetylcholine-induced relaxation or increased contraction of vessels, decreased nitric oxide (NO) synthesis in cultured endothelial cells (Grieve et al., 1998; Goulter et al., 2003; Ohara et al., 2003). *In vitro* experiments have shown that chylomicrons can induce increased expression of E-selectin and vascular cell adhesion molecule-1 (VCAM- 1) (Moers et al., 1997) and artificial chylomicron remnant-like particles strongly induce cyclooxygenase-2 (COX-2) expression in endothelial cells (Botham et al., 2005). In addition, these artificial particles can enhance endothelial production of the vasoconstrictor molecule thromboxane A2 (TXA2) (Botham et al., 2005), suggesting that these particles may promote an imbalance in the production of vasodilator and vasoconstrictor mediators and hence impact on the pro-atherogenic properties of the endothelium. These studies indicate that both TRL can directly modify inflammatory processes in endothelial cells *in vitro*.

Endothelial activation and impairment of endothelium-dependent vasodilation have been observed with fat-rich meals, mostly rich in saturated fats, even in subjects without clinical or laboratory evidence of risk factors for coronary heart disease (Nappo et al., 2002). The addition of antioxidant supplements (Nappo et al., 2002) or vegetables to the meal (Esposito et al., 2003) has been shown to reverse the increase in circulating adhesion molecules, proinflammatory cytokines, such as interleukin-6 (IL-6) and tumor necrosis factor-alpha (TNF-♋), and endothelial dysfunction induced by a single high-fat (saturated) meal consumption. Thus, both monounsaturated fats, such as olive oil rich in phenolic acid content, and vegetables may help prevent endothelial activation and dysfunction in the postprandial state. In this regard, TRL isolated from healthy males after consumption of meals rich in oleic acid increased NO release from human venous endothelial cells (HUVEC) (Perona et al., 2004).

Pacheco et al., (2008) found that the postprandial levels of serum intercellular ashesion molecuel-1 (ICAM-1) and VCAM-1 increased as triglyceride did in both hypertriglyceridemic and healthy subjects. However, a meal rich in refined olive oil induced lower net area under the curve for ICAM-1 and VCAM-1 than a meal rich in high-palmitic sunflower oil meal. These authors concluded that the challenge of a meal with olive oil appears to have a significant postprandial benefit on serum ICAM-1 and VCAM-1 as surrogate markers of endothelial activation and vascular inflammation in healthy and hypertriglyceridemic subjects.

Investigation of the postprandial effect of olive oil on endothelial function from a previous study, showed that 50 gr of olive oil caused a significant decrease on flow-mediated dilation (FMD), which lasted for 3 hours post-consumption, possibly through induced hypertriglyceridemia and increased oxidative stress (Vogel et al., 2000). This phenomenon was reversed by addition of antioxidant vitamins (C and E) from balsamic vinegar and salad. In that study, it was shown that antioxidants in red wine and olive oil not only prevented the possible deterioration of FMD, but they induced an improvement of endothelial function (Karatzi et al., 2008).

According to Cortes et al. (2006), the intake of walnuts reversed the impairment of endothelial function associated with eating a fatty meal to a greater extent than olive oil, confirming previous results in hypercholesterolemic subjects that showed that a walnut meal in a background walnut diet was associated with improved brachial artery vasoactivity (Ros et al., 2004). However, Cortes et al., (2006) did not find differences in the postprandial concentrations of adhesion molecules (soluble E-selectin, sICAM-1, and sVCAM-1) between meals rich in olive oil or walnuts. These findings were consistent with the evidence of decreased expression of adhesion molecules by endothelial cells exposed to marine n-3 PUFA or oleic acid (De Caterina et al., 2000).

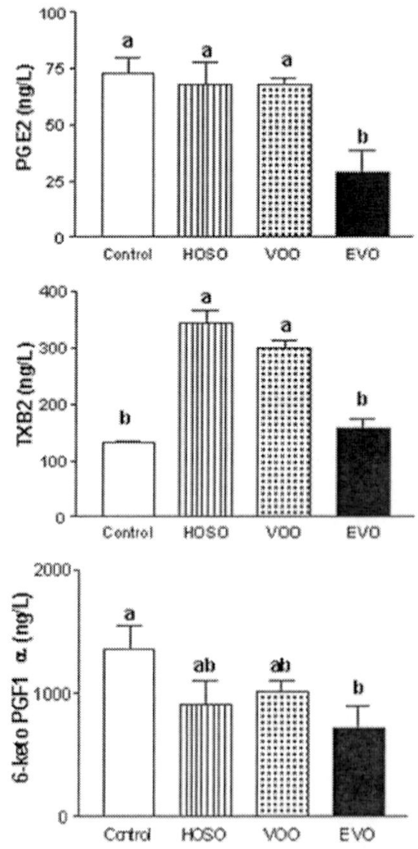

Figure 2. Effect of triglyceride-rich lipoprotein (TRL) on eicosanoid production. HUVEC were incubated (for 24 h) with TRL obtained 2 h after the ingestion of high-oleic sunflower oil (HOSO), virgin olive (VOO) or enriched-virgin olive (EVO) oils. Eicosanoid released to the medium were determined by EIAs. Results corresponding to PGE2, TXB2 and PGI2 (as 6-keto-PGF1α) are shown in panels A, B and C respectively. a: P<0.05, vs. control; b: P<0.05, vs. HOSO; c: P<0.05, vs. VOO. Data from Perona et al., (2004).

Minor components of olive oil have also shown some influence on the effect of postprandial lipoproteins on endothelial activation by improving the balance between vasoprotective and prothrombotic factors. Camargo et al., (2010) have recently shown that a virgin olive oil based breakfast is able to repress *in vivo* expression of several pro-inflammatory genes in a group of 20 patients suffering from metabolic syndrome, thereby switching activity of peripheral blood mononuclear cells to a less deleterious inflammatory profile. In our laboratory, we incubated endothelial cells with postprandial TRL derived from the intake by healthy subjects of meals containing virgin olive oil or virgin olive oil supplemented with its own unsaponifiable fraction. We found a reduction in the production of prostaglandin E2 (PGE2) and thromboxane B2 (TXB2) after the incubation with TRL obtained after the intake of the supplemented oil, with no effect on NO production, though (Perona et al., 2004) (Figure 2). However, we were unable to elucidate which minor components were responsible for the effects observed. We considered it very unlikely that phenolics were involved, because its concentration in VOO and EVO was very similar, and because due to their hydrophilic nature they are not transported in TRL. Therefore, we suggested that unsaponifiable components, like tocopherols, sterols or terpenoids might be responsible for the effects observed.

α-Tocopherol has shown an inhibitory effect on LDL- and cytokine-induced production and expression of adhesion molecules (Liu et al., 2003) and adhesion of monocytes to endothelial cells (Rodriguez-Rodriguez et al., 2004), although this effect does not seem to be mediated by NF-κB (Massaro and De Caterina, 2002). Vitamin E can also modulate eicosanoid metabolism in endothelial cells as it can restore reduced prostaglandin I2 (PGI2) synthesis (Moreno and Mitjavila, 2003) and inhibit 5-lipoxygenase (5-LOX) and COX-2 activities (Bayindir et al., 2002). Despite the increasing evidence of the hypocholesterolemic effect of phytosterols (Maclouf et al., 1998), very little is known about their effect on vascular function and dissenting results have been reported (Herrera et al., 2001; Benkhalti et al., 2003). The potential therapeutic importance of triterpenoids has not been extensively studied, but oleanolic acid can inhibit 5-LOX and COX-2 activities *in vitro* (de la Puerta et al., 1999; Bonanome et al., 2000), therefore reducing the production of PGE2 and leukotriene B4 (LTB4), as well as evoke an endothelium-dependent vasorelaxation in rat aorta.

Vacular Smooth Muscle Cells

The role of vascular smooth muscle cells (VSMC) in the stability of plaques in response to postprandial triglyceridemia is of key importance to understand the progression of atherosclerosis. During the development of atherosclerosis, phenotypically modified VSMC migrate from the media into the intima where they proliferate and secret growth factors, cytokines, and matrix metalloproteinases to contribute to atheroma formation (Ross, 1999 and Libby, 2002). Postprandial TRL have been shown to cause proliferation of VSMC, regardless of their oxidative state (Kawakami et al., 2001; Botham et al., 2005), which, together with foam cell formation, causes the appearance of fatty streaks, the first visible lesions in the vessel wall (Kadar and Glasz, 2001). Additionally, these lipoproteins have been suggested to participate in immune responses by inducing monocyte chemoattractant protein-1 (MCP-1) expression in VSMC (Domoto et al., 2003). Actually, these authors demonstrated that induction of MCP-1 expression in VSMC was much greater with chylomicron remnants than with oxidized-LDL. The exact mechanisms for the effects of postprandial TRL on VSMC proliferation have not been elucidated yet, but several signaling pathways seem to be involved (Kawakami and Yoshida, 2005).

Although the internalization of TRL in VSMC seems to be low, an effect of the origin of the fat transported has been observed. Pacheco et al., (2001) showed that in the presence of purified LPL, TRL from virgin olive oil were better taken up by VSMC than TRL from HOSO. It appeared that the VLDL receptor expression was the most important factor in VSMC for the cell processing of postprandial TRL, with no significant differences between TRL from virgin olive oil or HOSO.

Berhane et al., (2004) showed that expression of COX-2 and heme oxygenase-1 (HO-1) proteins are also induced by CRLPs containing n-6 PUFA, in contrast to CRLPs enriched in MUFA and SFA. There was also a clear trend for an increase in release of both PGI2 and TXA2 in response to n-6 PUFA particles, but only TXA2 in response to MUFA and SFA particles. These data demonstrate that the effects of artificial chylomicron remnants on VSMC are modulated by the fatty acid composition of the particles, with PUFA being more active than SFA.

More recently, Bermudez et al., (2008) prepared TRL from plasma of healthy volunteers after the ingestion of meals enriched in refined olive oil, butter or a mixture of vegetable and fish oils, which caused different transcriptional profiles in VSMC. The data revealed that TRL from butter and the plant and fish oil blend predominantly activated genes involved in the regulation of cell proliferation and inflammation, while TRL from refined olive oil promoted a less atherogenic gene profile.

Macrophages

It is known that monocyte-endothelial interaction plays a causative role in the early stage of atherosclerosis. Accumulation of lipid-laden macrophages and the proliferation of VSMC cause the appearance of fatty streaks, the first visible lesions in the vessel wall (Kadar and Glasz, 2001). It is well-known that LDL has a major role in macrophage foam cell formation, although modification of the particles either chemically or by oxidation, is compulsory before lipid accumulation is induced (Albertini et al., 2002). In contrast, postprandial TRL are able to induce macrophages to form foam cells without prior oxidation of the particles in several different experimental models, like the murine macrophage cell line J774 (Naplitano et al., 2001), mouse peritoneal macrophages (Fujioka et al., 1998), primary human monocyte derived macrophages (HMDM) (Yu and Mamo, 2000) and the human monocyte cell line THP-1 (Batt et al., 2004a).

The exact mechanisms mediating chylomicron uptake by macrophages still remain unclear. The LDL receptor (LDLr) was the main candidate but it is known to be saturable and down-regulated by the influx of cholesterol into cells, thus inhibiting further uptake of lipoprotein, and this is believed to be the reason why native-non modified LDL do not induce foam cell formation (Albertini et al., 2002). In addition, it has been shown that inhibition or down-regulation of the LDLr does not block chylomicron delivery to macrophages (Van Lenten et al., 1985; Fujioka et al., 1998; Batt et al., 2004b), indicating that chylomicron remnants can be taken up by other pathways. The other candidates are the LRP, which, like the LDL receptor, recognizes apoE and is expressed in macrophages; the apoB48 TRL receptor expressed in monocytes, macrophages and endothelial cells; and scavenger receptors, such as scavenger receptor A (SR-A) and CD36 (Yu and Cooper, 2001; Botham et al., 2005). Phagocytosis has also been suggested as a possible mechanism (Mamo et al., 1996). It is clear, therefore, that macrophages take up chylomicron remnants by multiple routes and this allows excessive amounts of lipid to accumulate in the cells.

Dietary lipids carried in postprandial TRL have the potential to induce and modulate macrophage foam cell formation, and the type of fat contained in the particles may modulate this effect. In experiments with CRLPs and THP-1 macrophages, we found that particles containing SFA cause increased accumulation of total lipid in the cells in comparison with those containing MUFA or PUFA, and that this is mainly due to raised triglyceride incorporation to the cell (De Pascale et al., 2006). Although CRLPs can be taken up by macrophages without the need of previous oxidation, the oxidative state of CRLPs influences their uptake (Moore et al., 2004). The MUFA-rich CRLPs, were less susceptible to oxidation that the other CRLP types, and this may partially explain their relatively rapid rate of uptake compared with PUFA-rich CRLPs (De Pascale et al., 2006). Another recent study demonstrated that the fatty acid content of chylomicrons can also affect NF-κB activity in macrophages, an thus inflammatory processes, but the effect of MUFA resulted to be lower than that of PUFA (De Pascale et al., 2009).

Despite a connection between TRL composition and lipid uptake by macrophages has been established, little is known about the influence of dietary fatty acids carried in these particles on macrophage receptors. We observed that incubation of two types of TRL obtained from olive oil intake but differing in their minor component composition, with THP-1 macrophages, led to a different mRNA expression of the scavenger receptors CD36, SR-A2 and SR-B1 (Cabello-Moruno et al., 2007). Minor lipid soluble antioxidants, that are transported in the blood in chylomicron remnants, have been shown to protect CRLP from oxidation, but surprisingly, they led to enhanced, rather than reduced, lipid accumulation in macrophages (Moore et al., 2003; 2004). The potential beneficial effects of dietary antioxidants, therefore, may be attenuated in conditions where blood chylomicron remnant levels are raised, and this may provide a part of the explanation for the failure to demonstrate anti-atherogenic effects of dietary antioxidants in large scale intervention studies (Clarke and Armitage, 2002).

CONCLUSION

The Mediterranean Diet, with olive oil as its characteristic fat source, is now widely considered the dietary pattern that best fulfills the need for nourishment, health and pleasure. The beneficial effects of olive oil on cardiovascular risk have been attributed to its high MUFA content, but new evidences are now suggesting that highly bioactive minor components have also an important role.

Chylomicrons, the natural carriers of dietary lipids are involved in promoting atherosclerosis in the postprandial state. During their transport to the liver, chylomicron remnant particles may enter the artery wall and are retained in the sub-endothelial space, where they have the opportunity to interact with cells involved in the formation of the atherosclerotic plaque: endothelial cells, VSMC and macrophages. The fatty acid composition of the diet determine the size and composition of chylomicrons, which could in turn determine differences in their metabolism. In general, diets containing or supplemented with MUFA and PUFA as compared to SFA have been found to cause a reduced response of postprandial triglyceridemia. Oleic acid has been regarded as the most potent fatty acid when it comes to stimulating chylomicron assembly and secretion, which may be explained by a more efficient absorption due to a higher preference of intestinal pancreatic lipase for monounsaturated fatty acids. However, the positional distribution of fatty acids within the triglyceride molecule are also relevant in both the process of chylomicron assembly and clearance. Probably due to its high oleic acid content, ingestion of olive oil results in a greater postprandial response in the Sf>400 fraction, leading to the formation of a greater number of large particles, which are more rapidly cleared.

The deleterious effect of postprandial particles in the first events of the development of atheroclerosis may be mitigated by olive oil components. The fatty acid composition, but more importantly, the presence of highly active minor components of olive oil in chylomicrons, may help to prevent endothelial dysfunction in the postprandial state by modulation of the secretion of endothelial reactive substances. This effect has been observed also in vascular smooth muscle cells. Another process occurring during atherogenesis is foam cell formation from macrophages. In *in vitro* experiments with chylomicron-like particles and THP-1 macrophages, MUFA-rich particles caused less triglyceride accumulation compared to SFA-rich particles and were less susceptible to oxidation that PUFA-rich particles. In addition, minor components influenced the gene expression of receptors involved in postprandial triglyceride-rich lipoprotein uptake.

Therefore, there is increasing evidence pointing towards the protective effects of olive oil components in the pathophysiology of atherosclerosis in the postprandial state. However, there is an urgent need of investigation of the mechanisms of these processes. In this regard, new tools are emerging and the new fields, like nutrigenomics, are rapidly being developed and applied to the olive oil and Mediterranean diet research. These new techniques will help to elucidate the pathways, today only envisaged, by which olive oil exerts its beneficial effect in the postprandial phase, but also to identify the components (major and minor) with a greater contribution. It is expected that when these components are fully revealed, new lines of "à la carte" olive oil-derived products, containing different concentrations of the desired proactive components, might be developed.

References

Abia, R; Pacheco, YM; Perona, JS; Montero, E; Muriana, FJ; Ruiz-Gutiérrez, V. The metabolic availability of dietary triacylglycerols from two high oleic oils during the postprandial period does not depend on the amount of oleic acid ingested by healthy men. *J Nutr.* 2001, 131(1), 59-65.

Albertini, R; Moratti, R; DeLuca, G. Oxidation of low-density lipoprotein in atherosclerosis from basic biochemistry to clinical studies. *Curr Mol Med* 2002, 2, 579-592.

Alipour, A; Elte, JWF; van Zaanen, HCT; Rietveld, AP; Castro Cabezas, M. Novel aspects of postprandial lipemia in relation to atherosclerosis. *Atheroscler Suppl,* 2008, 9, 39-44.

Bansal, S; Buring, JE; Rifai, N; et al. Fasting compared with nonfasting triglycerides and risk of cardiovascular events in women. *JAMA,* 2007, 298, 309-316.

Batt, KV; Avella, M; Moore, EH; Jackson, B; Suckling, KE; Botham, KM. Differential effects of low density lipoprotein and chylomicron remnants on lipid accumulation in human macrophages. *Exp Biol Med* 2004a; 229: 528-37.

Batt, KV; Patel, L; Botham, KM; Suckling, KE. Chylomicron remnants and oxidised low density lipoprotein have differential effects on the expression of mRNA for genes involved in human macrophage foam cell formation. *J Mol Med* (Berl) 2004b, 82(7), 449-458.

Bayindir, O; Ozmen, D; Mutaf, I; Turgan, N; Habif, S; Gulter, C; Parildar, Z; Uysal A. Comparison of the effects of dietary saturated, mono-, and n-6 polyunsaturated fatty acids on blood lipid profile, oxidant stress, prostanoid synthesis and aortic histology in rabbits. *Ann Nutr Metab* 2002, 46, 222– 228.

Benkhalti, F; Legssyer, A; Gomez, P; Paz, E; Lopez-Miranda, J; Perez- Jimenez, F ; el Boustani, ES. Effects of virgin olive oil phenolic compounds on LDL oxidation and vasorelaxation activity. *Therapie* 2003, 58, 133–137.

Benlian, P; De Gennes, JL; Foubert, L; Zhang, H; Gagné, SE; Hayden, M. Premature atherosclerosis in patients with familial chylomicronemia caused by mutations in the lipoprotein lipase gene. *N Engl J Med.,* 1996, 335(12), 848-854.

Bentley, C; Hathaway, N; DePascale, C; et al. Influence of dietary fats on human monocyte activation in vitro. *Atheroscler Suppl,* 2008, 9, 99-100.

Bergstedt, SE; Hayashi, H; Kritchevsky, D; Tso P. A comparison of absorption of glycerol tristearate and glycerol trioleate by rat small intestine. *Am J Physiol* 1990, 259, G386-G393.

Berhane, Y; Botham, KM; Elliott, J; Wheeler-Jones, CPD. Effect of chylomicron remnant-like particles (CRLP) of different fatty acid composition on endothelial and smooth muscle cell function. *Chem Phys Lipids* 2004, 130, 72.

Bermúdez, B; López, S; Pacheco, YM; Villar, J; Muriana, FJ; Hoheisel, JD; Bauer, A; Abia, R. Influence of postprandial triglyceride-rich lipoproteins on lipid-mediated gene expression in smooth muscle cells of the human coronary artery. *Cardiovasc Res* 2008, 79(2), 294-303.

Bester, D; Esterhuyse, AJ; Truter, EJ; van Rooyen, J. Cardiovascular effects of edible oils: a comparison between four popular edible oils. *Nutr Res Rev* 2010, 23(2), 334-348.

Bjorkegren, J; Packard, CJ; Hamsten, A; Bedford, D; Caslake, M; Foster, L; Shepherd, J; Stewart, P; Karpe, F. Accumulation of large very low density lipoprotein in plasma during intravenous infusion of a chylomicron-like triglyceride emulsion reflects competition for a common lipolytic pathway. *J Lipid Res* 1996, 37(1), 76-86.

Bonanome, A; Pagnan, A; Caruso, D; Toia, A; Xamin, A; Fedeli, E; Berra, B; Zamburlini, A; Ursini, F; Galli, G. Evidence of postprandial absorption of olive oil phenols in humans. *Nutr Metab Cardiovasc Dis* 2000, 10, 111–120.

Bosetti, C; Pelucchi, C; La Vecchia, C. Diet and cancer in Mediterranean countries: carbohydrates and fats. *Public Health Nutr* 2009, 12(9A):1595-1600.

Botham, KM. Oxidation of chylomicron remnants and vascular dysfunction. *Atheroscler Suppl* 2008,9, 57–61.

Botham, KM; Avella, M; Cantafora, A; Bravo, E. The lipolysis of chylomicrons derived from different dietary fats by lipoprotein lipase in vitro. *Biochim Biophys Acta* 1997, 1349(3), 257-263.

Botham, KM; Bravo, E; Elliott, J; Wheeler-Jones, CP. Direct interaction of dietary lipids carried in chylomicron remnants with cells of the artery wall: implications for atherosclerosis development. *Curr Pharm Des,* 2005, 11(28), 3681-3695.

Cabello-Moruno, R; Perona, JS; Osada, J; Garcia, M; Ruiz-Gutierrez, V. Modifications in postprandial triglyceride-rich lipoprotein composition and size after the intake of pomace olive oil. *J Am Coll Nutr* 2007b, 26(1), 24-31.

Cabello-Moruno, R; Perona, JS; Ruiz-Gutierrez, V. Influence of minor components of olive oils on the composition and size of TRLs and on macrophage receptors involved in foam cell formation. *Biochem Soc Trans* 2007a, 35, 470-471.

Camargo, A; Ruano, J; Fernandez, JM; Parnell, LD; Jimenez, A; Santos-Gonzalez, M; Marin, C; Perez-Martinez, P; Uceda, M; Lopez-Miranda, J; Perez-Jimenez, F. Gene expression changes in mononuclear cells in patients with metabolic syndrome after acute intake of phenol-rich virgin olive oil. *BMC Genomics* 2010, 11:253.

Cartwright, IJ; Higgins, JA. Increased dietary triacylglycerol markedly enhances the ability of isolated rabbit enterocytes to secrete chylomicrons: an effect related to dietary fatty acid composition. *J Lipid Res* 1999, 40, 1858-1866.

Clarke, R; Armitage, J. Antioxidant vitamins and risk of cardiovascular disease. Review of large scale randomised trials. *Cardiovasc Drugs Ther* 2002, 1, 411-415.

Cohn, JS; Marcoux, C; Davignon, J. Detection, quantification, and characterization of potentially atherogenic triglyceride-rich remnant lipoproteins. *Arterioscler Thromb Vasc Biol,* 1999, 19, 2474–2486.

Cohn, JS; McNamara, JR; Cohn, SD; Ordovás, JM; Schaefer EJ. Plasma apolipoprotein changes in the triglyceride-rich lipoprotein fraction of human subjects fed a fat-rich meal. *J Lipid Res* 1988, 29, 925-936

Cortés, B; Núñez, I; Cofán, M; Gilabert, R; Pérez-Heras, A; Casals, E; Deulofeu, R; Ros, E. Acute effects of high-fat meals enriched with walnuts or olive oil on postprandial endothelial function. *J Am Coll Cardiol* 2006, 48(8), 1666-1671.

Covas, MI. Olive oil and the cardiovascular system. *Pharmacol Res* 2007, 55(3), 175-186.

Covas, MI; Konstantinidou, V; Fitó M. Olive oil and cardiovascular health. *J Cardiovasc Pharmacol,* 2009, 54(6):477-482.

de Bruin, TW; Brouwer, CB; van Linde-Sibenius Trip, M; Jansen, H; Erkelens, DW. Different postprandial metabolism of olive oil and soybean oil: a possible mechanism of the high-density lipoprotein conserving effect of olive oil. *Am J Clin Nutr* 1993, 58(4), 477-483.

De Caterina, R; Liao, JK; Libby, P. Fatty acid modulation of endothelial activation. *Am J Clin Nutr* 2000, 71(1 Suppl), 213S-223S.

de Koning, EJP; Rabelink, TJ. Endothelial function in the postprandial state. *Atheroscler Suppl* 2002, 3, 11–16.

de la Puerta, R; Ruiz-Gutierrez, V; Hoult, JR. Inhibition of leukocyte 5-lipoxygenase by phenolics from virgin olive oil. *Biochem Pharmacol* 1999, 57, 445–449.

De Pascale, C; Avella, M; Perona, JS; Ruiz-Gutierrez, V; Wheeler-Jones, CP; Botham, KM. Fatty acid composition of chylomicron remnant-like particles influences their uptake and induction of lipid accumulation in macrophages. *FEBS J* 2006, 273(24), 5632-5640.

De Pascale, C; Graham, V; Fowkes, RC; Wheeler-Jones, CP; Botham, KM. Suppression of nuclear factor-kappaB activity in macrophages by chylomicron remnants: modulation by the fatty acid composition of the particles. *FEBS J* 2009, 276(19), 5689-5702.

Domoto, K; Taniguchi, T; Takaishi, H; Takahashi, T; Fujioka, Y; Takahashi, A;Ishikawa, Y; Yokoyama, M. Chylomicron remnants induce monocyte chemoattractant protein-1 expression via p38 MAPK activation in vascular smooth muscle cells. *Atherosclerosis* 2003, 171(2), 193-200.

Dubois, C; Beaumier, G; Juhel, C et al. Effects of graded amounts (0-50 g) of dietary fat on postprandial lipemia and lipoproteins in normolipidemic adults. *Am J Clin Nutr,* 1998, 67, 31-38.

Escrich, E; Moral, R; Grau, L; Costa, I; Solanas M. Molecular mechanisms of the effects of olive oil and other dietary lipids on cancer. *Mol Nutr Food Res* 2007, 51(10), 1279-1292.

Esposito, K; Nappo, F; Giugliano, F; Giugliano, G; Marfella, R; Giugliano, D. Effect of dietary antioxidants on postprandial endothelial dysfunction induced by a high-fat meal in healthy subjects. *Am J Clin Nutr* 2003, 77(1), 139-43.

Félétou, M; Vanhoutte, PM. Endothelial dysfunction: a multifaceted disorder (The Wiggers Award Lecture). *Am J Physiol Heart Circ Physiol* 2006, 291(3), H985-1002.

Field, FJ; Albright, E; Mathur SN. Regulation of triglyceride-rich lipoprotein secretion by fatty acids in CaCo-2 cells. *J Lipid Res,* 1988, 1427-1437.

Fielding, BA; Frayn, KN. Lipoprotein lipase and the disposition of dietary fatty acids. *Br J Nutr.,* 1998, 80(6), 495-502.

Fitó, M; de la Torre, R; Covas, MI. Olive oil and oxidative stress. *Mol Nutr Food Res* 2007, ;51(10), 1215-1224.

Fuentes, F; Lopez-Miranda, J; Perez-Martinez, P; Jimenez, Y; Marin, C; Gomez; et al. Chronic effects of a high-fat diet enriched with virgin olive oil and a low-fat diet enriched with alpha-linolenic acid on postprandial endothelial function in healthy men. *Br J Nutr,* 2008, 100, 159-165.

Fujioka, Y; Cooper, AD; Fong, LG. Multiple processes are involved in the uptake of chylomicron remnants by mouse peritoneal macrophages. *J Lipid Res* 1998, 39, 2339-2349.

Ginsberg, HN. New perspectives on atherogenesis: role of abnormal triglyceride-rich lipoprotein metabolism. *Circulation,* 2002, 106, 2137–2142.

Goldberg, IR; Kako, Y; Lutz EP. Responses to eating: lipoproteins, lipolytic products and atherosclerosis. *Curr Opin Lipidol,* 2000, 11, 235-241.

Goulter, AB; Avella, M; Botham, KM; Elliott, J. Chylomicron-remnant-like particles inhibit the basal nitric oxide pathway in porcine coronary artery and aortic endothelial cells. *Clin Sci* (Lond), 2003, 105, 363–371.

Grieve, DJ; Avella, MA; Elliott, J; Botham, KM. The influence of chylomicron remnants on endothelial cell function in the isolated perfused rat aorta. *Atherosclerosis* 1998, 139, 273–281.

Harris, WS; Muzio, F. Fish oil reduces postprandial triglyceride concentrations without accelerating lipid-emulsion removal rates. *Am J Clin Nutr* 1993, 58, 68-74.

Herrera, MD; Perez-Guerrero, C; Marhuenda, E; Ruiz-Gutierrez, V. Effects of dietary oleic-rich oils (virgin olive and high-oleic-acid sunflower) on vascular reactivity in Wistar-Kyoto and spontaneously hypertensive rats. *Br J Nutr* 2001, 86, 349 –357.

Higashi, K; Ishikawa, T; Shige, H; Tomiyasu, K; Yoshida, H; Ito, T; Nakajima, K; Yonemura, A; Sawada, S; Nakamura H. Olive oil increases the magnitude of postprandial chylomicron remnants compared to milk fat and safflower oil. *J Am Col Nutr* 1997, 16(5), 429-434.

Hu; FB. The Mediterranean Diet and mortality-olive oil and beyond. *N Engl J Med;* 2003; 348; 2595-2596.

Huang, CL; Sumpio, BE. Olive oil, the mediterranean diet, and cardiovascular health. *J Am Coll Surg* 2008, 207(3), 407-416.

Hunter, KA; Crosbie, LC; Horgan, GW; Miller, GJ; Dutta-Roy, AK. Effect of diets rich in oleic acid; stearic acid and linoleic acid on postprandial haemostatic factors in young healthy men. *Br J Nutr.,* 2001, 86(2), 207-215.

Hussain, MM. A proposed model for the assembly of chylomicrons. *Atherosclerosis,* 2000, 148, 1-15.

Hyson, D; Rutledge, JC; Berglund, L. Postprandial lipemia and cardiovascular disease. *Curr Atheroscler Rep,* 2003, 5, 437-444.

Jackson, KG; Robertson, MD; Fielding, BA; Frayn, KN; Williams, CM. Measurement of apolipoprotein B-48 in the Svedberg flotation rate (S(f))>400, S(f) 60-400 and S(f) 20-60 lipoprotein fractions reveals novel findings with respect to the effects of dietary fatty acids on triacylglycerol-rich lipoproteins in postmenopausal women. *Clin Sci* (London) 2002, 103(3), 227-237.

Kadar, A; Glasz, T. Development of atherosclerosis and plaque biology. *Cardiovasc Surg,* 2001, 9, 109-121.

Karatzi, K; Papamichael, C; Karatzis, E; Papaioannou, TG; Voidonikola, PT; Vamvakou, GD; Lekakis, J; Zampelas, A. Postprandial improvement of endothelial function by red wine and olive oil antioxidants: a synergistic effect of components of the Mediterranean diet. *J Am Coll Nutr* 2008, 27(4), 448-453.

Karpe, F. Postprandial lipoprotein metabolism and atherosclerosis. *J Int Med*, 1999, 246, 341-355.

Karpe, F; Steiner, G; Olivecrona, T; Carlson, A; Hamsten A. Metabolism of triglyceride-rich lipoproteins during alimentary lipemia. *J Clin Invest* 1993, 91, 748-758.

Kawakami, A; Tanaka, A; Nakano, T; Saniabadi, A; Numano, F. Stimulation of arterial smooth muscle cell proliferation by remnant lipoprotein particles isolated by immuno-affinity chromatography with anti-apo A-I and anti-apo B-100. *Horm Metab Res,* 2001, 33(2), 67-72.

Kawakami, A; Yoshida, M. Remnant lipoproteins and atherogenesis. *J Atheroscler Thromb* 2005, 12(2), 73-76.

Kelley, DS; Siegel, D; Vemuri, M; Mackey, BE. Docosahexaenoic acid supplementation improves fasting and postprandial lipid profiles in hypertriglyceridemic men. *Am J Clin Nutr 2007*, 86, 324- 333.

Kindel, T; Lee, DM; Tso, P. The mechanism of the formation and secretion of chylomicrons. *Atheroscler Suppl.* 2010, 11(1), 11-16.

Kuksis, A; Manganaro, F. Biochemical characterization and purification of intestinal acylglycerol acyltransferases. In: Kuksis A, editor. *Fat absorption.* Boca Raton: CRC Press; 1986; 233–259.

Lairon, D. Intervention studies on Mediterranean diet and cardiovascular risk. *Mol Nutr Food Res* 2007, 51(10), 1209-1214.

Lairon, D. Macronutrient uptake and modulation on chylomicron production and clearance. *Atheroscler Suppl,* 2008, 9, 45-48.

Libby, P. Inflammation in atherosclerosis. *Nature* 2002, 420, 868-874.

Lichtenstein, AH; Ausman, LM; Carrasco, W; Jenner, JL; Gualtieri, LJ; Goldin, BR; Ordovas, JM; Schaefer, EJ. Effects of canola; corn; and olive oils on fasting and postprandial plasma lipoproteins in humans as part of a National Cholesterol Education Program Step 2 diet. *Arterioscler Thromb Vasc Biol* 1993, 13(10), 1533-1542.

Liu, M; Wallmon, A; Olsson-Mortlock, C; Wallin, R; Saldeen, T. Mixed tocopherols inhibit platelet aggregation in humans: potential mechanisms. *Am J Clin Nutr* 2003, 77, 700 – 706.

Lopez-Miranda, J; Williams, C; Lairon, D. Dietary, physiological, genetic and pathological influences on postprandial lipid metabolism. *Br J Nutr* 2007, 98, 458-473 .

Maclouf, J; Folco, G; Patrono, C. Eicosanoids and isoeicosanoids: constitutive, inducible and transcellular biosynthesis in vascular disease. *Thromb. Haemost* 1998, 79, 691– 705.

Maggi, FM; Raselli, S; Grigore, L; Redaelli, L; Fantappie, S; Catapano, AL. Lipoprotein remnants and endothelial dysfunction in the postprandial phase. *J Clin Endocrinol Metab* 2004, 89, 2946–2950.

Mamo, JC. Atherosclerosis as a post-prandial disease. Endocrinol Metab, 1995, 2, 229-244.

Mamo, JC; Elsegood, CL; Gennat, HC; Yu K. Degradation of chylomicron remnants by macrophages occurs via phagocytosis. *Biochemistry* 1996, 35, 10210-10214.

Mamo, JC; Proctor, SD; Smith, D. Retention of chylomicron remnants by arterial tissue; importance of an efficient clearance mechanism. *Atherosclerosis* 1998, 141, S63-S69.

Martins, IJ; Mortimer, B-C; Miller, J; Redgrave, TG. Effects of particle size and number on the plasma clearance of chylomicrons and remnants. *J Lipid Res* 1996, 37, 2696-2705.

Massaro, M; De Caterina, R. (Vasculoprotective effects of oleic acid: epidemiological background and direct vascular antiatherogenic properties. *Nutr Metab Cardiovasc Dis* 2002, 12, 42–51.

Mekki, N; Charbonnier, M; Borel, P; Leonardi, J; Juhel, C; Portugal, H; Lairon, D. Butter differs from olive oil and sunflower oil in its effects on postprandial lipemia and triacylglycerol-rich lipoproteins after single mixed meals in healthy young men. *J Nutr* 2002, 132 (12), 3642-3649.

Moers, A; Fenselau, S; Schrezenmeir, J. Chylomicrons induce E-selectin and VCAM-1 expression in endothelial cells. *Exp Clin Endocrinol Diabetes* 1997, 105 Suppl 2, 35-37.

Moore, EH; Napolitano, M; Avella, M; Bejta, F; Suckling, KE; Bravo, E; Botham, KM. Protection of chylomicron remnants from oxidation by incorporation of probucol into the particles enhances their uptake by human macrophages and increases lipid accumulation in the cells. *Eur J Biochem* 2004, 271(12), 2417-2427.

Moore, EH; Napolitano, M; Prosperi, A; Avella, M; Suckling, KE; Bravo, E; Botham, KM. Incorporation of lycopene into chylomicron remnant-like particles enhances their induction of lipid accumulation in macrophages. *Biochem Biophys Res Commun* 2003; 312: 1216-1219.

Moreno, JJ; Mitjavila, MT. The degree of unsaturation of dietary fatty acids and the development of atherosclerosis. *J Nutr Biochem* 2003, 14, 182–195.

Napolitano, M; Avella, M; Botham, KM; Bravo, E. Chylomicron remnant induction of lipid accumulation in J774 macrophages is associated with up-regulation of triacylglycerol synthesis which is not dependent on oxidation of the particles. *Biochim Biophys Acta*, 2003, 1631, 255–264.

Napolitano, M; Rivabene, R; Avella, M; Botham, KM; Bravo, E. The internal redox balance of the cells influences the metabolism of lipids of dietary origin by J774 macrophages: implications for foam cell formation. *J Vasc Res* 2001, 38, 350-360.

Nappo, F; Esposito, K; Cioffi, M; Giugliano, G; Molinari, AM; Paolisso, G; Marfella, R; Giugliano, D. Postprandial endothelial activation in healthy subjects and in type 2 diabetic patients: role of fat and carbohydrate meals. *J Am Coll Cardiol* 2002, 39(7), 1145-1150.

Nguyen, P; Leray, V; Diez, M et al. Liver Lipid Metabolism. *J Anim Physiol Anim Nutr* (Berl), 2008, 92, 272-283.

Nordestgaard, BG; Benn, M; Schnohr, P; Tybjaerg-Hansen, A. Non fasting triglycerides and risk of myocardial infarction; ischemic heart disease; and death in men and women. *JAMA,* 2007, 298, 299-308.

Nordestgaard, BG; Ziversmit, DB. Large lipoproteins are excluded from the arterial wall in diabetic cholesterol-fed rabbits. *J Lipid Res* 1988, 29, 1491-1500.

O'Keefe, JH; Bell, DSH. Postprandial hyperglycemia/hyperlipidemia (postprandial dysmetabolism) is a cardiovascular risk factor. *Am J Cardiol,* 2007, 100, 899-904.

Ohara, N; Takeichi, S; Naito, Y et al. Remnant-like particles from subjects who died of coronary artery disease suppress NO synthase activity and attenuate endothelium-dependent vasorelaxation. *Clin Chim Acta* 2003, 338, 151–156.

Pacheco, YM; Abia, R; Perona, JS; Reina, M; Ruiz-Gutiérrez, V; Montero, E; Muriana, FJ. Triacylglycerol-rich lipoproteins interact with human vascular cells in a lipid-dependent fashion. *J Agric Food Chem* 2001, 49(11), 5653-5661.

Pacheco, YM; López, S; Bermúdez, B; Abia, R; Villar, J; Muriana, FJ. A meal rich in oleic acid beneficially modulates postprandial sICAM-1 and sVCAM-1 innormotensive and hypertensive hypertriglyceridemic subjects. *J Nutr Biochem* 2008, 19(3), 200-205.

Panagiotakos, D; Pitsavos, C; Chrysohoou, C; Palliou, K; Lentzas, I; Skoumas, I, et al. Dietary patterns and 5-year incidence of cardiovascular disease: a multivariate analysis of the ATTICA study. *Nutr Metab Cardiovasc Dis* 2008.

Patsch, JR; Miesenböck, G; Hopferwieser, T; Mühlberger, V; Knapp, E; Dunn, JK; Gotto, AM Jr; Patsch, W. Relation of triglyceride metabolism and coronary artery disease. Studies in the postprandial state. *Arterioscler Thromb.,* 1992, 12(11), 1336-1345.

Perez-Jimenez, F; Alvarez de Cienfuegos, G; Badimon, L; Barja, G; Battino, M; Blanco, A, et al. International conference on the healthy effect of virgin olive oil. *Eur J Clin Invest,* 2005, 35, 421-424.

Pérez-Jiménez, F; Ruano, J; Perez-Martinez, P; Lopez-Segura, F; Lopez-Miranda, J. The influence of olive oil on human health: not a question of fat alone. *Mol Nutr Food Res* 2007, 51(10), 1199-1208.

Pérez-López, FR; Chedraui, P; Haya, J; Cuadros, JL. Effects of the Mediterranean diet on longevity and age-related morbid conditions. *Maturitas* 2009, 64(2):67-79.

Perez-Martinez, P; Lopez-Miranda, JL; Perez-Jiminez, F; Ordovas, JM. Influence of genetic factors in the modulation of postprandial lipemia. *Atheroscler Suppl,* 2008, 9, 49-55.

Perez-Martinez, P; Ordovas, JM; Garcia-Rios, A; Delgado-Lista, J; Delgado-Casado, N; Cruz-Teno, C; Camargo, A; Yubero-Serrano, EM; Rodriguez, F; Perez-Jimenez, F; Lopez-Miranda, J. Consumption of diets with different type of fat influences triacylglycerols-rich lipoproteins particle number and size during the postprandial state. *Nutr Metab Cardiovasc Dis* 201, 21(1), 39-45.

Perona, JS; Cabello-Moruno, R; Ruiz-Gutierrez, V. The role of virgin olive oil components in the modulation of endothelial function. *J Nutr Biochem* 2006, 17(7), 429-445.

Perona, JS; Martinez-Gonzalez, J; Sanchez-Dominguez, JM; Badimon, L; Ruiz-Gutierrez, V. The unsaponifiable fraction of virgin olive oil in chylomicrons from men improves the balance between vasoprotective and prothrombotic factors released by endothelial cells. *J Nutr* 2004, 134, 3284-3289.

Proctor, SD; Vine, DF; Mamo, JC. Arterial retention of apolipoprotein B(48)- and B(100)-containing lipoproteins in atherogenesis. *Curr Opin Lipidol* 2002, 13(5), 461-470.

Psaltopoulou, T; Naska, A; Orfanos, P; Trichopoulos, D; Mountokalakis, T; Trichopoulou, A. Olive oil; the Mediterranean Diet; and arterial blood pressure: the Greek European Prospective Investigation into Cancer and Nutrition (EPIC) study. *Am J Clin Nutr* 2004, 80, 1012-1018.

Raederstorff, D. Antioxidant activity of olive polyphenols in humans: a review. *Int J Vitam Nutr Res* 2009, 79(3), 152-165.

Redgrave, TG. Formation and metabolism of chylomicrons. *Int Rev Physiol* 1983, 28, 103-130.

Rein, P; Saely, CH; Aczel, S; Patsch, B; Drexel, H. Omega-3 fatty acids significantly reduce postprandial triglyceridemia in male smokers: a pilot study. *Nutr Metab Cardiovasc Dis* 2009, 19, e3-4.

Roche, HM; Zampelas, A; Knapper, JM; Webb, D; Brooks, C; Jackson, KG; Wright, JW; Gould, BJ; Kafatos, A; Gibney, MJ; Williams CM. Effect of long-term olive oil dietary intervention on postprandial triacylglycerol and factor VII metabolism. *Am J Clin Nutr* 1998, 68(3), 552-560.

Roche, HM; Zampelas, A; Knapper, JM; Webb, D; Brooks, C; Jackson, KG; Wright, JW; Gould, BJ; Kafatos, A; Gibney, MJ; Williams, CM. Effect of long-term olive oil dietary intervention on postprandial triacylglycerol and factor VII metabolism. *Am J Clin Nutr* 1998, 68(3); 552-560.

Rodriguez-Rodriguez, R; Herrera, MD; Perona, JS; Ruiz-Gutierrez, V. Potential vasorelaxant effects of oleanolic acid and erythrodiol, two triterpenoids contained in "orujo" olive oil, on rat aorta. *Br J Nutr* 2004, 92, 635– 642.

Ros, E; Núñez, I; Pérez-Heras, A; Serra, M; Gilabert, R; Casals, E; Deulofeu, R. A walnut diet improves endothelial function in hypercholesterolemic subjects: a randomized crossover trial. *Circulation* 2004, 109(13), 1609-1614.

Ross R. Atherosclerosis--an inflammatory disease. N Engl J Med, 1999, 340(2), 115-126.

Sanderson, P; Olthof, M; Grimble, RF. Dietary lipids and vascular function: UK Food Standards Agency workshop report. *Br J Nutr*, 2004, 91, 491–500.

Sato, K; Takahashi, T; Takahashi, Y; Shiono, H; Katoh, N; Akiba, Y. Preparation of chylomicrons and VLDL with monoacid-rich triacylglycerol and characterization of kinetic parameters in lipoprotein lipase-mediated hydrolysis in chickens. *J Nutr* 1999, 129(1), 126-131.

Schneeman, BO; Kotite, L; Todd, KM; Havel RJ. Relationship between the responses of triglyceride-rich lipoproteins in blood plasma containing apolipoproteins B-48 and b-100 to a fat-containing meal normolipidemic humans. *Proc Nat Acad Sci US.* 1993,90, 2069-2073.

Sharrett, AR; Heiss, G; Chambless LE, et al. Metabolic and lifestyle determinants of postprandial lipemia differ from those of fasting triglycerides. *Arterioscler Thromb Vasc Biol,* 2001, 21, 275-281.

Silva, KD; Kelly, CN; Jones, AE; Smith, RD; Wootton, SA; Miller, GJ; Williams, CM. Chylomicron particle size and number, factor VII activation and dietary monounsaturated fatty acids. *Atherosclerosis* 2003, 166, 73–84.

Silva, KD; Kelly, CN; Jones, AE; Smith, RD; Wootton, SA; Miller, GJ; Williams, CM. Chylomicron particle size and number; factor VII activation and dietary monounsaturated fatty acids. *Atherosclerosis,* 2003, 166(1), 73-84.

Silva, KDRR; Jones, AE; Smith, RD; Kelly, CNM; Lovegrove, JA; Wootton, SA and Williams, CM. Different postprandial responses of larger and smaller chylomicrons and remnant particles. *Proc Nutr Soc,* 2001, 60, 44A.

Sofi, F; Cesari, F; Abbate, R; Gensini, GF; Casini, A. Adherence to Mediterranean Diet and health status: meta-analysis. *BMJ,* 2008, 337, a1344.

Stender, S; Zilversmit, DB. Transfer of plasma lipoprotein components and of plasma proteins into aortas of cholesterol-fed rabbits: molecular size as a determinant of plasma lipoprotein influx. *Arteriosclerosis* 1981, 1, 38-49.

Storch, J; Thumser, AE. The fatty acid transport function of fatty acid-binding proteins. *Biochim Biophys Acta,* 2000, 1486, 28-44.

Tholstrup, T; Sandstrom, B; Bysted, A; Holmer, G. Effect of 6 dietary fatty acids on the postprandial lipid profile; plasma fatty acids; lipoprotein lipase; and cholesterol ester transfer activities in healthy young men. *Am J Clin Nutr* 2001, 73(2), 198-208.

Thomsen, C; Rasmussen, O; Lousen, T; Holst, JJ; Fenselau, S; Schrezenmeir, J; Hermansen, K. Differential effects of saturated and monounsaturated fatty acids on postprandial lipemia and incretin responses in healthy subjects. *Am J Clin Nutr* 1999, 69(6), 1135-1143.

Thomson, ABR. Influence of site and unstirred layers on the rate of uptake of cholesterol and fatty acids into rabbit intestine. *J Lipid Res* 1980, 21, 1097-1107.

Trichopoulou, A; Bamia, C; Trichopoulos, D. Mediterranean Diet and survival among patients with coronary heart disease in Greece. *Arch Intern Med,* 2005a, 165, 929-935.

Trichopoulou, A; Costacou, T; Bamia, C; Trichopoulos, D. Adherence to a Mediterranean Diet and survival in a Greek population. *N Engl J Med,* 2003, 348, 2599-2608.

Trichopoulou, A; Orfanos, P; Norat, T; Bueno-de-Mesquita, B; Ocke, MC; Peeters, PH; et al. Modified Mediterranean Diet and survival: EPIC-elderly prospective cohort study. *BMJ,* 2005b, 330, 991.

Tso, P; Drake, DS; Black, DD; Sabesin, SM. Evidence for separate pathways of chylomicron and very low-density lipoprotein assembly and transport by rat small intestine. *Am J Physiol,* 1984, 247, G599-G610.

Vallot, A; Bernard, A, Carlier H. Influence of the diet on the portal and lymph transport of decanoic acid in rats Simultaneous study of its mucosal catabolism. *Comp Biochem Physiol* 1985, 82, 693-699.

van Greevenbroek, MM; Erkelens, DW; de Bruin, TW. Caco-2 cells secrete two independent classes of lipoproteins with distinct density: effect of the ratio of unsaturated to saturated fatty acid. *Atherosclerosis*, 149, 25-31.

Van Greevenbroek, MM; Robertus-Teunissen, MG; Erkelens, DW; de Bruin, TW. Participation of the microsomal triglyceride transfer protein in lipoprotein assembly in

Caco-2 cells: interaction with saturated and unsaturated dietary fatty acids. *J Lipid Res,* 1998, 39, 173-185.

van Greevenbroek, MM; van Meer, G; Erkelens, DW; de Bruin TW. Effects of saturated; mono-; and polyunsaturated fatty acids on the secretion of apo B containing lipoproteins by Caco-2 cells. *Atherosclerosis,* 1996, 121(1), 139-150.

Van Lenten, BJ; Fogelman, AM; Jackson, RL; Shapiro, S; Haberland, ME; Edwards, PA. Receptor-mediated uptake of remnant lipoproteins by cholesterol-loaded human monocyte macrophages. *J Biol Chem* 1985, 260, 8783-8788.

Vogel, RA; Corretti, MC; Plotnick, GD. The postprandial effect of components of the Mediterranean diet on endothelial function. *J Am Coll Cardiol* 2000, 36, 1455–1460.

Waterman, E; Lockwood, B. Active components and clinical applications of olive oil. *Altern Med Rev* 2007, 12(4), 331-342.

West, SG. Effect of diet on vascular reactivity: an emerging marker for vascular risk. *Curr Atheroscler Rep* 2001, 3, 446–455.

Westphal, S; Orth, M; Ambrosch, A; Osmundsen, K; Luley, C. Post- prandial chylomicrons and VLDLs in severe hypertriacylglycerolemia are lowered more effectively than are chylomicron remnants after treatment with n-3 fatty acids. *Am J Clin Nutr* 2000, 71, 914-920.

Wilhelm, MG; Cooper, AD. Induction of atherosclerosis by human chylomicron remnants: a hypothesis. *J Atheroscler Thromb,* 2003, 10, 132-139.

Williams, CM; Bateman, PA; Jackson, KG and Yaqoob, P. Dietary fatty acids and chylomicron synthesis and secretion. *Biochem Soc Trans* 2004,32,55-58.

Williams, CM; Moore, F; Morgan, L; Wright, J. Effects of n-3 fatty acids on postprandial triglyceride and hormone concentrations in normal subjects. *Br J Nutr* 1992, 68, 655-666.

Yang, LY; Kuksis, A; Myher JJ. Lipolysis of menhaden oil triacylglycerols and the corresponding fatty acid alkyl esters by pancreatic lipase in vitro: a reexamination. *J Lipid Res* 1990, 31(1),137-147.

Yu, KC; Cooper, AD. Postprandial lipoproteins and atherosclerosis. *Front Biosci,* 2001, 6, D332-D354.

Yu, KC; Mamo, JCL. Chylomicron remnant-induced foam cell formation and cytotoxicity: a possible mechanism for cell death in atherosclerosis. *Clin Sci* 2000, 98, 183-192.

Zilversmit, DB. Atherogenesis: A postprandial phenomenon. *Circulation,* 1979, 60, 473-485.

In: Olive Consumption and Health
Editors: C. A. Savalas and S. M. Nicolau

ISBN: 978-1-62100-774-6

Chapter 5

MATRIX-ASSISTED LASER DESORPTION/IONIZATION TIME-OF-FLIGHT (MALDI–TOF) MASS SPECTROMETRY FINGERPRINTING AS A NEW TOOL FOR QUALITY CONTROL AND HEALTH RISK ASSESSMENT OF VIRGIN OLIVE OIL

Cosima Damiana Calvano,[1,*] Cristina De Ceglie,[1] Antonio Monopoli[1] and Carlo Giorgio Zambonin[1,2]

[1]Dipartimento di Chimica, Università degli Studi di Bari Aldo Moro, Bari, Italy
[2]Centro Interdipartimentale di Ricerca S.M.A.R.T.,
Università degli Studi di Bari Aldo Moro, Bari, Italy

ABSTRACT

Over the past thirty years the knowledge of the nutritional properties of olive oil has deeply improved and olive oil is presently considered as a basic element of the "Mediterranean diet". Olive oil contains important nutrients, such as essential and monounsaturated fatty acids in addition to other particular compounds useful in a healthy diet. The quality of olive oil depends on several aspects such oxidation stability, absence of contaminants (pesticides, solvents or adulterants), nutritional values expressed as the amount of saturated fatty acids, monounsaturated and polyunsaturated fats, presence of phytosterols, vitamins and natural antioxidants. For these reasons, olive oil is one of the most expensive and is often object of frauds involving replacement of high-cost ingredients with lower grade and cheaper substitutes. For example, adulteration of virgin olive oil with different seed oils, such as hazelnut and almond oils, represents a serious problem for regulatory agencies, oil suppliers, and consumers. Moreover, in addition to economic implications, adulteration is a serious health problem related to the possible presence of carcinogenic mycotoxins. Further, many seeds, such as hazelnut (Corylus avellana L.) and peanuts, are among the major food allergens in the dried fruit shell. The

* Corresponding author: Cosima Damiana Calvano, Phone number : +39-080-5443589, Fax number: +39-080-5442026. E-mail: calvano@chimica.uniba.it.

presence of protein residues of hazelnut oil used for adulteration can trigger allergic reactions in the respiratory tract such as oral allergy syndrome (OAS), rhinoconjunctivitis or, in severe cases, anaphylactic shock. Adulterated olive oil becomes a source of hidden allergens very dangerous to the health of consumers. Another potential health hazard can be represented from the exposure of consumers to oxidized oils since the oxidation mechanism occurring during processing and storage can have effects on palatability, nutritional quality, and toxicity. This chapter resumes the use of an analytical technique based on a new type of ion source, Matrix-Assisted Laser Desorption /Ionization (MALDI) coupled to a time-of-flight mass spectrometer (TOF-MS) analyzer for the comprehensive assessment of olive oil quality in terms of absence of contaminants, adulterants and oxidation processes. The main advantages of MALDI-TOF-MS in comparison to other analytical methods consist of a fast and easy sample preparation and no need for analyte derivatization.

1. Introduction

Food safety is defined from European Union and World Health Organization (WHO) as a responsibility to be shared *from farm to fork.* This fact implies the existence of a control over the whole food processing chain; the raw used materials should be wholesome and all the operations of processing, transport, preparation, preservation and consumption must be correctly managed step by step.

The quality control and assurance should be organized and executed by competent authorities; when the process goes out of control and sanitary emergencies occur, the population should be readily alerted and a plan of action ordered.

Specific institutions are involved in consumer protection for the prevention of the adulteration of beverages and foodstuffs. In Italy, for example, the most important offices are the Central Inspectorate for the control of food quality (ICQ), coastguard, forest warden, Customs Agencies and the Ministry for Agricultural and Forestry Policies, for Health and for Social Policies.

Food adulterations are alterations intentionally introduced in food to realize unlawful earnings and they can be applied in different points of the food chain at level of process, documentation or product. As far as concern adulterations at product level they are classified in adulterations, sofistications, falsifications, forgeries, alterations, denaturations and dangerous imitations [1].

Adulteration includes all the actions aimed at modifying the analytical composition of food such as the addition or the removal of some components in food to obtain a larger profit without significantly changing the product resulting in commercial and sanitary consequences. Examples of common adulterations are dilution of wine, use of casein or powdered milk in cheese production, addition of water in meat or fish to increase their weight, selling of skimmed milk and semi-skimmed milk instead of full-cream milk.

One of the most common mistake is the abuse of the term *adulteration* to indicate a generic food fraud; for example, differently to adulteration, the sofistication consists in the addition of extraneous substances into the food in order to improve the appearance of the product, to mask defects or to facilitate the partial changing of a food with another one. Sofistication diverges from adulteration since at least one of the added substances is unrelated to the real composition of the product. Examples of sofistication are the methanol addition into the wine to increase the alcoholic degree or the addition of antioxidants in oils for retarding growing rancidity.

According to the European Union Regulation EC 1531/2001 an olive oil labeled as *virgin olive oil* is obtained from olive fruits only by mechanical pressing or other physical means (washing, settling, centrifugation, filtration) under conditions that do not alter its characteristic properties responsible for nutritional and health benefits and pleasant flavor. An exception is made for the oils obtained by solvent extraction, chemical/biochemical action, addition of esters or by mixture with different source of oils. As it is well known, the virgin olive oils are then classified according to the free acidity (expressed as oleic acid) as *extra-virgin olive oils* (free acidity ≤ 0.8%), *virgin olive oil* (free acidity ≤ 2%) and *lamp olive oil* (free acidity > 2%). A *refined olive oil* is an oil obtained by the refining of virgin olive oil with a free acidity minor than 0.3%. *Olive oils* are mixtures of refined olive oils and virgin olive oils with a free acidity ≤ 1%. *Crude pomace olive oil* is obtained from pomace by solvents or physical means and *refined pomace olive oil* is obtained by the refining of crude pomace olive oil with a free acidity ≤ 0.3%. *Pomace olive oil* is the combination of refined pomace olive oil and virgin olive oil with a free acidity ≤ 1%.

However, the content of free fatty acids cannot be considered, of course, as the only parameter for quality classification. In fact, the principal factors determining the food quality are nutritional values, food safety, sensory and technological values [2].

In particular, the quality of olive oil depends on several aspects such as oxidation stability, absence of contaminants (pesticides, solvents or adulterants), nutritional values expressed as saturated, monounsaturated and polyunsaturated fatty acids content, presence of phytosterols, vitamins and natural antioxidants.

Due to the presence of important nutrients, such as essential and monounsaturated fatty acids, olive oil appears to be an example of a functional food, with a components variety that may contribute to its overall therapeutic characteristics [3,4]. In this perspective, it is easy to understand why olive oil has gained a large development on the market. Usually, olive oil is sold as virgin (VOO) or extra-virgin type (EVOO), which corresponds to the purest and most expensive on sale. The different price between EVOO and other vegetable oils implies that large amounts of money are involved and can be gained adding cheaper components such as seed oils to the more expensive olive oil.

As an example, in Italy, common fraudulent activities are the *falsification* as the selling of olive oils or lamp olive oils of foreign origin (Spanish or Tunisian) as Italian oils or the *adulteration* of Italian olive oils by foreign oils cheaper because of minor beneficial effects or minor labor force costs. Other frequent adulterations in this field are the addition to the olive oil of pomace-olive oils or esterified oils, of chlorophill as coloring agent, of cheaper seed oils (maize, soy, palm, sunflower) and of moldy or discarded hazelnut oil (at low percentages).

The evaluation of olive oil quality is carried out by an organoleptic test that considers the olive oil on the basis of olfactory, visual and taste properties and by chemical-physical analyses that estimate fat content and acidity. Organoleptic test is based on *Panel test*. In this analysis a group of selected people tastes various types of oil and expresses a sensory opinion. At the end of the test each oil, receives a score corresponding to a specific merceologic category (CEE 2568/91). An olive oil that is considered extra-virgin on the basis of chemical parameters, must be also acceptable from an organoleptic point of view.

The analyses generally performed on olive oil samples belong to the following three categories:

1) analyses relevant to olive oil quality as for example evaluation of acidity, peroxides, fatty acids, sterols and halogenated solvents content, UV and gas chromatographic analyses;
2) analyses of the olive oil storability as peroxide number, UV, acidity, panel test, induction time;
3) analyses of the olive oil authenticity as fatty acids, sterols, waxes and stigmastadiens content, UV, halogenated solvents residues, TAGs analyses.

The main analytical parameters to be determined are free acidity (free fatty acids amount), peroxide number, tocopherols and polyphenols content, sterols content, glycerides fatty acids, UV parameters [5]. The determination of free fatty acids is not an absolute index of quality oil since the saponifiable fraction composition of olive oils depends on the geographical origin and often it is unlikely to detect adulteration by hazelnut oil, rapeseed oil and sunflower oil. On the other hand, the composition of the sterols in the unsaponifiable fraction is related to the vegetable species and it is less affected by geographical origin, and then can be liable for adulteration detection [5].

As said before, another parameter of olive oil quality is the stability to oxidation processes. Due to the high content in unsaturated fatty acids vegetable oils are susceptible of autooxidation; this process leads to the formation of undesired compounds that affect oil aromatic profile and influence the oil nutritional properties. Also olive oil can undergo oxidation in spite of the presence of antioxidants molecules and the low amount of polyunsaturated fats [6, 7]. Another problem relevant to food safety is the presence of extraneous substances [8]. These contaminants can derive from the industrial processing operations; they include pesticides and solvents that represent a risk for human health.

Thus, there is an increasing need of analytical methods able to allow a simple, fast and cost effective quality control of oils in order to detect trace amounts of residues, contaminants, allergens, trans-fatty acids and other undesired components such as oil decomposition products in rancid oils. The following chapter resumes the use of a new type of ion source, Matrix-Assisted Laser Desorption/Ionization (MALDI) coupled to a time-of-flight mass spectrometer (TOF-MS) analyzer for the comprehensive assessment of olive oil quality in terms of absence of adulterants, sofistications, allergenic compounds and oxidation by-products.

2. From Traditional Techniques to MALDI Mass Spectrometry

Vegetable oils contain almost every class of lipid compounds, therefore, lipid analysis involves the characterization of triacylglycerols (TAGs), sterols, squalene, carotenoids and phospholipids (PLs). With such a naturally occurring complexity, complete characterization of lipid mixtures in oils must still involve the combination of several analytical approaches. Analytical methods allow the qualitative and quantitative determination of the main components of food products but can also be selective and sensitive enough to permit the detection of minor components, often very important for the assessment of quality and detection of adulteration. Several reviews have outlined the multiple-step approach necessary for complete structural characterization of lipids in particular of TAGs and PLs [9-12]. TAGs have been separated using different chromatographic techniques such as gas chromatography (GC), supercritical fluid chromatography (SFC), thin layer chromatography (TLC)[13], and high performance liquid chromatography (HPLC) [14] with a reverse phase or silver ion HPLC [12], often coupled with UV detection. The prevalent problem in this latter case was linked to the poor reproducibility of the detection system. In fact, in these compounds the substituted fatty acids can strongly vary from completely saturated to highly unsaturated, leading a high difference in polarity, hydrophobicity and absorption properties. The use of UV spectroscopy leads to considerable differences in the detectability of PLs and TAGs containing fatty acids with different degree of saturation and different UV absorbance. Moreover, these methods are quite tedious and time-consuming [15]. For these reasons, mass spectrometry (MS) coupled to either gas or liquid chromatography, with its characteristic high sensitivity and specificity, is becoming increasingly popular for determining these compounds. In particular, the use of LC-MS separation techniques became more useful than GC because it was possible to analyze TAGs and PLs in their intact form. By MS it is possible to identify, with high mass resolution and remarkable sensitivity, overlapped or non-resolved TAGs and PLs in chromatographic peaks, making this method the most effective for their qualitative detection. In addition, another advantage of mass spectrometric methods, regarding lipid analysis, is the minimal need for sample preparation and the short time of analysis, allowing large numbers of samples to be daily analyzed [16]. Therefore, as reviewed by Careri et al. [17], most investigators have preferred MS techniques as the methods of choice for the analysis of intact lipid species from different fat and oil systems.

Briefly, a mass spectrometer consists of an ion source, in which the sample molecules are ionized, a mass analyzer, which separates the ions according to their mass-to charge-ratios, before they are registered by a detector. In addition, a computer system can be connected to the mass spectrometer for the computing of mass spectra from the output data. There are several ionization techniques; among them, the conventional techniques as electron impact (EI) [18,19] and chemical ionization (CI) [20] are limited in the study of lipids field because of their intense fragmentation and low mass range detection. In the last decades, new ionization techniques like field desorption (FD), field ionization (FI), plasma desorption (PD), fast atom bombardment (FAB) and laser desorption were introduced. These techniques were applied extensively in lipid analysis, even if most of them give rise to unwanted fragmentation. In the '80s two new "soft-ionization" techniques emerged: electrospray ionization (ESI) [21,22] and matrix assisted laser desorption ionization (MALDI) [23,24], becoming the favorite ionization techniques for biological samples. In fact, in these ionization processes large molecules can be analyzed without major degradation, enabling the molecular ion detection. Moreover, large mass ranges can be investigated up to hundred kDa.

3. MALDI MASS SPECTROMETRY

Although ESI-MS is strongly used in lipid field, the interest is now increasing toward the use of MALDI technique because of some advantages respect to the other one.

The concept for UV MALDI was developed between 1984 and 1986 and summarized in 1987 by Karas and Hillenkamp [25]. At the same time, an alternative approach was studied by Tanaka in 1987 and published in 1988. Both of them started from the principle of the already known laser desorption ionization (LDI) technique where the molecules were ionized by direct irradiation with lasers [26]. The idea developed from Karas was the introduction of a specific matrix consisting of a small organic compound exhibiting a strong resonance absorption at the laser wavelength used. The matrix was simply mixed with the sample in a large excess and the resultant solution was deposited on a microtiter plate and allowed to crystallize. The matrix introduction limited the fragmentation for large non-volatile biomolecules making possible to desorb protein molecules of several hundred kDa as intact ions, largely increasing the mass range upper limit of LDI; then MALDI became the preferred ionization technique for their analysis [23,25,27]. The mechanism behind the ionization process in MALDI is still unknown, likely because a single mechanism cannot describe all ions generated in one single experiment. In general, the matrix molecules are believed to aid in the ionization process in several ways; in particular, the matrix was described to have three main functions. First, a controllable energy transfer to the condensed-phase matrix-analyte mixture induces a *"uniform and soft desorption"*: the matrix molecules absorb laser light at a wavelength different from the analyte molecules. As a consequence of the energy absorption, they excite, and the successive thermal relaxation of these, results in the decomposition of the matrix molecules in addition to the transfer of analyte molecules into the gas phase (sublimation). Since the latter do not absorb the laser light directly, fragmentation is minimized. Secondly, a promotion of ionization by chemical reactions: the matrix molecules functions as a proton donor (in positive ion mode) and a proton acceptor (in negative ion mode). Thirdly, it generates "favorable prerequisites" by isolating analyte molecules in the excess matrix: the matrix molecules are added in large molecular excess (100-1000 fold molar excess), which separates the analyte molecules from each other and prevents analyte cluster formation. Several different matrices are used in MALDI MS and there are also numerous different sample preparation techniques. Looking at the reported applications in literature, it is evident that this technique has been applied mainly to peptides and proteins analysis [28-30]; however, in the past few years it became a method of choice for analyzing any kind of non-volatile labile compound. Some of the obvious advantages using MALDI MS are the rapid sample preparation and analysis. The sample-matrix mixture is applied directly on the sample probe tip, enabling the simultaneous investigation of numerous samples. It is a very sensitive method and requires a low amount of sample, ranging from pico-moles to atto-moles. MALDI MS has also a high tolerance towards salts. The technique is suited for analysis of heterogeneous and semi-complex samples that are analyzed as solid samples because of the crystallization process after solvent evaporation. It is potentially possible to couple this ionization technique with any type of mass analyzer; however, due to the pulsed generation of ions, the MALDI technique lent itself to a combination with time-of-flight (TOF) mass analyzers, which until then only played a little role. A schematic description of the process is given in the figure 1.

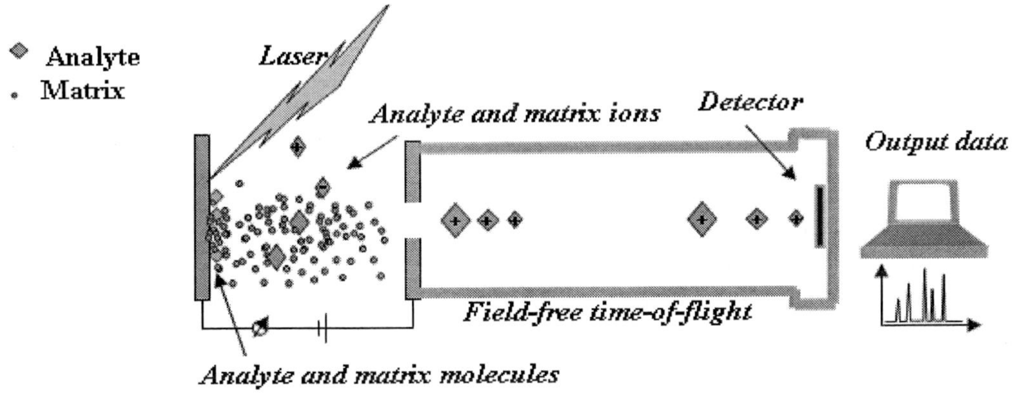

Figure 1. Scheme of the basic processes occurring during MALDI-TOF analysis.

In summary, a laser beam, typically originated by a nitrogen UV-laser, with a wavelength at 337 nm, hits the spot being absorbed from the matrix. Due to the laser energy, a part of the matrix is vaporized and carries the analyte into the gaseous phase. In this process a "plume" or expanding gas [23] cloud is formed with molecules that leave the target at velocities of about 500 m/s.

The sample ions formed in the ion source are extracted and accelerated in an electric field with voltages of about 20 kV. After passing the charged grid, the ions fly into the TOF mass analyzer, consisting of a 'drift tube' typically 0.5-3 m long. The velocity reached by an ion is constant in the field free space and it is inversely proportional to the square root of its m/z ratio. Since the distance from the source to the detector is fixed, the time taken to traverse the analyzer is directly proportional to the square root of its m/z ratio. Thus, each m/z value has its characteristic time–of–flight from the source to the detector.

The capability to produce separate signals from ions of similar mass measures the mass resolution of a spectrometer [23]. As result, the length of the field-free path influences the mass resolution, since the separation of ions is achieved over this distance. The traditional tube of TOF mass analyzers was characterized by a linear configuration, with a length around 0.7 m. The resolution obtained was poor, therefore, an improvement was reached using longer flight tubes called also "electrostatic mirror", where ions are reflected (reflectron mode) at the end of the flight tube and reach another detector at the opposite direction [31]. MALDI-TOF mass spectra of "small" molecules, like lipids, should be recorded in the reflectron mode since this approach enhances the achievable resolution significantly in comparison to the linear mode.

4. MALDI-TOF-MS Analysis of Lipid Classes in Edible Oils

As can be inferred by the previous paragraph, both sample preparation and spectra acquisition in MALDI-TOF-MS experiments are very fast. In fact, one sample can be analyzed in less than one minute, often with no need of sample pre-treatment. Moreover, the configuration of the microtiter plates for MALDI-TOF targets allow the simultaneous (even often automated) analysis of many samples [31].

The low number of applications that MALDI-TOF MS has experienced in the field of lipid analysis is then quite surprising, if one considers that lipids and matrices are both readily soluble in organic solvents and all manipulations can be performed in a single organic phase, in contrast with more polar molecules that require solvent mixtures. This aspect is very important because implies a co-crystallization of the analyte and the matrix, allowing a good sample preparation reproducibility. Lipid amounts in the range of a few nanograms are sufficient for MS analysis.

One disadvantage of MALDI is that the use of matrix gives rise to interfering peaks in the spectra below 1000 Da, which can suppress the signals of compounds in the low-molecular-weight range. These interferences vary among different matrices. Moreover, sometimes it is proved a lack of shot-to-shot and sample-to-sample reproducibility as a result of lack of homogeneity in the matrix-sample crystals. The choice of the matrix is crucial for the success of a MALDI experiment. In general, derivatives of benzoic acid, cinnamic acid, and related aromatic compounds have been recognized as good MALDI matrices for proteins, peptides and lipids [32], while 3-hydroxypicolinic acid (3-HPA) [33,34] and succinic acid [35] are used as matrices in the UV and in the infrared, respectively, for the analysis of oligonucleotides. New matrices have been proposed for lipid analysis as lumazine [36], 9-aminoacridine [37], proton sponge [38,39] and ionic liquids [40,41]. Unfortunately, all analytical problems are different, and this implies that specific guidelines for an ideal matrix selection do not exist; thus, a choice can be made only after the screening of a large number of candidate compounds [42,34]. MALDI is generally characterized by little fragmentation, caused essentially by the extraction field, because ions are pulled through the neutral plume and suffer collisions. The matrix choice is important for the control of fragmentation. Matrices are classified as "hot" or "cold", depending on the degree of fragmentation they cause to the sample. Matrices like 2,5 dihydroxybenzoic (DHB), that does not induce much fragmentation, are considered to be "cold", whereas matrices like α-Cyano-4-hydroxycinnamic acid are essentially "hot".

The analysis of food products may be directed to the assessment of food quality and authenticity, the control of technological processes, the determination of nutritional value and the detection of molecules with a possible beneficial effect on human health. Since lipids are among the major components of vegetable oils, accurate and precise analysis is important for determining constituting components and nutritive value, preparing nutritional material, promoting and understanding the effects of fats and oils on food functionality. Moreover, a deep knowledge of the structural characteristics of lipids may help the development of new products designed for particular functions or applications.

5. Olive Oil Adulteration by Seed Oils

Very recently, MALDI-TOF MS has been increasingly applied [43-52] to the determination of TAGs in oils, offering some advantages in comparison to other analytical methods, e.g. fast and easy sample preparation and no need for analyte derivatization. However, to overcome intrinsic problems in MALDI measurements as interferences of matrix peaks in the low-mass region, and lack of shot-to-shot and sample-to-sample reproducibility, an interesting approach has been demonstrate to be the complete avoidance of the matrix

[53,54]. This approach could further simplify the sample preparation step, completely eliminate the presence of matrix peaks in the spectra, and, in principle, improve reproducibility due to the absence of the crystallization step.

Table 1. Main ions observable in the spectra of figure 2A

m/z	Relative Abundance (%)	Attribution
575.47	32	$[PL]^+$
577.55	25	$[PO]^+$
599.51	52	$[LL]^+$
601.50	56	$[OL]^+$
603.56	46	$[OO]^+$
615.55	9	$[dg(PL)+Na]^{+\,**}$
617.54	17	$[dg(PO)+Na]^{+\,**}$
639.50	9	$[dg(LL)+Na]^{+\,**}$
641.55	16	$[dg(OL)+Na]^{+\,**}$
643.54	41	$[dg(OO)+Na]^{+\,**}$
659.54	18	$[dg(OO)+K]^{+\,**}$
661.54	100	$[LaLaLa+Na]^+$
677.51	74	$[LaLaLa+K]^+$
855.78	10	$[POP+Na]^+$,$[PPO+Na]^+$
871.18	5	$[POP+K]^+$,$[PPO+K]^+$
877.78	3	$[PLL+Na]^+$, $[POLn+Na]^+$
879.77	16	$[PLO+Na]^+$,$[POL+Na]^+$,$[OPL+Na]^+$
881.79	53	$[POO+Na]^+$,$[OPO+Na]^+$
883.78	18	$[POS+Na]^+$,$[SPO+Na]^+$, $[PSO+Na]^+$
893.78	6	$[PLL+K]^+$, $[POLn+K]^+$
895.74	8.7	$[PLO+K]^+$,$[POL+K]^+$,$[OPL+K]^+$
897.75	20	$[POO+K]^+$,$[OPO+K]^+$
899.74	7	$[POS+K]^+$,$[SPO+K]^+$, $[PSO+K]^+$
901.78	38	$[LLL+Na]^+$, $[OLLn+Na]^+$, $[OLnL+Na]^+$, $[LOLn+Na]^+$
903.79	52	$[OLL+Na]^+$, $[LOL+Na]^+$, $[OOLn+Na]^+$, $[OLnO+Na]^+$
905.78	23	$[OLO+Na]^+$,$[OOL+Na]^+$
907.77	73	$[OOO+Na]^+$,$[SOL+Na]^+$
909.78	19	$[SOO+Na]^+$
917.75	9	$[LLL+K]^+$,$[OLLn+K]^+$, $[OLnL+K]^+$, $[LOLn+K]^+$
919.76	14	$[OLL+K]^+$, $[LOL+K]^+$, $[OOLn+K]^+$, $[OLnO+K]^+$
921.74	12	$[OLO+K]^+$,$[OOL+K]^+$
923.73	28	$[OOO+K]^+$,$[SOL+K]^+$,$[SLO+K]^+$,$[LSO+K]^+$
925.75	13	$[SOO+K]^+$

Legend: P=palmitic acid; O=oleic acid; S=stearic acid; L=linoleic acid; La=lauric acid; Ln=linolenic acid **dg = diacylglycerol.

(MA)LDI-TOF-MS has been employed for the analysis of TAGs in different oils [53]. Figure 2 shows, for instance, the LDI-TOF mass spectrum relevant to the analysis of a commercial extra-virgin olive oil sample (A) and a sunflower seed oil (B). Table 1. reports the main ions observable in the spectra of figure 2A, their relative abundance and attribution.

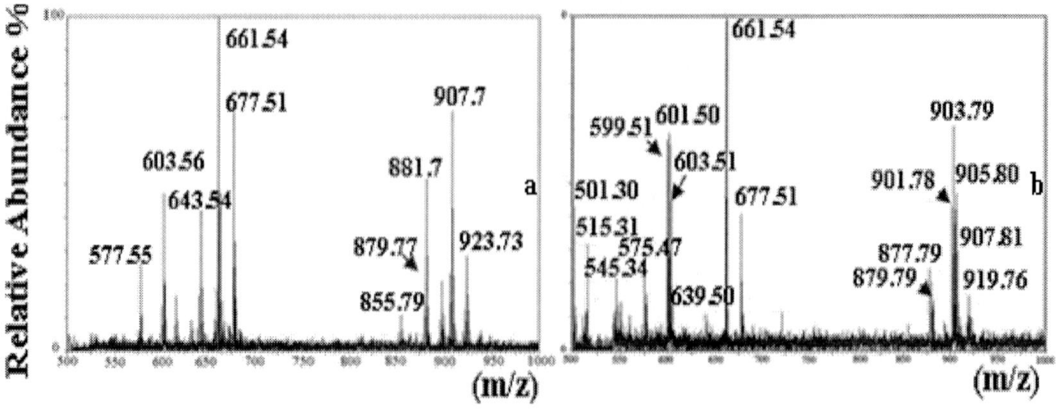

Figure 2. LDI-TOF mass spectrum relevant to the analysis of a commercial extra-virgin olive oil sample. (a) and a commercial sunflower oil sample (b) dissolved in an acetonitrile:tetrahydrofuran (75:25, v:v) mixture.

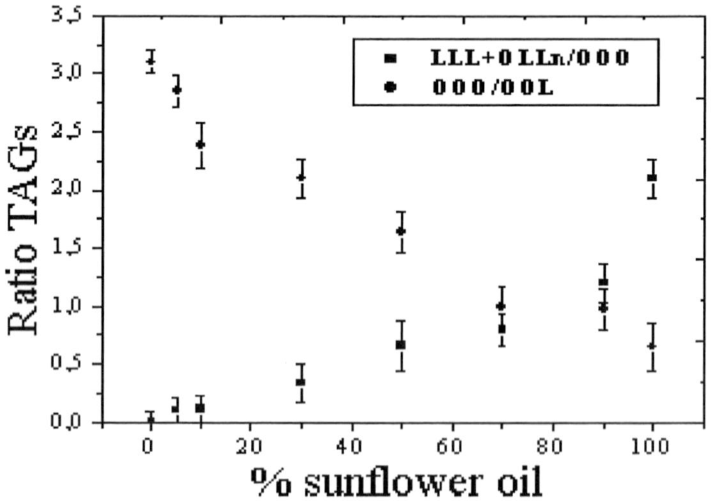

Figure 3. Plot of the OOO/OOL and LLL+OLLn/OOO ratios versus the percentage composition of sunflower/extra-virgin olive oils mixture.

As can be seen, the spectra revealed the presence of Na^+ and K^+ adducts of major TAGs and their fragments, in both oils and of the internal standard trilaurin at m/z 661.54. In the low-mass range peaks attributable to the fragmentation of the most abundant TAGs, corresponding to losses of a sodiated or potassiated fatty acid molecule, are clearly distinguishable at the m/z values 577.55, 601.54, and 603.56 in olive oil and at m/z 575.47, 599.51 and 601.50 in sunflower oil. Obviously, no interfering peaks arising from the matrix were observed.

A careful inspection of the mass spectra revealed that different oils produced different spectra. For instance, the most intense triacylglycerols observed in the spectrum of sunflower oil are the ions at m/z 903.79 (OLL) and 901.78 (LLL/OLLn), while the TAGs most abundant in olive oils are observed at m/z 907.77 (OOO) and m/z 881.77 (POO) as expected from the free fatty acids content. These evidences bring to the observation that the present method could be potentially used to obtain a rapid, fast and simple TAGs fingerprint that could allow an easy recognition of the analyzed oil and/or of an olive oil adulteration. In order to demonstrate these potentialities, an extra-virgin olive oil sample was progressively adulterated with increasing quantities of sunflower oil, and subjected to LDI-MS analysis. Then, diagnostic ions for sunflower (903.79 and 901.78) and olive (907.77) oils were selected, and the intensity ratios of OOO/OOL and LLL+OLLn/OOO were calculated for each spectrum and used as markers for the adulteration. Figure 3 reports the plot of the OOO/OOL and LLL+OLLn/OOO ratios versus the percentage composition of sunflower /extra-virgin olive oils mixture.

As apparent, the value of the ratio OOO/OOL decreases with the percentage increase of sunflower oil, while the value of the ratio LLL+OLLn/OOO increases with the percentage increase of sunflower oil, clearly showing that the present approach can be used for the proposed aim.

Regarding the potential healthy problems, olive and canola are nonallergenic, corn and coconut are rarely allergenic, sunflower, sesame, and cottonseed belong to the group of foods that are less commonly allergenic while peanuts, soybeans, and tree nuts belong to the group of allergenic foods [55]. If peanut or soybean oils are used in olive oil adulteration they could be a source of hidden allergens and a concern for human health because of the allergenicity of residual proteins. Soybean contains different allergens such as the seed storage proteins glycinin and beta-conglycinin, Kunitz trypsin inhibitor, and Gly m Bd 30K, a thiol protease [56].

Soy is a food involved in food allergy and causes severe reactions in allergic individuals, even anaphylaxis. It seems that fully refined soybean oils are safe for allergic consumers; Taylor et al.[57] show that hot pressed, bleached and deodorized soybean oil is not allergenic even if Errahali et al [58] have shown that both cold pressed and fully refined soybean oils contain allergens and they have found in soy oil two allergenic proteins (56 and 20 kDa) minor proteins in soybean.

However, proteins are minor compounds of oils, they are solubilized during oil extraction and their content depends on the oil processing. Therefore the procedure of oil extraction influences the number and the typology of proteins detectable in oils.

Peanuts, belonging to the same family of soybean (legumes), are considered one of the most allergenic food. Main allergens are vicilin Ara h1 (63.5 kDa), conglutin Ara h2 (17 kDa), glycinin Ara h3 (57 kDa) and Ara h4 that is an isoallergen of Ara h3, followed by the minor allergens Ara h5 (profilin, 15 kDa), Ara h6 (15 kDa) and Ara h7 (15 kDa) [55].

6. Olive Oil Adulteration by Hazelnut Oils

Hazelnut oil (HO) is obtained from Corylus avellana L.seeds. Hazelnut kernels have an high lipid content (60%), a good amount of proteins (16%) and of carbohydrates (14%). More than 90% of the fat content is constituted by oleic and linoleic acids that are the most abundant fatty acids also in olive oil. The crude fat content of hazelnut oil samples (Table 2) accounted for up to 56% of the dried weight of seed. Besides oleic (72.8-83.5%) and linoleic (7.6-16.6%) acids HO also contains low quantities of palmitic (4.1-6.8%), stearic (1.9-2.8%) and linolenic acids (0.1-0.6%).

Table 2. Fatty acids composition of hazelnut and olive oil

Fatty acids content of olive oil		Fatty acids content of hazelnut oil	
Oleic acid (C18:1)	60-85%	Oleic acid (C18:1)	72.8- 83.5%
Linoleic acid (C18:2)	5-15%	Linoleic acid (C18:2)	7.6-16.6%
Linolenic acid (C18:3)	traces	Linolenic acid (C18:3)	0.1-0.6%
Stearic acid (C18:0)	1.5-3%	Stearic acid (C18:0)	1.9-2.8%
Palmitic acid (C16:0)	9-15%	Palmitic acid (C16:0)	4.1-6.8%

Table 3. Chemical composition of olive oil

Unsaponifiable matter 2%	• hydrocarbons (squalene) • alcohols • polyphenols • tocopherols • sterols • pigment, enzyme, vitamins	30-50% 19-34% 18-37% 2-3%
Saponifiable matter 98%	• triacylglycerols • partial glicerides (mono- e diglicerides) • free fatty acids	

Table 4. Chemical composition of hazelnut oil

Unsaponifiable matter	• alcohols • tocopherols • sterols • hydrocarbons (squalene)	
Saponifiable matter	Non polar lipids: triacylglycerols Polar lipids: • glycolipids • phospholipids (PC,PE,PI)	98.4% 1.4% 0.2%

The top world producer of hazelnuts is Turkey followed by Italy, Spain and USA. Hazelnut oil is consumed raw (generally obtained from roasted hazelnut) or refined. The chemical composition of HO depends on geographical origin, on variety of hazelnut tree and on oil extraction process. The major components are triacylglycerols and fatty acids; the minor ones are waxes, sterols, methyl sterols, aliphatic and terpenic alcohols, tocopherols, tocotrienols and hydrocarbons. Hazelnut oil is often used in adulteration of extra virgin olive oil because of their similar chemical composition with respect to both major and minor compounds (Tables 3 and 4).

This high level of similarity makes very difficult the detection of low percentages of hazelnut oil in extra virgin olive oil, especially below 20%. This adulteration causes a big economical loss and has also sanitary consequences due to the possible presence of carcinogenic mycotoxins or traces of hazelnut allergenic proteins in the olive oil. Tree nuts (almond, walnut, hazelnut) are among the most common allergenic foods together with soybean and peanuts. Hazelnut allergens are proteins with molecular masses ranging from 10 to 60 kDa. The main allergen is known as Cor a1 (17kDa); other potential allergens are Cor a2 (14 kDa), Cor a8 (12 kDa), a lipid transfer protein (LTP), Cor a9 (known as globulin 11S) and Cor a11 (known as globulin 7S) [59,60]. More recently, two oleosin isoforms, Cor a12 and Cor a13, have been identified as new allergens in hazelnut. Olive oil adulterated by hazelnut oil becomes a probable source of *hidden allergens* and this is a serious risk for hazelnut allergic consumers; the presence of traces of hazelnut proteins in the oil used for the adulteration can provoke severe responses in sensitive patients such as the oral allergy syndrome (OAS), rhinoconjunctivitis and anaphylactic reactions [60].

Hazelnut oil can be considered a *protein free* food but the presence of residual proteins depends on the method of manufacture and processing of hazelnut oil used in adulteration of extra virgin olive oil. Crude hazelnut oils have a fair protein amount and their presence in olive oil can provoke allergic reactions in sensitive individuals; refined hazelnut oils should have a lower protein content and it should be a safe product for consumers while partially refined oils, containing residual hazelnut proteins, are a great risk to the human health. Arlorio et al. [59] compare the protein content of extra virgin olive oil adulterated by raw cold-pressed hazelnut oil and by solvent-extracted hazelnut oil demonstrating the presence of hazelnut proteins in solvent extracted hazelnut oil.

Many scientific papers argue about the allergenicity of refined seed oils and their real protein content [61]. Some studies report cases of allergic reactions to oils which are presumed to be refined; probably the cause relies in processing procedures of the oils.

A few methods are available for the detection of residual hazelnut proteins in adulterated olive oils. On this point an important study [62] concerns the use of a biosensor immunoassay for traces of hazelnut proteins in olive oil. It is necessary to consider that the protein concentration in hazelnut oil depends on the kernels employed; hazelnut can be raw or roasted and generally roasting lowers the amount of residual proteins even if the process conditions are important. Data show that protein content of crude oils is of the order of 100-300 μg and that refining results in levels up to about 100-fold lower. On the other hand, polar components of hazelnut oil, as glycolipids and phospholipids, have been little studied compared to those of olive oil [63]. Therefore, the search for new techniques and/or new hazelnut markers is still an open issue.

Chemical markers usually employed for adulteration detection are free fatty acids [47, 64], triacylglycerols [49, 65], sterols [66], volatile organic compounds (VOC) [67] and filbertone [68], a ketone absent in olive oils. The presence of filbertone in olive oils is detected by gas chromatography or liquid and gas chromatography (LC-GC) coupled to mass spectrometry. The use of a refined hazelnut oil instead of a crude oil in the adulteration makes difficult the filbertone detection because of its partial or full degradation during refining process.

More recently, a method of solid phase microextraction (μSPE) based on hydrophilic interaction chromatography (HILIC) coupled with MALDI-TOF mass spectrometry for the detection of the polar component in hazelnut and olive oil has been developed [69]. The pre-treatment with HILIC columns has enabled the enrichment of some hazelnut polar compounds. A deep examination of the *m/z* range 450–600 of the spectra relevant to the HILIC micro-columns elution fractions of EVOO (Figure 4A) and HO (Figure 4B) has been performed.

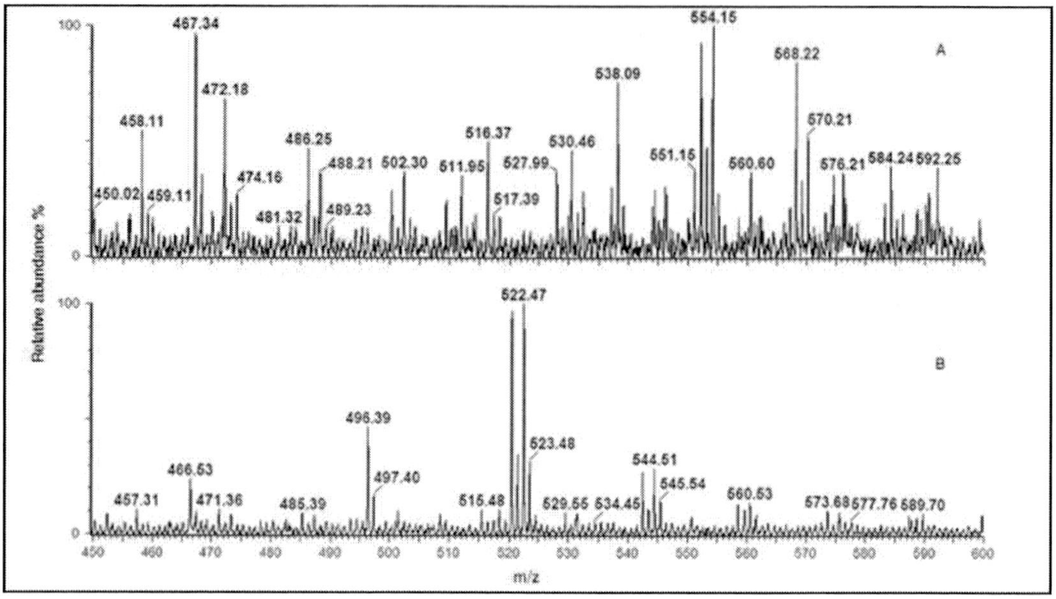

Figure 4. MALDI-ToF- MS spectra (m/z range 450-600) relevant to the enriched polar fraction eluted from HILIC micro-columns of (A) an extra-virgin olive oil and (B) a hazelnut oil sample.

Some peaks were present in both spectra while some others were peculiar of a specific oil sample. In particular, the *m/z* ions 496.39, 520.46, 522.47, 542.50, 544.51, 558.52 and 560.53 were found in all pressed HOs at concentration levels higher than that of the other constituents of its polar fraction and were totally absent in EVOO, indicating that they could be diagnostic for the presence of HO in EVOO. Consecutive analysis by tandem mass spectrometry has allowed to indentify these markers as lysophosphatydilcholines. In fact, phospholipids are usually present in seed oils at a concentration range of 10-20 g/kg [70], while their amount in virgin olive oil is 300-400 times lower than those in seed oils [71]. These markers were found at level of adulteration up to 5%.

7. Olive Oil Oxidation

Besides the absence of *adulterants*, an healthy olive oil should not contain *oxidized components*.

Oils begin to decompose from the moment they are isolated from their natural environment, mainly for atmospheric oxidation [72].The initial compounds produced by autoxidation are hydroperoxides and cyclic peroxides. The mechanisms of the reactions and the implications of the autoxidation reactions with vegetable oils have been thoroughly reviewed [73,74].

Oxidation is accelerated by heat, humidity and presence of transition metals. The intense heating of oils during industrial (deodoration) or domestic processes such as frying, boiling or microwave heating causes oxidative thermal degradation of beneficial compounds (essential fatty acids, phenolic components). The main phenolic compounds of olive oil (oleuropein, oleocanthal, hydroxytyrosol, tyrosol) have important antioxidant and anti-inflammatory functions and they reduce the risk of cancer and heart diseases [75].

Moreover, oxidation can produce toxic compounds and oxidized polymers, so the exposure of consumers to oxidized oils is a potential health hazard.

The analytical methods used to study the effects of oil oxidation during thermal stressing of edible oils are liquid chromatography coupled to UV [76,77] or mass spectrometry [78-80] or gas chromatography with flame-ionization detection (FID) [81,82].

More recently, matrix-assisted laser desorption ionization time-of-flight mass spectrometry (MALDI–TOF MS) has emerged as a useful tool for TAG oxidation determination in oils [49, 65, 83,84] since it offers fast and easy sample preparation without the need for analyte derivatization.

In particular, Schiller and co-workers [84] proposed the use of MALDI-TOF MS in combination with ^{1}H and ^{31}P NMR for monitoring the changes on saturated and unsaturated TAGs in selected oils during the thermal stressing. In some cases, the use of a matrix produces several background signals in the low m/z range, that has limited the application of the technique for the analysis of relatively low molecular weight compounds. A possible alternative is provided by direct laser desorption ionization (DLDI) on a standard stainless steel target plate [83].

Figure 5A and 5B report the LDI–TOF mass spectra obtained for the same commercial extra-virgin olive oil sample, incubated at 200 °C for 2 and 6 h, respectively. Both figures show a progressive decrease in TAG peak intensity and the simultaneous appearance of oxidation products at +16 Da or + 32 Da indicating the incorporation of one or two oxygen atoms.

More interesting information can be retrieved lasting the incubation time at 200 °C up to 48 hours.

The LDI spectra of an olive oil heated 48 h show the occurrence of new signals in the m/z ranges 700–860 (Figure 6, Inset B) and 850–980 (Figure 6, Inset A), mainly due to oxidation reactions, can be observed.

Comparison of both spectra with fresh samples clearly shows that two major changes occur upon ageing, leading to the formation of oxidized TAGs (mass shift of +16 or +32 Da) and to by-products containing a shorter acyl fatty acid (mass shift to lower m/z) likely formed through a β-cleavage mechanism [72]. For instance, in the TAGs mass window (m/z 850–980) of Figure 6A, the signal at m/z 881.67 (corresponding to the sodiated adduct of palmitoyl-diolein TAG, $[POO+Na]^{+}$) is practically absent, whereas Na^{+} adducts of its oxidation products are clearly distinguishable at m/z values 897.70 (mono-oxidized oleic acid residue–mass shift +16 Da) and 913.69 (hydroperoxidized oleic acid residue and/or two mono-oxidized oleic acid residues–mass shift +32 Da), respectively. This behavior can be generalized for all the detected TAGs. It is worth noting that typically, the higher the unsaturation degree the higher was the extent of conversion to oxidized species.

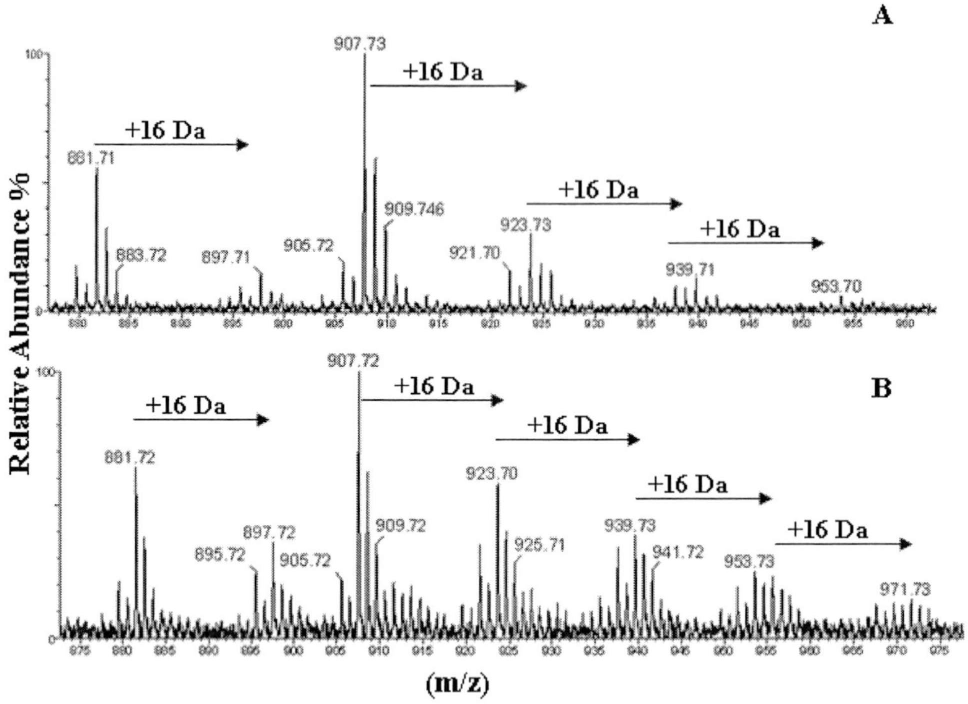

Figure 5. LDI-ToF- MS spectra of a commercial extra-virgin olive oil sample incubated at 200 °C for 2 h (A) and 6 h (B) respectively.

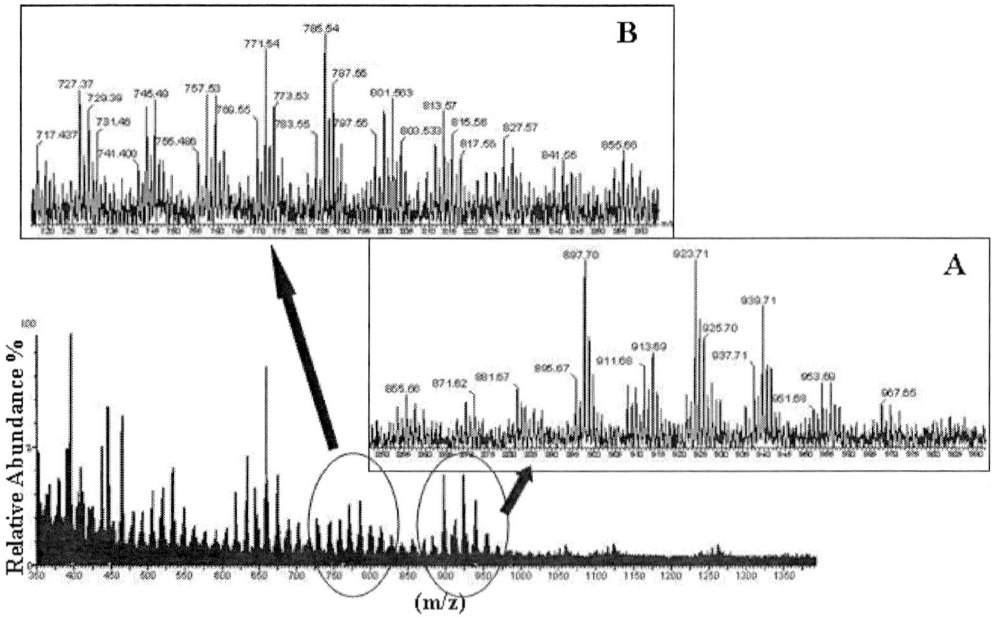

Figure 6. LDI-ToF- MS spectrum of a commercial extra-virgin olive oil sample incubated at 200 °C for 48 h. Insets are zoom in the mass range m/z 860-960 (A) and m/z 710-860 (B).

As can be seen in Figure 6B, additional ions in the range m/z 700-800 were observed in heated samples. These can probably be attributed to short-chain aldehydic or carboxylic oxidized TAGs originating from β-cleavage oxidation processes [83, 84] of the unsaturated fatty acyl residues. For instance, POL may generate short-chain products due to β-scission of the linoleic or oleic acid residues (the saturated palmitic acid is not expected to undergo radical oxidation). Linoleic and oleic acids can be oxidized to hydroperoxide that are then readily decomposed, through a β-scission break-down mechanism, into short-chain TAG products bearing aldehydic and dicarboxylic functions (see Scheme 1).

For instance, the peak at m/z 771.54 could be attributed to the sodium ion adduct of the aldehyde resulting from the scission of the intermediate hydroperoxide of the triacylglycerol LOP if the cleavage involves the C9 of the linoleic acid residue. This residue is further oxidized as can be seen in the spectrum where the m/z ion at 787.55 is observed. If the cleavage occurs at C10 in the linoleic acid residue then thermal β-scission will lead to the formation of different aldehydes. For instance, the m/z ion 783.54 could be explained as the sodium ion adduct of the aldehyde resulting from the scission at C10 of the LOP formed hydroperoxide. In the same way, most of the peaks observed in the m/z range 700-850 of the spectrum of figure 6 can be easily attributed.

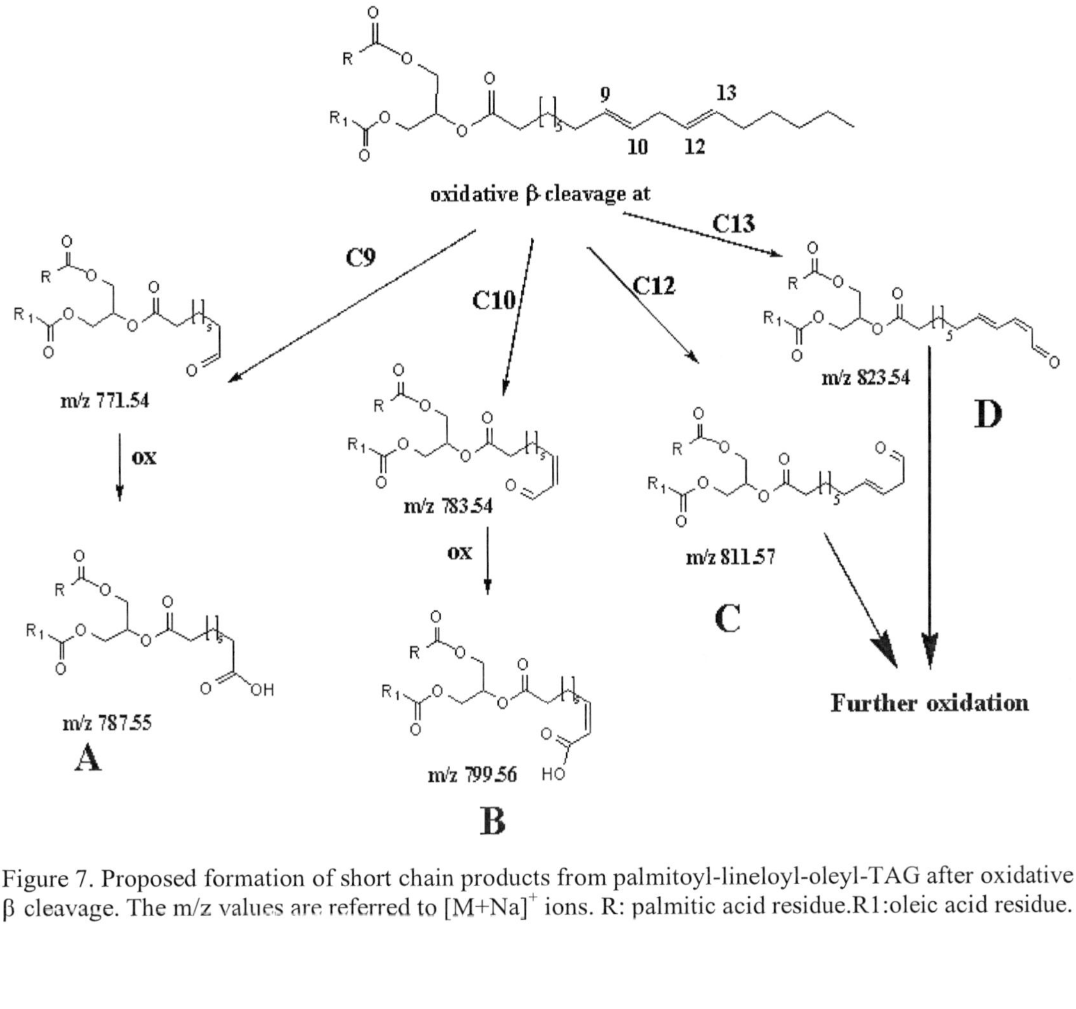

Figure 7. Proposed formation of short chain products from palmitoyl-lineloyl-oleyl-TAG after oxidative β cleavage. The m/z values are referred to $[M+Na]^+$ ions. R: palmitic acid residue.R1:oleic acid residue.

All these experimental evidences clearly indicate that the present approach represents a simple and fast method for the detection of olive oil rancidity.

Laser desorption/ionization on a stainless steel target plate was successfully used as a tool for easy and fast detection of edible oil rancidity. The advantages of this approach are: no matrix interference peaks in the spectra; the absence of a sample preparation step; the ability to obtain TAG and oxidized TAG fingerprints, allowing easy individuation of oil degradation/oxidation. This approach could potentially be applied as a rapid screening method for oil quality control.

8. Olive Oil Contaminants

In conclusion, high quality olive oil has to be free from contaminants and residues. These compounds are often present at low levels so the analytical methods developed for their detection should be very sensitive.

Their presence in food is related to the production process or to the storage and processing of food [2]. The first group of contaminants is composed by synthetic chemical compounds as for example hexachlorobenzene (HCB), dichlorodiphenyltrichloroethane (DDT) and many other polychlorinated biphenyls (PCBs). They are toxic to organisms and persistent in the environment and their presence in food can be caused by negligence or fraud [85].

A second class of residues is represented by halogenated solvents (bromodichloro methane, dibromochloromethane, chloroform, bromoform, tetrachloroethene, trichloroethene, vinyl chloride and ethylenedichloride) [86]. Their limits are established at 0.1 mg/kg (individual compounds) and 0.2 mg/ kg (total content) by the Commission Regulation (EC) No. 1989/2003.

A great number of mono- and polyaromatic hydrocarbons (PAH) can also contaminate olive oils. Examples of these compounds are benzene, toluene, ethylbenzene and xylenes that belong to the group of BTEX. These molecules derive from biological processes in olives, from production technology, from plastics used to realize containers for food products. Their presence must be monitored especially in virgin olive oils because of the absence of the refining process that removes most of the volatile compounds. The recent methods used to detect BTEXs in virgin olive oils are headspace solid-phase microextraction (HS-SPME), coupled with GC–MS analysis [8, 87].

A serious concern for human health is also the detection in olive oils of phytosanitary products as insecticides, fungicides, and herbicides used to control pests, diseases, weeds. 3-Chloropropane-1,2-diol (3-MCPD) esters form a class of contaminants present in food as a consequence of high temperature processing of fat-based matrices. Therefore the refining process (especially the deodorisation step) used to improve taste and appearance of different oils led to the formation of these compounds.

As far as concern polluting substances, Codex Alimentarius Commission, European Union, Food and Agriculture Organization of the United Nations (FAO) and World Health Organization (WHO) have established the Maximum Residues Limits (MRLs) relevant to the residues of pesticides in olives and in olive oils.

The methods mostly employed for the detection of residues of pesticides in olive oil are based on gas chromatography coupled with ionization detectors (FID, NPD, ECD, PID) or Electron Impact (EI) Mass Spectrometry and on various analyte extraction procedures.

There are a lots of analytical problems for this detection in fat-based matrices [88,89]. Olive oil, in particular, is difficult to analyze because of the high lipid concentration; lipids are extracted together with the analyte and they cause interferences during the instrumental analysis [90]. The pesticides extraction methods from olive oils are based on Liquid-Liquid Extraction (LLE) with hexane and acetonitrile [91,92], adsorption chromatography [93,94], gel permeation chromatography [95], low temperatures for lipids precipitation [96]. Each of these techniques is time consuming and need of huge amount of solvents but has also advantages (precision and deftness).

An open issue is still the need of new, economic and simple methods to detect residues of pesticides (organophosphorus pesticides, triazine) in extra-virgin olive oil.

CONCLUSION

In this paper the great potential of MALDI-TOF mass spectrometer as a new tool for quality control and health risk assessment of virgin olive oil has been discussed. Few MALDI applications in the lipid field have been reported compared to proteomic, since an intrinsic disadvantage of MALDI experiments is the presence of interfering matrix peaks in the spectra in the relatively low mass range investigated for lipids.

In order to avoid these interferences, an alternative interesting approach could be the complete matrix avoidance, performing the so-called laser desorption ionization (LDI) analysis using a stainless steel target plate. This approach further simplifies the sample preparation step and completely eliminates the presence of matrix peaks in the spectra.

As far as the oil TAG content is concerned, it varies with the oil type, the extraction method, the geographical origin and some others fraudulent manipulations such as the adding of cheaper oils to more expensive ones. Therefore, it can be used as a measurement for oil authentication, for the identification of oil adulteration and for the individuation of rancid oils.

The MALDI approach is useful to obtain simple and rapid fingerprintings of different oils. Moreover, it proved able to detect simulated olive oil adulterations, obtained after the addition of small aliquots of sunflower oil or hazelnut oil, and to check the olive oil oxidation status after thermal stressing, i.e. heating oil at 200°C ~~for~~ at different times. In synthesis, MALDI MS demonstrated to be a fast and easy method to assess the quality and purity of vegetable oils, considering its ability to perform analyses of many samples in few minutes and without any particular pre-treatment.

REFERENCES

[1] Storelli, M. (2006). Le frodi alimentari: classificazione, tipologie, metodi di contrasto. Corso di aggiornamento in sicurezza e lotta alle frodi dei prodotti delle filiere agroalimentari pugliesi.

[2] Muller, A.; Steinhart, H. *Food Chem.* 2007, 102, 436-444.

[3] Stark, A.H.; Madar, P.Z. *Nutrition reviews* 2002, 60, 170-176.

[4] Kafatos A.; Comas G.; In El Aceite de Oliva Edited by Kiritsaki, Madrid: Madrid Vicente, 1991, pp. 199-223.

[5] Ranalli A.; Modesti G.; Patumi M.; Fontanazza G. *Food Chem.* 2000, 69, 37-46.

[6] Bendini, A.; Cerretani, L.; Salvador, M.D.; Fregapane, G.; Lercker, G. *Italian Food and Beverage Technol.* 2010, N.60

[7] FRYING OF FOOD: Oxidation, Nutrient and Non-Nutrient Antioxidants, Biologically Active Compounds and High Temperatures. Dimitrios Boskou and Ibrahim Elmadfa, eds.

[8] Gilbert-Lopez, B.; Robles-Molina, J.; Garcia-Reyes, J.F.; Molina-Diaz, A. *Talanta* 2010, 83, 391-399

[9] Kuksis, A.; Myher, J.J. *J Chromatogr. B. Biomed. Appl.* 1995, 671, 35-70.

[10] Myher, J.J.; Kuksis,A. *J. Chromatogr. B*, 671, 1995, 3-33.

[11] Ruiz-Gutierrez, V.; Barron, L.J. *J.* Chromatogr. *B. Biomed. Appl.* 1995, 671, 133-168.

[12] Laakso, P. *Food Rev. Int.* 1996, 12, 199-250.

[13] Ackman, R.G.; In: Analyses of Fats, Oils and Lipoproteins, ed. E.G. Perkins, American Oil Chemists' Society, Champaign, U.S.A., 1991, pp. 97-121.

[14] Aitzetmuller, K. *Fat Sci. Technol.* 1991, 93, 501-510.

[15] Christie, W.W. Lipid Analysis; Oily Press: Bridgwater, U.K., 2003.

[16] Kurvinen, J.P.; Rua, P.; Sjovall, O.; Kallio, H. *Rapid Comm. Mass Spectrom.* 2001, 15, 1084-1091.

[17] Careri, M.; Bianchi, F.; Corradini,C. *J. Chromatogr. A.* 2002, 970, 3-64.

[18] Klein, R.A. *J. Lipid Res.* 1971, 12, 628-634.

[19] Klein, R.A. *J. Lipid. Res.* 1971, 12, 123-131.

[20] Crawford, C.G.; Plattner, R.D. *J. Lipid Res.* 1983, 24, 456-460.

[21] Lorenz, S.A.; Maziarz, E.P.; Wood, T.D. *Appl. Spectro.* 1999, 53, 18-36.

[22] Whitehouse, C.M.; Dreyer, R.N.; Yamashita, M.; Fenn, J.B. *Anal. Chem.* 1985, 57, 675-679.

[23] Hillenkamp, F.; Karas, M.; Beavis, B.T.; Chait, B.T. *Anal. Chem.* 1991, 63, 1193-1203.

[24] Tanaka, K.; Waki, H.; Ido, Y.; Akita,S.; Yoshida, Y.; Yoshida, T. *Rapid Comm. Mass Spectrom.* 1988, 2, 151-153 .

[25] Karas, M.; Hillenkamp, F. *Anal. Chem.* 1988, 60, 2299- 2301.

[26] Posthumus, M.A.; Kistemaker, P.G.; Meuzelaar, H.L.C. *Anal. Chem.* 1978, 50, 985-991.

[27] Karas, M.; Kruger, R. *Chem. Rev.* 2003, 103, 427-439.

[28] Domon, B.; Aebersold R. *Science* 2006, 312, 212-217.

[29] Wang, H.; Clouthier, S. G.; Galchev, V.; Misek, D. E.; Duffner, U.; Min, C.-Ki; Zhao, R.; Tra, J.; Omenn, G. S.; Ferrara, J. L. M.; Hanash S.M. *Mol. Cell. Prot.* 2005, 4, 618-625.

[30] Hu, S.; Michels, D. A.; Fazal, Md. A.; Ratisoontorn, C.; Cunningham, M. L.; Dovichi, N. J.; *Anal. Chem.* 2004, 76, 4044-4049.

[31] Schiller, J.; Arnold, K. In Encyclopedia of analytical chemistry; Meyers, R.A.; Wiley: Chichester, 2000; pp 559-585.

[32] Beavis, R.C.; Chait, B.T.; *Rapid Comm. Mass Spectrom.* 1989, 3, 233-237.

[33] Wu, K.J.; Shaler, T.A.; Becker, C.H. *Anal. Chem.* 1994 , 66, 1637-1645.

[34] Wu, K.J.; Steding, A.; Becker, C.H. *Rapid Comm. Mass Spectrom.* 1993, 7, 142-146.

[35] Nordhoff , E.; Cramer, R.; Karas, M.; Hillenkamp, F.; Kirpekar, F.; Kristiansen, K.; Roepstorff, P. *Nucl. Acid Res.* 1993, 21, 3347-3357.

[36] Calvano, C.D.; Carulli, S.; Palmisano, F. *Anal. Bioanal. Chem.* 2010, 398(1), 499-507.

[37] Eibisch, M.; Schiller, J. *Rapid Comm. Mass Spectrom.* 2011, 25, 1100-1106.

[38] Shroffand, R.; Svatos, A. *Anal. Chem.* 2009, 81 (19), 7954–7959

[39] Calvano, C.D.; Zambonin, C.G.; Palmisano, F. *Rapid Comm. Mass Spectrom.* 2011, 25, 1757-1764.

[40] Armstrong, D.W.; Zhang, L.-K.; He, L.; Gross, M. *Anal. Chem.* 2001, 73, 3679-3686.

[41] Calvano, C.D.; Carulli, S.; Palmisano, F. *Rapid Comm. Mass Spectrom.* 2009, 23, 1659–1668.

[42] Fitzgerald, M. C.; Parr, G. R.; Smith, L. M. *Anal. Chem.* 1993, 65, 3204-3211.

[43] Asbury, G.R.; Al-Saad, K.; Siems, W.F.; Hannan, R.M.; Hill, H.H. *J. Am. Soc. Mass Spectrom.* 1999, 10, 983-991.

[44] Ayorinde, F.O.; Elhilo, E.; Hlongwane, C. *Rapid Comm. Mass Spectrom.* 1999, 13, 737-739.

[45] Ayorinde, F.O.; Eribo, B.E.; Balan, K.V.; Johnson, J.H.; Wan, L.W. *Rapid Comm. Mass Spectrom.* 1999, 13, 937-942.

[46] Ayorinde, F.O.; Keith, Q.L.; Wan, L.W. *Rapid Comm. Mass Spectrom.* 1999, 13, 1762-1769.

[47] Ayorinde, F.O.; Garvin, K.; Saeed, K. *Rapid Comm. Mass Spectrom.* 2000, 14, 608-615.

[48] Hlongwane, C.; Delves, I.G.; Wan, L.W.; Ayorinde, F.O. *Rapid Comm. Mass Spectrom.* 2001, 15, 2027-2034.

[49] Jakab, A.; Nagy, K.; Heberger, K.; Vekey, K.; Forgacs, E. *Rapid Comm. Mass Spectrom.* 2002, 16, 2291-2297.

[50] Robins, C.; Limbach, P.A. *Rapid Comm. Mass Spectrom.* 2003, 17, 2839-2845.

[51] Al-Saad, K.A.; Zabrouskov, V.; Siems, W.F.; Knowles, N.R.; Hannan, R.M.; Hill, H.H. *Rapid Comm. Mass Spectrom.* 2003, 17, 87-96.

[52] Calvano, C. D.; Zambonin, C. G.; Foti, C.; Cassano, N.; Vena, G. A. *Food Chem. Toxicol.* 2008, 46, 3580-3585.

[53] Calvano, C.D.; Palmisano, F.; Zambonin, C.G. *Rapid Commun. Mass Spectrom.* 2005, 19, 1315-1320.

[54] Zambonin, C.G.; Calvano, C.D.; D'Accolti L.; Palmisano F. *Rapid Comm. Mass Spectrom.* 2006, 20, 325–327.

[55] Hidalgo, F.J.; Zamora, R. *Trends Food Sci. Technol.* 2006, 17, 56-63.

[56] Thelen, J.J. *Regul. Toxicol. Pharm.* 2009, 54, S41-S45.

[57] Taylor, S.L.; Nordlee, J.A.; Sicherer, S.H.; Sampson, H.A.; Levy, M.B.; Steinman, H. *J All. Clin. Immunol.* 2004, 113, S99.

[58] Errahali, Y.; Morisset, M.; Moneret-Vautrin, D.A.; Kanny, G.; Metche, M.; Nicolas, J.P.; Fremont, S. *Allergy* 2002, 57, 648-649.

[59] Arlorio, M.; Coisson, J.D.; Bordiga, M.; Travaglia, F.; Garino, C.; Zuidmeer, L.; Van Ree, R.; Giuffrida, M.G.; Conti, A.; Martelli, A. *Food Add. Contam.* 2010, 27, 11-18.
[60] Rigby, N.M.; Marsh, J.; Sancho, A.I.; Wellner, K.; Akkerdaas, J.; van Ree R.; Knulst, A.; Montserrat, F.R.; Brettlova, V.; Schilte, P.P.; Summer, C.; Pumphrey, R.; Shewry, P.R.; Mills, E.N.C. *Mol. Nutr. Food Res.* 2008, 52, S251-S261.
[61] Martin-Hernandez, C.; Benet, S.; Obert L. *J. Agric. Food Chem.* 2008, 56, 4348-4351.
[62] Bremer, M.G.E.G.; Smits, N.G.E.; Haasnoot, W. *Anal. Bioanal. Chem.* 2009, 395, 119-126.
[63] Gordon, M.H.; Covell C.; Kirsch N. *JAOCS* 2001, 78, 621-624.
[64] Park, K.H.; Kim H.J. *Rapid Comm. Mass Spectrom.* 2001, 15, 1494-1499.
[65] Cozzolino, R.; De Giulio, B. *Eur. J. Lipid Sci Technol.* 2011,113, 160-167.
[66] Cercaci, L.; Rodriguez-Estrada, M.T.; Lercker, G. *J. Chromatogr.* A 2003, 985, 211-220.
[67] Bail,S.; Stuebiger, G.; Unterweger, H.; Buchbauer, G.; Krist, S. *Eur. J. Lipid Sci Technol.* 2009, 111, 170-182.
[68] Pavon, J.L.P.; del Nogal Sanchez, M.; Fernandez Laespada E.M.; Cordero, B.M.; *Anal. Bioanal. Chem.* 2009, 394, 1463-1470.
[69] Calvano,C.D.; Aresta, A.; Zambonin, C.G. *J. Mass Spectrom.* 2010, 45, 981-988.
[70] Bernardini, E. Oilseeds, oils and fats; Oil Publishing House: Rome, Italy (IT), 1983; 1, pp 173-178
[71] Koidis, A.; Boskou, D. *Eur. J. Lipid Sci. Technol.* 2006, 108, 323-328.
[72] Choe, E.; Min, D.B. *Compr. Rev. Food Sci. Food Safety* 2006, 5, 169–186.
[73] Velasco, J.; Dobarganes, C *Eur. J. Lipid Sci. Technol.* 2002, 104, 661–676.
[74] Porter, N.A.; Caldwell, S.E.; Mills, K.A. *Lipids* 1995, 30, 277–290.
[75] Grignaffini, P.; Roma, P.; Galli, C.; Catapano, A. L. *Lancet* 1994, 343, 1296–1297.
[76] Miyashita, K.; Frankel, E.N.; Neff, W.E.; Awl R.A. *Lipids* 1990, 25, 48–53.
[77] Bauer-Plank, C.; Steenhorst-Slikkerveer L *J. Am. Oil. Chem. Soc.* 2000, 77, 477–482.
[78] Sjövall, O.; Kuksis, A.; Kallio, H. *J. Chromatogr. A* 2001, 905, 119–132.
[79] Sjövall, O.; Kallio, H. *Lipids* 2002, 37, 81–94.
[80] Giuffrida, F.; Destaillats, F.; Skibsted, L.H.; Dionisi, F. *Chem. Phys. Lipids* 2004, 131,41–49.
[81] Velasco, J.; Berdeaux, O.; Marquez-Ruiz, G.; Dobarganes, C. *J. Chromatogr. A* 2002, 982:145–152.
[82] Lagarda, M.J.; Manez, J.G.; Manglano, P., Farré, R. *Eur. J. Lipid Sci. Technol.* 2003, 105, 339–345.
[83] Calvano, C.D.; Aresta A.; Palmisano F.; Zambonin, C. G. *Anal. Bioanal. Chem.* 2007, 389, 2075–2084.
[84] Schiller, J.; Suss, R.; Petkovic, M.; Arnold, K. *Eur. Food Res. Technol.* 2002, 215, 282-286 .
[85] Brambilla, G.; Cherubini,G.; De Filippis, S.; Magliuolo, M.; Di Domenico, A. *Anal. Chim. Acta* 2004, 514, 1-7.
[86] Arrebola, F.J.; Gonzalez-Rodriguez, M.J.; Garrido Frenich, A.; Marin-Juan, A.; Martinez Vidal, J.L. *Anal. Chim. Acta* 2005, 552, 60-66.

[87] Vichi, S.; Pizzale, L.; Conte, L. S.; Buxaderas, S.; Lopez-Tamames E. *J. Chromatog. A,* 2005, 1090,146–154.

[88] Walters, S.M. *Anal. Chim. Acta* 1990, 236, 77-82.

[89] Armishaw, P.; Millar, R.G. *J. AOAC Int.* 1993, 76, 1317-1322.

[90] Lentza-Rizos, Ch.; Avramides, E.J. *Rev. Environ. Contam. Toxicol.* 1995, 141, 111-134.

[91] Cabras, P.; Angioini, A.; Melis, M.; Minelli, E.V.; Pirisi, F.M. *J. Chromatogr. A* 1997, 761, 327-331.

[92] Hiskia, A.E.; Atmajidon, M.E.; Tsipi, D.F. *J. Agric. Food Chem.* 1998, 46, 570-574.

[93] Tekel, J.; Hatrik, S. *J. Chromatogr. A.* 1996, 754, 397-410.

[94] Rastrelli, L.; Totano, K.; De Simone, F. *Food Chem.* 2002, 79, 303-305.

[95] Steinwandter, H.; *Fresenius' J. Anal. Chem.* 1988, 331, 499-502.

[96] Lentza-Rizos, Ch.; Avramides, E.J.; Cherasco, F. *J. Chromatogr. A* 2001, 919, 135-142.

In: Olive Consumption and Health
Editors: C. A. Savalas and S. M. Nicolau
ISBN: 978-1-62100-774-6

Chapter 6

LAST ADVANCES IN THE STUDY OF OLIVE AIRBORNE POLLEN DYNAMIC

M. A. Hernández-Ceballos*[*1,3], H. García-Mozo[2], J. A. Adame[1] and C. Galán[2]

[1] National Institute of Aerospace Technology (INTA), Atmospheric Research and Instrumentation Branch, Spain Atmospheric Sounding Station "El Arenosillo". Crta. Huelva-Matalascañas km 34. 21130. Mazagón – Huelva, Spain

[2] Departamento de Botánica, Ecología y Fisiología Vegetal, Universidad de Córdoba, 14071 Córdoba, Spain

[3] Department of Applied Physics, University of Huelva, Huelva, Spain

ABSTRACT

The genus *Olea L.* is represented in the Mediterranean region by the species *Olea europaea L.* with two varieties, *O. europaea* var. *sylvestris* (wild olive), which forms part of the natural vegetation, and *O. europaea* var. *europaea*, cultivated primarily for olive and oil production. Nowadays, Andalusia (Spain) is the world's leading olive-oil-producing region. Due to its great land cover extensions and to the high flower production, high levels of olive pollen are detected in the air of southern Spain during springtime, being the most abundant pollen type and causing severe pollinosis problems among population. This fact, together with the considerable economic importance, makes the study of olive-pollen characteristics over this area of a high relevance.

Olive-pollen season in south Spain runs from April to June, being the timing and severity of the pollen curve highly controlled by weather conditions. This work represents a paper review on the olive pollen studies, paying special attention to its relationship with meteorological parameters and the usefulness of back-trajectory analysis, due to they provide information about synoptic conditions responsible for high pollen counts, the origin of airborne pollen, and the type of pollen transport (local or regional). With the present review we sought 1) to determine potential pollen sources, 2)

---

* Corresponding Author: Hernández-Ceballos, M.A. INTA, Carretera Huelva-Matalascañas, Km 31.3, E-21130. Mazagón, Huelva, Spain e-mail: hernandezma@inta.es Telephone: 959-20-88-56. Fax: 959-20-88-57.

to describe pollen transport dynamic and 3) to clarify the real contribution of the different olive-growing areas to airborne pollen counts in Cordoba province.

1. Introduction

Olive tree cultivation probably started about 5000 years ago in the eastern Mediterranean region, due to mediterranean basin is a region characterised by a dry summer subtropical climate (Koeppen's classification), where olive tree can adapt well to drought and high temperature. The genus *Olea* is represented in this region by the species *Olea europaea* L. and two varieties, *Olea europaea* var. *sylvestris* (wild olive), which forms part of the natural vegetation, and *Olea europaea* var. *europaea*, mainly cultivated for oil.

Nowadays, olive cultivation constitutes a major economic activity in the Mediterranean basin. Spain has the largest surface area given over to this crop, leading the world in olive production. Andalusia region (southern Spain) devotes more than 60% of their total surface area to olive cultivation, accounting over the 60% of the total Spanish olive crop. This cultivation is concentrated mainly in the provinces of Córdoba and Jaén, pointing out that province of Jaén dedicates more than 90% of its surface area to this crop, becoming the zone with the highest olive oil production in the world.

The abundance of this crop as well as the intense flowering of this anemophilous species, which produce abundant pollen during springtime, make olive pollen the most abundant type in South Europe, registering extremely high levels in Andalusia (Recio et al., 1996; Alba et al., 1998; Fornaciari et al., 2000; Orlandi et al., 2010). Moreover, *Olea* pollen is the major cause of allergy in the Mediterranean area, (Bousquet et al., 1985; Licardi et al., 1996; Cariñanos et al., 2002; Sánchez-Mesa et al., 2005; De Linares et al., 2007). In southern Spain, it is the principal cause of seasonal allergic rhinitis and bronchial asthma, with high percentages of the population being allergic: 46% in Málaga (Burgos 1991), 72% in Córdoba (Domínguez et al., 1993), 77% in Granada (Martínez Cañavate et al., 1995) and 89% in Jaén (Florido et al., 1999).

The characterization of the olive pollen dynamic, pollen emission and transport through the atmosphere, the influence of meteorological parameters on pollen content in the air, and their influence on human health, has an important relevancy in this region. In this sense, the analysis of phenological data has allowed to identify how plants have adapted to their local climate and how they respond to climatic change (Galán et al., 2005; Garcia-Mozo et al., 2006, 2009; Geßler et al., 2007).

Phenology is developing rapidly as a world-wide discipline, and its value as an indicator assumes even greater importance in cases where phenological processes greatly affect biodiversity, agriculture, forestry and human health (Chuine et al., 1999; Fornaciari et al., 2005). Atmospheric pollen is a valuable aerobiological tool to obtain floral phenological data in anemophilous plants. In Spain, the airborne pollen is continuously registered by the Spanish Aerobiology Network (Red Española de Aerobiologia, REA, (www.uco.es/rea).This monitoring network was created in 1991, with the aim to satisfy the growing public demand for information, coupled with the need to coordinate and standardise the methodology used by each network member, prompted a move towards consolidating an aerobiological network covering a wide geographical area. From the origin, the University of Córdoba Aerobiological Monitoring Unit is the REA's National Coordinating Centre, which is the responsible for receiving, storing and processing data obtained at the various sampling sites, and for providing the media with data on airborne pollen counts. Nowadays, the pollen counts recorded at the current 47 Aerobiological Monitoring Units (Figure 1) are fully standardised, thus enabling the generation of strictly comparable information (Galán et al., 2007).

The creation of a growing number of Monitoring Units has been accompanied by an increasing range of activities intended to publicise the information generated, first at local level and then nationally and internationally (http://www.uco.es/rea/publicaciones /publicaciones.html). In this sense, the available of long-term and daily airborne pollen forecasts provide a great deal of information that can be useful to understand the dependence between pollen concentrations in the atmosphere and pollination of local flora.

As regards daily *Olea* pollen variations, several papers have highlighted the influence of heat-related variables such as temperatura and hours of sunlight on pollen emission and dispersion, as well as, rainfall, wind speed and direction, depending on the geographical location (Domínguez et al., 1993; Recio et al., 1996, 1997; Vázquez et al., 2003; De la Guardia et al., 2003, García-Mozo et al., 2008).

Other studies in the Mediterranean area have been focused on long-term *Olea* pollen forecasts, reporting that monthly rainfall during the month prior to the pollen season is the main variable for forecasting total pollen output, while temperature during the period prior to the pollen season (from the end of the chilling period) is the main factor for forecasting the start of the pollen season (Frenguelli et al., 1989; González-Minero et al., 1996; Fornaciari et al., 1997, 1998; Galán et al., 2001a, b).

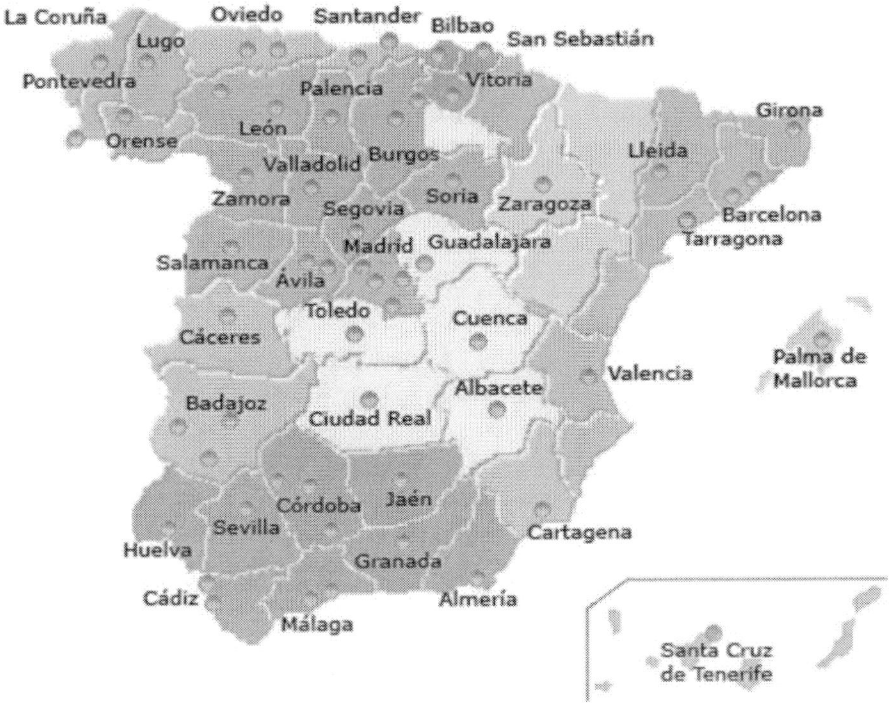

Figure 1. Map of REA Stations and Working Groups (http://www.uco.es/rea/infor_rea/estaciones.htm).

All of these factors are crucial to analyse the atmospheric transport of pollen taxa from adjacent and distant regions (Sofiev et al., 2006a; Vogel et al., 2008). In addition, the use of atmospheric dispersion models allow us to evaluated the pollen transport. The back-trajectory calculation has also become in a common tool both for understanding the general characteristics of air masses that affect a specific area (Miller, 1981; Jorba et al., 2004; Hondula et al., 2010). Also it is an interesting tool for air quality applications due to it computation enables us to know the pathway that an air mass has followed over a previous time period (Borge et al., 2007; Petzold et al., 2009; Lozano et al., 2011).

In Aerobiology, recent studies have been able to provide detailed data on the long and regional origin of a number of pollen types in various climatic areas by using back-trajectory analysis, including *Ambrosia* pollen in central Poland (Stach et al., 2007) and central northern Italy (Cecchi et al., 2007); *Betula* pollen in Denmark (Skjoth et al., 2008) and Lithuania (Šaulienė and Veriankaite 2006), grass pollen in the United Kingdom (Smith et al., 2005) or Cannabis in South Spain (Cabezudo et al., 1997). In this sense, HYSPLIT model has been used to study the contribution of upwind pollen sources to the characterization of *Juniperus ashei* J. Buchholz phenology (Van de Water and Levetin 2001), to analyse the long range transport of *Celtis* and *Nothofagus* pollen in the southeast of Buenos Aires province (Argentina) (Gassmann and Pérez 2006). The peculiarities of airborne birch pollen dispersion were analyzed in Lithuania (Šaulienė and Veriankaite 2006) and also to observe the contributions from remote source to the elevated birch pollen episodes in Denmark (Mahura et al., 2007). In addition, the adjoint dispersion option included in the air quality and emergency dispersion modelling system SILAM has recently been used in the analysis of the dispersion of pollen (Sofiev et al., 2006a, b; Siljamo et al., 2008). This model is based on numerical solution of the adjoint (inverse) dispersion equation (Marchuk 1982), and allows the analysis of the observational footprints of pollen, computing explicitly the sensitivity of the observed values to emission fluxes, chemical transformations and meteorological processes that can affect the particular observation. In the south of Spain, there was a lack in the application of meteorological models to evaluate and understand the olive pollen concentrations. Previous studies in the province of Cordoba, based on field phenological and aerobiological data, have sought to clarify the real contribution of the various olive-growing areas to airborne pollen counts. The results obtained suggest that crops located in the south may contribute to the pollen curve registered in Cordoba city, located in the center of the province (50-100 km far from the south sources), on days with favourable winds during the flowering period (Fornaciari et al., 2000). Our most recent studies have been focused in the used of this kind of modelling tools with the goal of providing a detailed analysis of olive-pollen transport dynamics along the province of Cordoba, that allow us to determine potential pollen sources and to clarify the real contribution of the different olive-growing areas to airborne pollen counts in Cordoba province (Hernández-Ceballos et al., 2011a).

2. Study Area

Cordoba province is situated in the central Andalusia region of southern Spain. The local climate is Mediterranean with continental influence, marked by considerable differences between the warm and cold seasons. The province is divided by the Guadalquivir valley, where oaks are scarce and cereal and olive are the predominant crops. The valley is bounded to the north by the Sierra Morena mountains, where *Quercus* forests and ''dehesas'' are the main vegetation, and to the south by the Subbética Mountains, where olive groves predominate.

As it was mentioned before this province is one of the most important regions in the world related with olive production. Figure 2 shows the spatial distribution of olive population in the province of Córdoba, pointing out the south-north gradient of *Olea* pollen sources across the province, with minimal presence in the north and an important population located in the south.

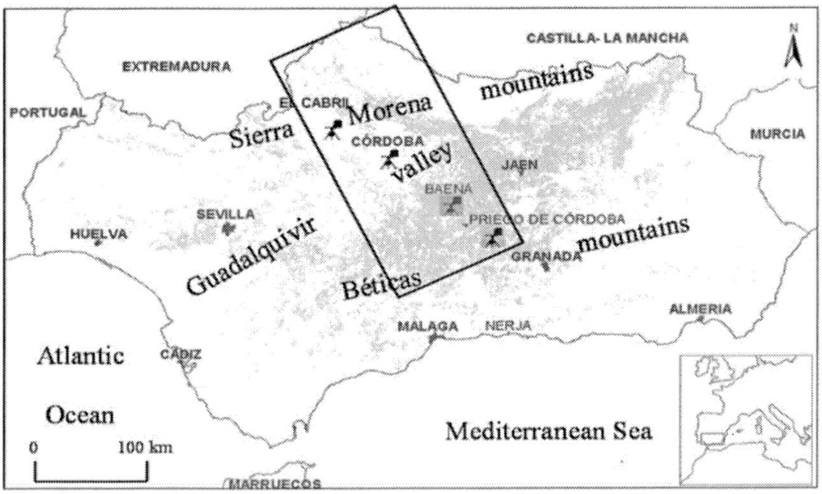

Figure 2. Location of the study sites and meteorological stations in Andalusia, representing grey areas the olive crop distribution (Hernández-Ceballos et al., 2011a).

Table 1. Geographical coordinates of the pollen monitoring sites used in this study. (a.m.s.l indicates above mean sea level)

Sites	Latitude	Longitude	Altitude (a.m.s.l)
Cordoba (COR)	37° 50' N	4° 45' W	123
Baena (BAE)	37° 37' N	4° 19' W	363
Priego de Córdoba (PRI)	37° 26° N	4° 11' W	650
El Cabril (CAB)	38° 4' N	5° 24' W	450

With the aim to cover the maximum area of the province, and, therefore, to obtain information from source areas of olive pollen and from others in where the olive population is scarce, four pollen sites have been taken as reference for this work: Cordoba, in the Guadalquivir river valley, Baena and Priego, to the south, in the Subbética Mountain Chain, and the "El Cabril" reserve in the northern part of the Hornachuelos Natural Park, Sierra Morena Mountain Chain (Figure 2, Table 1).

3. Field Phenology and Airbone Pollen Counts

Daily and bi-hourly airborne pollen data obtained from the four reference traps located in the province of Córdoba in 2007, together with field phenological data of the areas around the traps, have been used to provide a detailed analysis of olive-pollen counts in this province.

Weekly field phenological data were recorded for olive-groves surrounding the traps at Córdoba, Baena and Priego de Córdoba. The phenological key developed by Maillard (1975) was used to identify the main stages in floral phenology. Olive-pollen counts have been obtained using Hirst-type volumetric spore traps (Hirst 1952). Standardized data management procedures followed the rules laid down by the Spanish Aerobiology Network (REA) (Galán et al., 2007).

The curve for daily average airborne olive-pollen counts at each monitoring stations during 2007 is shown in Figure 3. As is observed in this figure, olive pollen season occurs from May to beginning of June. In general, curves displayed an irregular pattern, with peaks that tended to coincided in time but vary in magnitude. The main flowering period at each site, as identified using field phenological data, is also shown (horizontal bars). This flowering period has a temporal evolution along the province, being firstly observed in the olive population located in the surroundings of Cordoba city, and then in the south areas, starting in Baena area and, afterwards in Priego de Córdoba.

As it was expected, the mean pollen counts were higher at sites located in the south of the province, Baena and Priego, coinciding with the large olive-pollen source area. The Cordoba site may be seen as intermediate, recording occasional high counts and also low values. At the El Cabril site, in the north of the province, pollen-count peaks were lower due to the scarce olive crop areas in the vicinity of the trap.

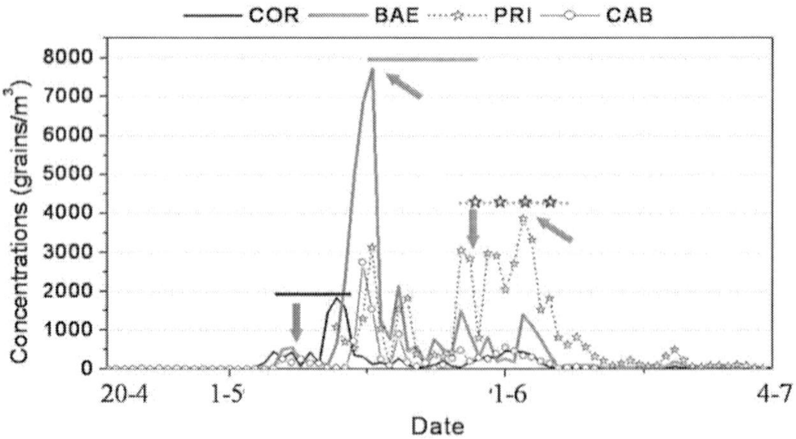

Figure 3. Daily average evolution of olive pollen count in Cordoba (COR), Baena (BAE), Priego de Córdoba (PRI) and El Cabril (CAB) monitoring site in 2007. Horizontal bars mean the time period of full flowering in each area detected from field phenological observations. Grains/m3: daily average pollen grains per m^3 of air (Hernández-Ceballos et al., 2011a).

With regard to pollen curve dynamics, monthly differences are shown, highlighting the temporal evolution of the maximum concentrations observed in each site. In Cordoba site, olive pollen peaks were mainly observed during the first days of May, coinciding with the flowering time of this area (from 1-15 May), with daily peaks of nearly 2000 grains/m^3, decreasing after that period until the final of May, when a progressive tendency to higher values (500 gr/m^3 per day) was shown. In Baena, the maximum concentrations were reached in the mid-May, with record concentrations of nearly 8000 gr/m^3, registering then, daily peaks occasionally exceeding 1500 gr/m^3 until the beginning of June. As happened in Córdoba, the higher concentrations were observed during the flowering period. On the other hand, in Priego de Córdoba higher daily olive pollen counts were recorded from late May to the beginning of June, reaching concentrations more than 2000 gr/m^3. In addition, higher daily peaks were observed coinciding with the intensive concentrations registered in Baena in the mid-May. At last, the evolution of the olive pollen concentrations at El Cabril showed the higher counts in the mid-May, with peaks more than 2500 gr/m^3, decreasing after that to lower values.

4. Air Mass Classification: Hysplit Model

The most common method for tracing the transport of airborne pollen is forward or backward trajectory modelling using various Lagrangian trajectory models, such as the Hybrid Single Particle Lagrangian Integrated Trajectory (HYSPLIT) model (Draxler and Hess 1998; Draxler et al., 2009) or FLEXPART (Stohl et al., 1998a). The HYSPLIT model, developed by the Air Resources Laboratory of the National Oceanic and Atmospheric Administration, has been used in this work due to it has proved highly effective in aerobiological works, focused on defining the pathway and possible long-range transport of air pollutants.

As it is reflected in Veriankaite et al. (2010) the accuracy of the HYSPLIT results is mainly conditioned by the horizontal spatial resolution of the meteorological data used to calculate back trajectories. For this reason, it is necessary to take into account the relationship between the spatial resolution of the meteorological data and the scale of the atmospheric transport distance consider in each study. In this case, the use of GDAS files, maintained by the ARL, with a resolution of 111 km, could be considered suitable to study the regional (up to 100 km) and long-range (more than 100 km) transport, defined in Seinfeld and Pandis (2006), of olive pollen along Cordoba province.

These files are generated from the GDAS (Global Data Analysis System) model, which is run four times a day at 00, 06, 12 and 18 UTC. GDAS files have a temporal resolution of three hours, being the data gridded to 1° x 1° in latitude and longitude, including the upper level information in 23 pressure levels with more resolution than FNL files below 500 hPa with twelve sigma pressure levels.

In addition, it has to be considered the difficult and complex to quantify the airflow patterns over mountains, the anabatic or katabatic flows that have this type of atmospheric transport model (Pérez-Landa et al. 2007a,b). Both mountain winds are mainly observed under fair-weather conditions and denote an upslope (downslope) wind driven by heating (cooling) at the slope surface with respect to the surrounding air, respectively, having a wind speeds range often between 3–5 m/s and a spatial development conditioned by the characteristic of the mountain, such a high and cover. Taking into account the orographic conditions of this area, with mountains with height less than 1,000 m, the influence of these flows over air-mass transport is limited. Moreover, the use of GDAS files to calculate back trajectories does not allow to consider these mountains flows, due to its spatial resolution is not enough to detect the development and behaviour of these.

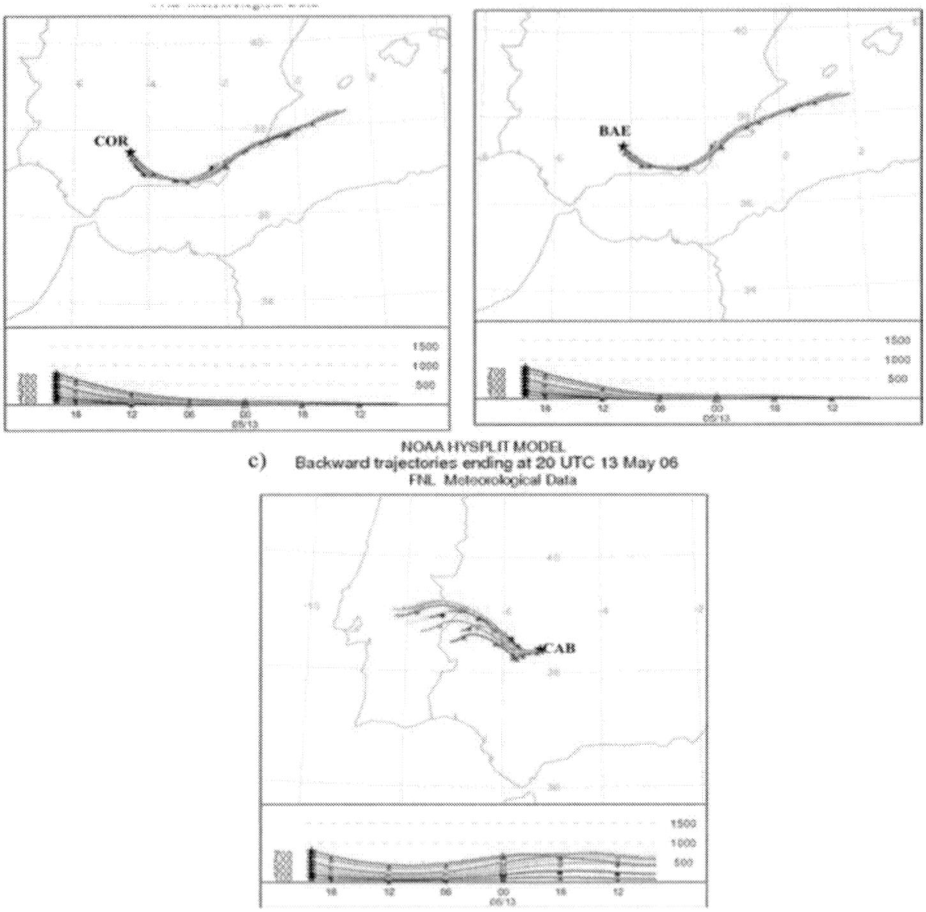

Figure 4. 36-h Back trajectories at 100-m intervals, from 100 m above ground level (a.g.l) to 700 m a.g.l., at a) Córdoba, b) Baena and c) El Cabril sites.

Motivated by these limitations, the topography of the area and the need to calculate trajectories close to the ground due to the low height of pollen displacement, a preliminary study was performed to determine any anomalies in the back-trajectory calculation with respect to height. Back trajectories were plotted at all sites during each episode at heights ranging from 100 m a.g.l to 700 m a.g.l., at 100-m intervals (Figure 4). The results showed that a single trajectory at 500 m a.g.l. could be taken as representative.

It should be noted that, despite this validation, differences might still exist between air mass arrival and the wind direction registered at ground level due to the spatial resolution of the model and the particular topography of the area (Figure 1). However, these potential differences did not alter the value of the trajectories, which in this study were intended to provide information on possible pollen routes rather than on wind conditions at a particular point.

Taking all into account, kinematic three dimensional back-trajectories at a height of 500 m a.g.l have been calculated using the vertical wind component information given by the meteorological files, which is more accurate than other operational methods contained in the model such as the isobaric or isentropic ones (Stohl, 1998b). Back-trajectories of 36 hours with a time-step of 6 hours were computed at different hours at all sites on episode days, in order to detect possible links between the variability and pathways of air mass trajectories and the pollen counts recorded. This temporal coverage of each back-trajectory was decided after testing a range from 24 to 96 hours. The results obtained suggested that the most suitable tool for charting local/regional transport from nearby pollen sources was a back-trajectory of 36 hours.

In Hernández-Ceballos et al. (2011b), by the use of the HYSPLIT model, an air-mass classification over Cordoba city from May to June during the period 2006-2008 was obtained applying a temporal duration of 48-h. Despite the use of 48-h instead of 36-h the increase in computational error is minimal. Considering the representative period of this classification, the set of air masses identified can be taken as reference for 2007.

This classification shows how six air-mass types are mainly influenced, coming from different areas, i.e. expanse in which the air mass was located 48 h prior its arrival over Córdoba city at 500 m.a.g.l (Figure 5) (Hernández-Ceballos et al., 2011b).

Two air masses originating in the Northwest were distinguished between them by the distance covered and by the speed of movement, since the time period was the same in both cases. One was associated with a long distance displacement designated ''Faster Northwest'', whilst the other is coming from an intermediate area closer to the Iberian Peninsula and was designated ''Slower Northwest''.

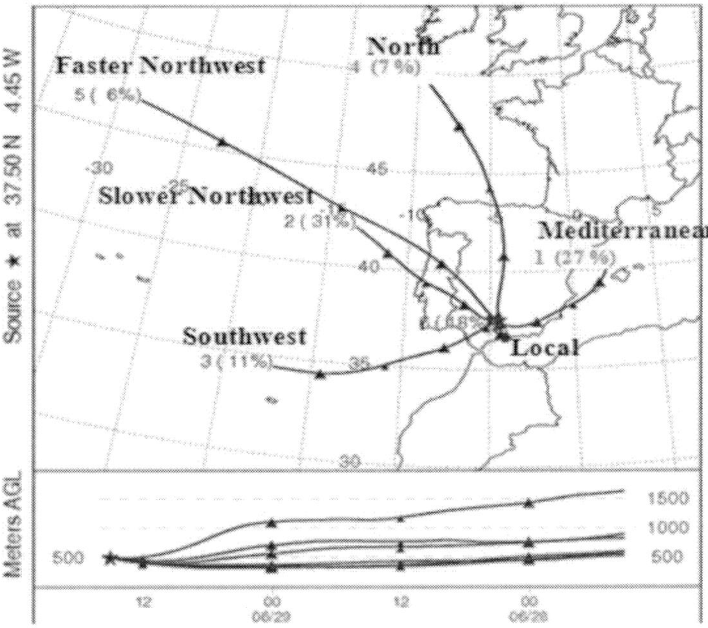

Figure 5. Horizontal and vertical average displacement of the air mass types identified over Cordoba city from May to June during 2006-2008.(Hernández-Ceballos et al., 2011b).

The other faster advection type, designated ''Northern'', originated below the British Isles, with a trajectory from North to South of the Iberian Peninsula. Two air-mass clusters were discerned along the west–east axis of the Iberian Peninsula, one coming in from Atlantic and another one from the Mediterranean, designated ''Southwest'' and "Mediterranean". Finally, the smallest air-mass movement—travelling slowly over Córdoba province— was designated ''Local''. From this set of air masses, the two most persistent are the "Mediterranean" and "Slower Northwest" movements, while the "Faster Northwest" and "Northern" are the least persistent.

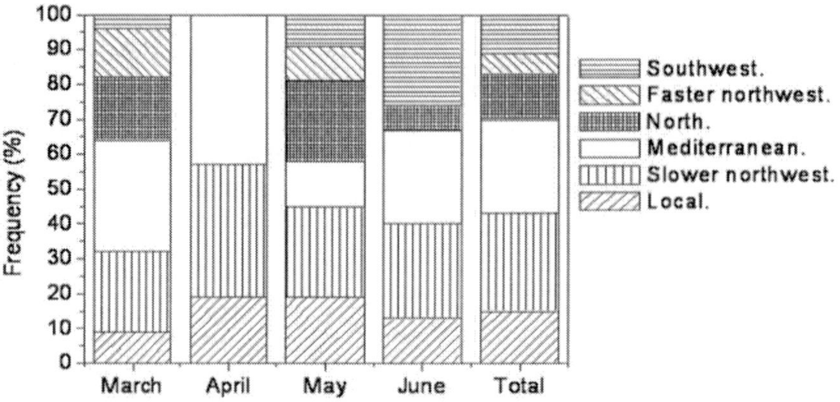

Figure 6. Monthly and total frequency for each type of air mass identified over Cordoba city during 2007.

Figure 6 reveals the monthly and total frequency for each type of air mass identified during 2007 over Cordoba city. Their monthly occurrence from March to June shows how the influence of the Slower Northwest Mediterranean group was clearly marked during the whole months, whilst the Mediterranean had a high frequency with the exception of May. On the other hand, Southwest circulations had a minimum influence in March and April, thereafter increasing from May. Local trajectories displayed a virtually constant frequency all months, whilst the North air-mass was more frequent in March and May and the Faster Northwest occurrence was not detected in April and June.

This air mass behaviour during this period is in agreement with the synoptic configurations prevailing from March to June over the Iberian Peninsula (López Ontiveros 2003). In this sense, the great variation in frequency of the air mass movements with a greater displacement, as North or Faster Northwest, and the tendency to register higher frequency the shorter-range movements, as "Local", "Mediterranean" or "Southwest", is determined by the progressive minimisation of unstable synoptic conditions and the increasing prevalence of stable conditions as summer approaches. Similar air mass monthly behaviour has been reported by Jorbá et al. (2004) and by Toledano et al. (2009).

Taking May as reference to observe the relationships between olive pollen counts and air masses identified over Córdoba city, the results showed that one of the least frequent air-masses movements (Mediterranean) were associated with the highest daily pollen counts (more than 600 pollen grains/m^3), while the rest of circulations were associated with daily counts of less than 200 gr/m^3, excepting the "North" and "Slower Northwest" air masses with daily counts of nearly 250 gr/m^3.

7. Analysis of Episodes

A set of "episode days" have been chosen and analyzed in order to determine the dynamic transport of olive pollen in the province of Cordoba and to trace the potential origin of non-typical intradiurnal patterns. For this purpose, "episode days" included days on which peak pollen counts were chosen, and also days on which high pollen counts were recorded outside the typical hours reported by Galán et al (1991) in a study of the intradiurnal pattern for airborne olive pollen counts in Cordoba, which noted maximum values between 11:00 UTC and 17:00 UTC.

Five episode days were analyzed in order to determine which weather conditions might favour higher pollen counts, and to trace the potential origin of non-typical intradiurnal patterns. Kinematic 3D back-trajectories, isobaric surface maps and bi-hourly pollen measurements at each site during episode days have been used to characterize each episode.

The back trajectory analysis has shown a relationship between travel by air masses and *Olea* pollen concentrations recorded throughout the province of Cordoba. The study of the five episodes has allowed identifying two main types of moving air masses, which are associated with two synoptic configurations on the southern Iberian Peninsula. These two air mass pathways associated with high pollen counts of olive are mainly from the south and the west.

7.1. South Air Mass Movement

Under the influence of anticyclonic conditions or scarce isobaric gradient over the Iberian Peninsula, a slow-moving stream at low altitude from the southern to the central areas of the province has been observed. Three episodes are examples of this type of air mass circulation.

Episode May 9th 2007

The highest pollen counts during this day were recorded at Córdoba (441 gr/m^3) and Priego de Córdoba (340 gr/m^3), with two major peaks, at 10:00 UTC (225 gr/m^3) in Córdoba and at 16:00 UTC (150 gr/m^3) in Priego (Figure 7a).

In addition, from 16:00 UTC the evolucion of the concentrations was opposite, with increasing in Córdoba and decreasing in Priego. In the rest of the emplacement, the olive pollen evolutions were lower, highlighting the increase registered at Baena site during the last hours of the day (Figure 7a).

During this day the backtrajectories reflected a progressive change of the air mass pathways over the province (Figures 7b-d). In the morning a northerly arrival is clearly detected showing a movement from north to south across the Iberian Peninsula, although all of them registering a short displacement from east to west along the province of Córdoba. This movement tended to change along the day, decreasing the displacement of the air masses that affected the south of the province and registering a pathway from the south. It is necessary to point out that this entrance of air masses from the south showed a progressive displacement from west to east.

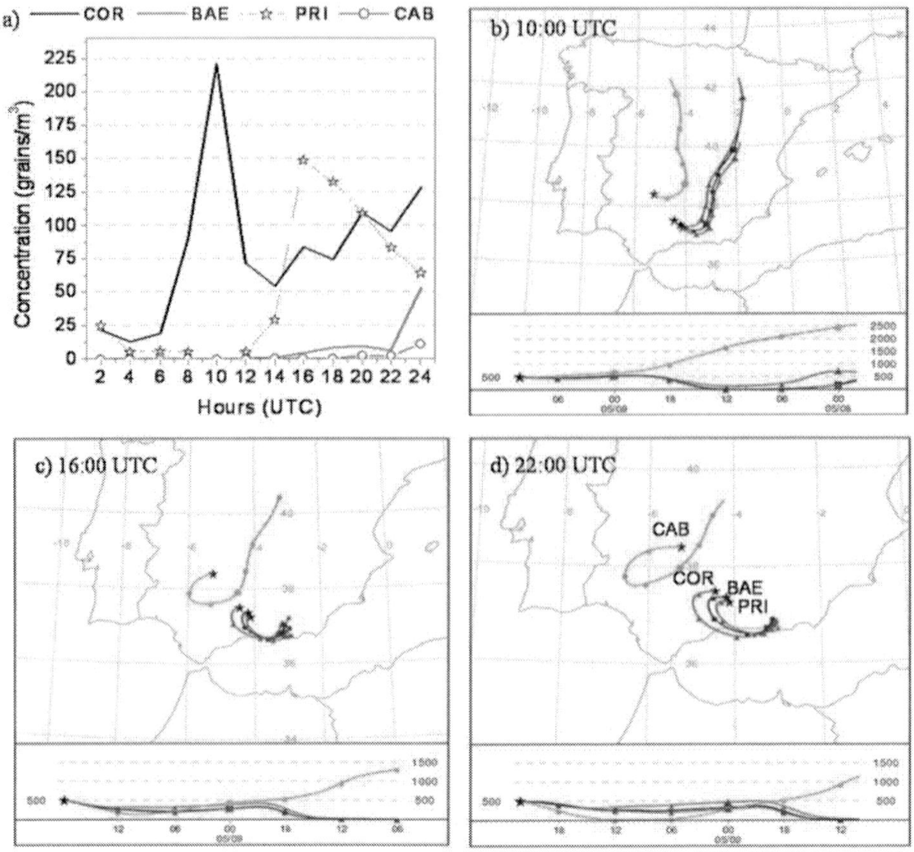

Figure 7. a) Bihourly Olive pollen counts registered at Córdoba (COR), Baena (BAE), Priego de Córdoba (PRI) and El Cabril (CAB) stations in average pollen grains per m^3 of air, 36-h backtrajectory analysis at a height of 500 m at b) 10:00, c) 16:00 and d) 22:00 UTC on 09/05/07 in Córdoba (COR), Baena (BAE), Priego de Córdoba (PRI) and El Cabril (CAB) sites (Hernández-Ceballos et al., 2011a).

Taking into account the peak recorded in Cordoba and in Priego de Córdoba on 9 May 2007 (Figure 7a) could be attributed to local pollen sources, since there were no matching peaks at other stations. However, the temporal evolution of the pollen concentrations in both sites from 16:00 UTC could be revealed a relationship between both sites. In this sense, the decreased in Priego and the following increased in Córdoba could be related with pollen transport from south to north of the province.

Episode May 20th 2007

The highest pollen count of all the episodes studied was recorded at Baena (7724 gr/m^3) (Figure 3) where two major peaks were observed in a single day at 8:00 UTC and 14:00 UTC (Figure 8a). Elsewhere, counts were considerably lower (3123 gr/m^3 at Priego, 1540 gr/m^3 at El Córdoba and 124 gr/m^3 at El Cabril. However, while in El Cabril no intensive peak was detected (Figure 8a), in Cordoba higher counts were recorded during the early hours and in the late afternoon. In addition, similar pollen counts to those registered in Baena were also recorded in Priego de Córdoba but of a lower magnitude.

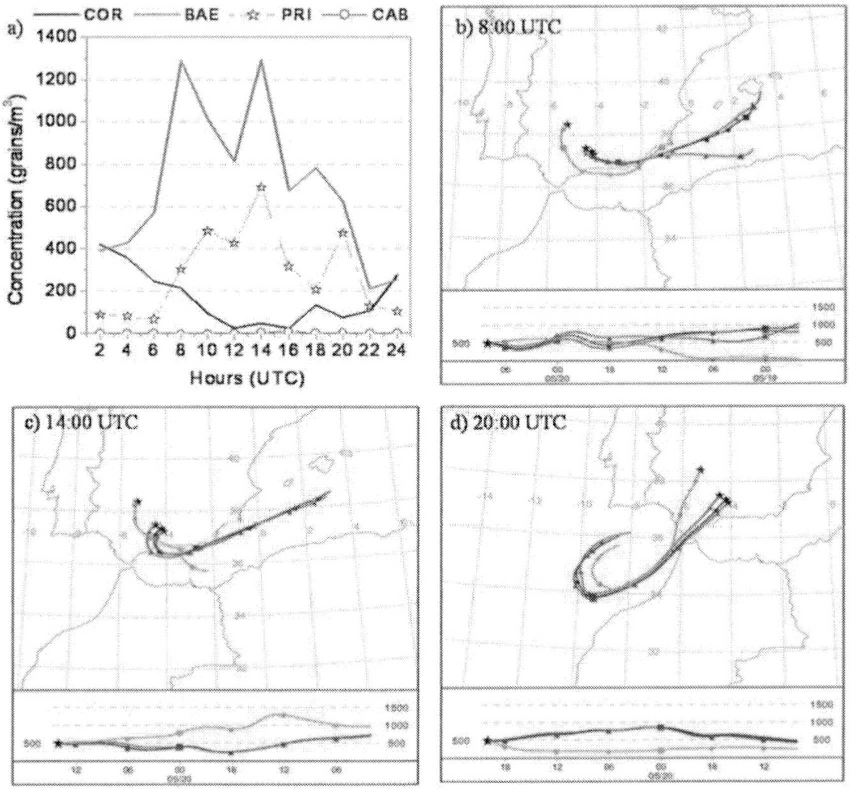

Figure 8. a) Bihourly Olive pollen counts registered at Córdoba (COR), Baena (BAE), Priego de Córdoba (PRI) and El Cabril (CAB) stations in average pollen grains per m^3 of air, 36-h backtrajectory analysis at a height of 500 m at b) 08:00, c) 14:00 and d) 20:00 UTC on 20/05/07 in Córdoba (COR), Baena (BAE), Priego de Córdoba (PRI) and El Cabril (CAB) sites (Hernández-Ceballos et al., 2011a).

Back trajectories originated mainly over the Mediterranean, arriving though the valleys that connect the Guadalquivir valley and the Mediterranean area; the height of air mass movement varied considerably, generally remaining relatively far from the ground except over El Cabril (Figure 8b-d). By the afternoon of that day, however, a strong southwesterly wind prevailed over the whole province. This progressive change reveal the modification in the synoptic configuration along the day, being modified from a weak surface pressure gradient over the Iberian Peninsula, together with relatively unstable conditions at higher levels, to an incipient westerly synoptic wind led to a sharp drop in pollen counts across the whole province.

Given these weather conditions, there are two possible explanations for the high pollen counts and the difference in their timing from one site to another. Due to the progressive increase in pollen counts during the preceding days, the elevated counts recorded in the course of the morning (until 10:00 UTC in Cordoba, at 8:00 UTC in Baena and at 10:00.

UTC in Priego) were probably due to residual airborne pollen from local sources, counts being higher in Baena and Priego owing to the presence of larger local pollen sources. At the same time, there was evidence of regional pollen transport from south to north; a correlation was apparent between the drop in counts in Baena and Priego at 12:00 UTC, and an increase in counts in Córdoba during the afternoon. Later in the day, this correlation disappeared due to the southwesterly synoptic wind, which probably transported pollen from other sources; this would account for the sharp decrease in pollen counts in Baena and Priego.

Episode June 6th 2007

Probably associated with the full flowering period in olive groves to the south of the province, pollen counts ranged from 3800 gr/m^3 in Priego to 1387 gr/m^3 in Baena, while values were considerably lower in Cordoba and El Cabril, At 442 gr/m^3 and 343 gr/m^3, respectively (Figure 9a). Different intensive pollen peaks were registered along the day, at 6:00 UTC (300 gr/m^3) in Baena, and at 10:00 UTC (375 gr/m^3) and 18:00 UTC (475 gr/m^3) in Priego, while in Córdoba the concentrations showed a increased from 6:00 to 20:00 UTC (Figure 9a).

The considerable difference between the amount of pollen recorded at Priego de Córdoba and Baena with the other sites may be due to the proximity of both sites to olive-pollen sources, coinciding with the flowering time of olive trees in this area. In this sense, the higher concentrations in the south of the province may be associated to local flow regimes at different times during the day. However, taking into account the constant air mass pathway from south to center of the province, and the increased in the pollen concentrations registered in Córdoba city along the day, a pollen transport may be identified.

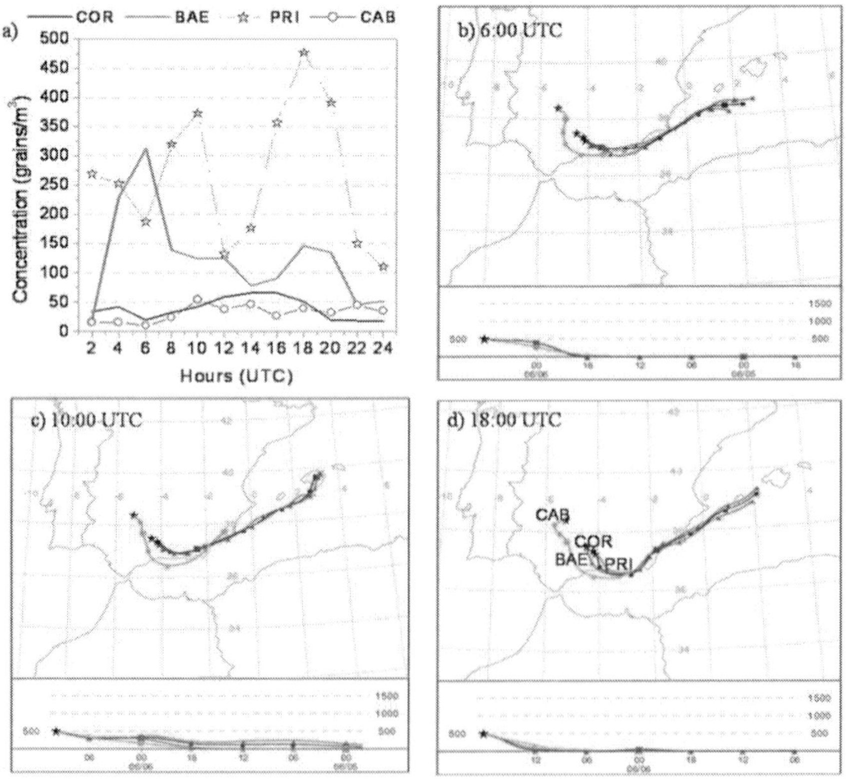

Figure 9. a) Bihourly Olive pollen counts registered at Córdoba (COR), Baena (BAE), Priego de Córdoba (PRI) and El Cabril (CAB) stations in average pollen grains per m^3 of air, 36-h backtrajectory analysis at a height of 500 m at b) 06:00, c) 10:00 and d) 18:00 UTC on 06/06/07 in Córdoba (COR), Baena (BAE), Priego de Córdoba (PRI) and El Cabril (CAB) sites(Hernández-Ceballos et al., 2011a).

As it shown in these examples, this air mass movement is in favour of encouraging entrainment of biological particles near the ground level, and therefore, favored the transport of olive pollen across the province. For this reason, this movement of air masses is associated with high daily levels of pollen in both the southern stations (Baena, Priego de Córdoba), and the city of Cordoba.

These results confirm the hypothesis of Fornaciari et al. (2000) who suggest that crops located in the south may contribute to the pollen curve registered in Cordoba city during the flowering period.

In this sense, this type of analysis should be taken into account when producing pollen forecasts for Cordoba city, since episodes of this kind are to be expected when weather conditions favour wind flows from the south, mainly with stable synoptic configurations. On the other hand, the El Cabril station is mainly subject to the arrival of air masses in the range west / southwest causing that this region is decoupled from the rest of the province. In this sense, the origin of the olive concentrations at El Cabril would not be related with the olive sources located in the south of the province.

7.2. West Air Mass Movement

A second pattern of transport is associated with the influence of atmospheric conditions that favour the advection of synoptic flows from the west. Two episodes are examples of this type of air mass circulation.

Episode May 11th 2007

The progressive change to instability atmospheric conditions over the Iberian Peninsula, associated with the progressive approach of a low pressure centre in the north was reflected by the change in the air mass movement, having on 11 May a constant entrance of winds blowing in from the Atlantic (Figure 10b-d).

During this day, the olive pollen concentration in the province were higher at Córdoba city (419 gr/m^3) and Priego de Córdoba (1200 gr/m^3) sites. However, while in Córdoba there was a peak at 12:00 UTC (300 gr/m^3) in Priego de Córdoba there were two intensive peaks of Olive concentration during the day, at 14:00 UTC (450 gr/m^3) and at 20:00 UTC (400 gr/m^3) (Figure 10a).

On the other hand, the concentrations at Baena were lower than 100 gr/m^3 during the day whilst at El Cabril were insignificant.

Taking into account the prevalence of westerly winds along the day in addition with the pollen evolution, a probable transport could be identified from the center to the south of the province, as shown the peaks in Cordoba at 12:00 UTC and in Priego de Córdoba at 14:00 UTC.

In addition, this hypothesis is supported due to this time coinciding with the flowering season of olive trees in the center of the province. On the other hand the peaks observed in Priego de Córdoba and Baena at 20:00 UTC may be due to local pollen contributions or pollen sources from outside the province, given the air-mass data and the fact that peaks occurred simultaneously at the two sites.

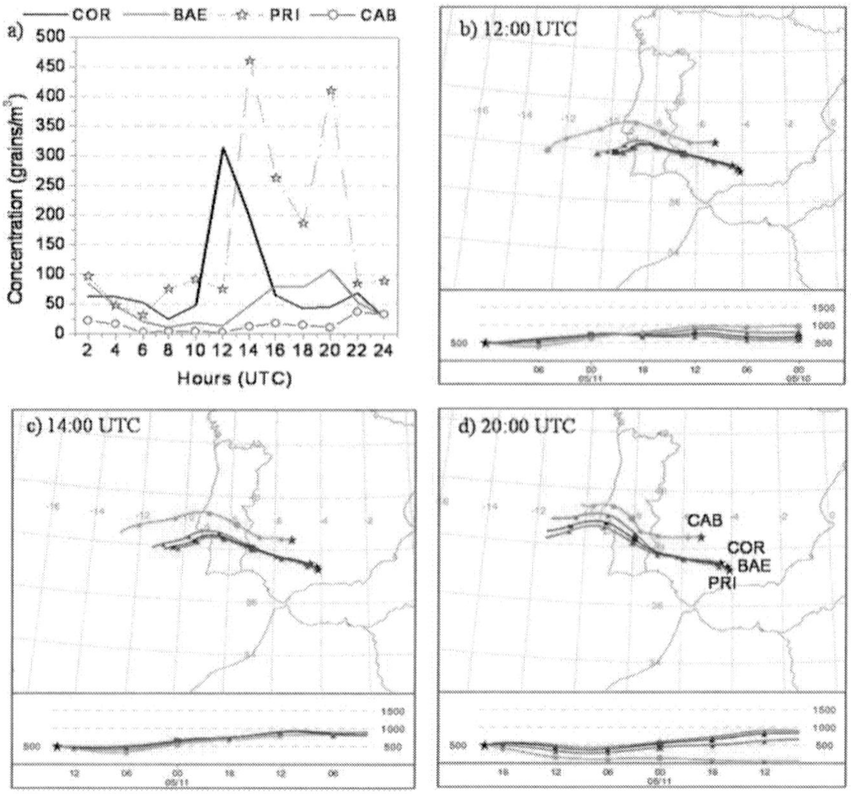

Figure 10. a) Bihourly Olive pollen counts registered at Córdoba (COR), Baena (BAE), Priego de Córdoba (PRI) and El Cabril (CAB) stations in average pollen grains per m^3 of air, 36-h backtrajectory analysis at a height of 500 m at b) 12:00, c) 14:00 and d) 20:00 UTC on 11/05/07 in Córdoba (COR), Baena (BAE), Priego de Córdoba (PRI) and El Cabril (CAB) sites (Hernández-Ceballos et al., 2011a).

Episode May 30th 2007

The outstanding feature of the 30 May episode was the high pollen count recorded at Priego (3,044 gr/m^3), which was twice that at Baena (1,497 gr/m^3) and much higher than the count recorded in El Cabril (478 gr/m^3) and Cordoba (51 gr/m^3) (Figure 11a). Significantly, these high values were the result of a sudden and rapid change in daily pollen counts, coinciding with the flowering season (Figure 3).

The back-trajectory revealed an air mass moving in from the west of the Iberian Peninsula, gradually falling towards the end of the day (Figure 11b-d), due to the confluence of two pressure centres, a ridge of high pressure in the east and a low in the north-western Iberian Peninsula.

In view of the synoptic wind regime, the marked increase in pollen counts at 16:00 UTC in Priego was probably caused by the arrival of air masses from external sources, probably from near Baena, containing a considerable amount of pollen. However, this external input was probably supplemented by pollen from local sources, coinciding with the full flowering period in phenological surveys. Similar causes may account for the peak recorded at El Cabril at 20:00 UTC, which was lower than that observed in the south of the province. However, pollen counts in Córdoba were very low, with no marked intradiurnal curve.

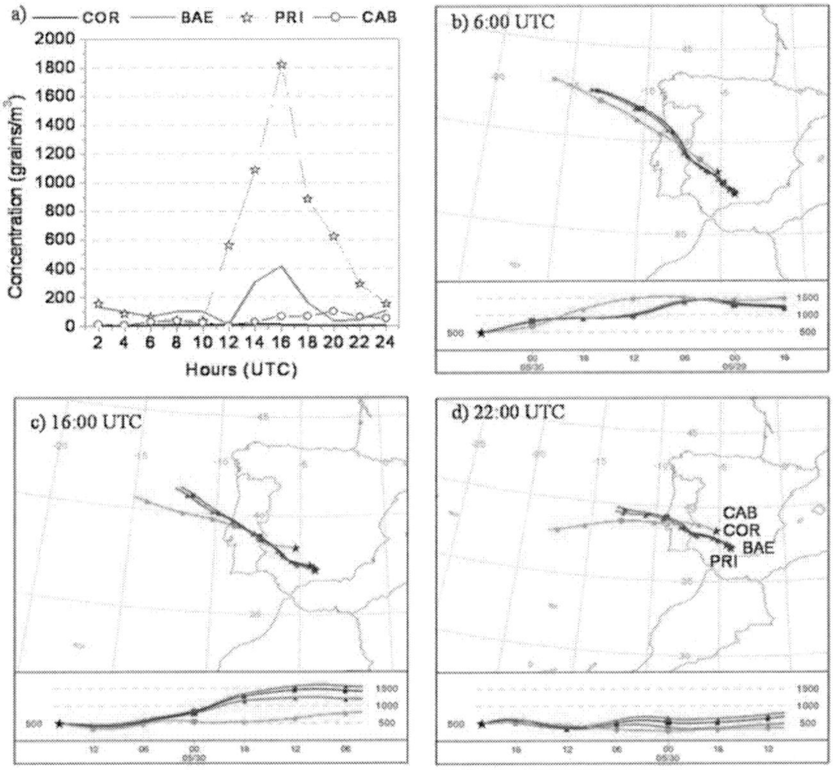

Figure 11. a) Bihourly Olive pollen counts registered at Córdoba (COR), Baena (BAE), Priego de Córdoba (PRI) and El Cabril (CAB) stations in average pollen grains per m^3 of air, 36-h backtrajectory analysis at a height of 500 m at b) 06:00, c) 16:00 and d) 22:00 UTC on 30/05/07 in Córdoba (COR), Baena (BAE), Priego de Córdoba (PRI) and El Cabril (CAB) sites (Hernández-Ceballos et al., 2011a).

During these episode days, as the backtrajectories analysis shown, the prevailing winds in each of the sites are similar, limiting the development of transport phenomena. This air mass movement are related with higher concentrations in the south of the province, in the stations of Baena and Priego de Córdoba. However, when this kind of circulation is detected coinciding with the flowering time in the centre of the province, it is possible to observe pollen transport to the south.

Conclusions

This review analyzes the first results of applying back-trajectory analysis in the characterization of olive-pollen transport dynamics along the Cordoba province, one of the main olive crop areas of the world. In this sense, the use of the HYSPLIT model allow to determine potential pollen sources, to describe pollen transport dynamic and to clarify the real contribution of the different olive-growing areas to airborne pollen counts in Cordoba province.

Five episode days were analyzed in order to determine which weather conditions might favour higher pollen counts, and to trace the potential origin of non-typical intradiurnal patterns. The results obtained show how high pollen counts in stations across Cordoba province are influenced mainly by large pollen sources situated in the south of the province and, to a lesser extent, by small external sources located to the west, prompting a gradient from south to north.

Two main air-mass paths have been identified in relation with intensive pollen peaks: winds from the south exerted greater influence on pollen counts in Baena, Priego and Cordoba city, while southwest/west flows were the prevailing influence at El Cabril. The other air mass movement is pointed out by westerly synoptic flows under unstable conditions. This circulation is related with higher concentrations in the south of the province, in the stations of Baena and Priego de Córdoba, and, in some cases, with transport from centre to south of the province.

Acknowledgments

The authors are grateful to the European Social Fund for co-financing with the Spanish Science Ministry. Dr. García Mozo was supported by a "Ramón y Cajal" contract, and the Andalusia Regional Government funded the project entitled "Modelización y analisis de la influencia de la variación genética en la fenología reproductiva de especies vegetales" (PO6-RNM-02195).

References

Alba, F., Díaz de la Guardia, C. (1998). The effect of air temperature on the starting dates of the Ulmus, Platanus and *Olea* pollen seasons in the SE Iberian Peninsula. *Aerobiologia* 14: 191 – 194.

Borge, R., Lumbreras, J., Vardoulakis, S., Kassomeno, P., Rodríguez, E. (2007). Analysis of long-range transport influences on urban PM10 using two-stage atmospheric trajectory clusters. *Atmospheric Environment*, 41, 4434-4450.

Bousquet, J., Guerin, B., Hewitt, B., Lim, S., Michel, F.B. (1985). Allergy in the Mediterranean area. III: cross-reactivity among Oleaceae pollens. *Clinical and Experimental Allergy*, 15, 439-48.

Burgos, F. (1991). Pólenes y Medio ambiente: sensibilizaciones polínicas en Andalucía. *In: 20e Reun. Asoc. Alergo. Inmuno. Sur Huelva 1991. Actas (ed. Org.Comm.)*, 134- 141. AAIS, Seville.

Cabezudo, B., Recio, M., Sánchez-Laulhé, J.M., Trigo, M.M., Toro, F.J., Polvorines, F. (1997). Atmospheric transportation of marihuana pollen from North Africa to the Southwest of Europe. *Atmospheric Environment* 31: 3323-3328.

Cariñanos, P., Sánchez-Mesa, J.A., Prieto-Baena, J.C., Lopez, A., Guerra, F., Moreno, C., Domínguez, E., Galan, C. (2002). Pollen allergy related to the area of residence in the city of Córdoba, south-west Spain. *Journal of Environmental Monitoring*, 4, 734-738.

Cecchi, L., Torrigiani Malaspina, T., Albertini, R., Zanca, M., Ridolo, E., Usberti, I., Morabito, M., Dall'Aglio, P., Orlandini, S. (2007). The contribution of long-distance transport to the presence of *Ambrosia* pollen in central northern Italy. *Aerobiologia*, 23, 145-151.

Chuine, I., Cour, P., Rousseau, D.D. (1999). Selecting models to predict the timing of flowering of temperate trees: implications for tree phenology modelling. *Plant, Cell and Environment*, 22, 1-13.

De la Guardia, C., Alba, F., Trigo, M.M., Galán, C., Ruíz, L., Sabariego, S. (2003). Aerobiological analysis of *Olea* europaea L. pollen in different localities of southern Spain. *Grana*, 42, 234-243.

De Linares, C., Nieto-Lugilde, D., Alba, F., Díaz de la Guardia, C., Galán, C., Trigoz, M.M. (2007). Detection of airborne allergen (Ole e 1) in relation to *Olea* europaea pollen in S Spain. *Clinical and Experimental Allergy*, 37, 125-132.

Domínguez, E., Infante, F., Galán, C., Guerra, F., Villamandos, F. (1993). Variations in the concentrations of airborne *Olea* pollen and associated pollinosis in Córdoba (Spain): A study of the 10- years period 1982 – 1991. *Journal of Investigational Allergology and Clinical Immunology*, 3, 121-129.

Draxler, R. R., and Hess, G. D. (1998). An overview of the HYSPLIT_4 modelling system for trajectories, dispersion, and deposition. *Australian Meteorology Magazine*, 47, 295-308.

Draxler, R.R., Stunder, B., Rolph, G., Taylor, A. (2009). HYSPLIT_4 User's Guide. NOAA Air Resources Laboratory. http://www.arl.noaa.gov/ documents/reports/hysplit_user_guide.pdf.

Florido, J. F., González Delgado, P., Saenz de San Pedro, B., Quiralte, J., Arias de Saavedra, J. M., Peralta, V., Ruiz Valenzuela, L. (1999). High levels of Olea europaea pollen and relation with clinical findings. *International Archives of Allergy and Immunology*, 119, 133-137.

Fornaciari, M., Galán, C., Mediavilla, A., Domínguez, E., Romano, B. (2000). Aeropalynological and phenological study in two different olive Mediterranean areas: Córdoba (Spain) and Perugia (Italia). *Plant Biosystems*, 134, 199-204.

Fornaciari, M., Orlandi, F., Romano, B. (2005). Yield forecasting for olive trees: a new approach in a historical series (Umbria, Central Italy). *Journal of Agronomy and Crop Science*, 97,1537-1542.

Fornaciari, M., Pieroni, L., Cichi, P., Romano, B. (1997). A statistical model for correlating airborne pollen grains (*Olea europaea* L.) with some meteorological parameters. *Mediterranean Agriculture*, 27, 134-137.

Fornaciari, M., Pieroni, L., Giuchi, P., Romano, B. (1998). A regresion model for the start of the pollen season in *Olea* europaea L. *Grana*, 37,110-113.

Frenguelli, G., Bricchi, E., Romano, B., Mincigrucci, G., Spieksma, FThM. (1989). A predictive study on the beginning of the pollen season for Gramineae and *Olea europaea* L. *Aerobiologia*, 1, 64-70.

Galán, C., Cariñanos, P., Alcázar, P., Domínguez, E. (2007). *Management and Quality Manual. Spanish Aerobiology Network (REA)*. Servicio Publicaciones Universidad de Córdoba, Córdoba, Spain. ISBN 978-84-690-6353-8.

Galán, C., Cariñanos, P., García-Mozo, H., Alcázar, P., Domínguez- Vilches, E. (2001a). Model for forecasting *Olea* europaea L. airborne pollen in the South-West Andalucía, Spain. *International Journal of Biometeorology*, 45, 59-63.

Galán, C., García-Mozo, H., Cariñanos, P., Alcázar, P., Domínguez- Vilches, E. (2001b) The role of temperature in the onset of the *Olea europaea* L. pollen season in southwestern Spain. *International Journal of Biometeorology*, 45, 8–12.

Galán, C., García-Mozo, H., Vázquez, L., Ruiz, L., Díaz de la Guardia, C., Trigo, M.M. (2005). Heat requirement for the onset of the *Olea europaea* L. pollen season in several sites in Andalusia and the effect of the expected future climate change. *International Journal of Biometeorology*, 49,184-188.

Galán, C., Tormo, R., Cuevas, J., Infante, F., Domínguez, E. (1991). Theoretical daily variation patterns of airbone pollen in the southwest of Spain. *Grana*, 30, 201-209.

García-Mozo, H., Galán, C., Jato, V., Belmonte, J., Díaz de la Guardia, C., Fernández, D., Gutiérrez, M., Aira, M.J., Roure, J.M., Ruiz, L., Trigo, M.M., Domínguez-Vilches, E. (2006). Quercus pollen season dynamics in the Iberian Peninsula: response to meteorological parameters and possible consequences of climate change. *Annal of Agricultural and Environmental Medicine*, 13, 209-224.

Garcia-Mozo, H., Orlandi, F., Galán, C., Fornaciari, M., Romano, B., Ruiz, L., Diaz de la Guardia, C., Trigo, M.M., Chuine, I. (2009). Olive flowering phenology variation between different cultivars in Spain and Italy: modeling analysis. *Theoretical and Applied Climatology*, 95, 385-395.

García-Mozo, H., Perez-Badía, R., Galán, C. (2008). Aerobiological and meteorological factors' influence on olive (*Olea* europaea L.) crop yield in Castilla-La Mancha (Central Spain). *Aerobiologia*, 24, 13-18.

Gassmann, I. M., and Pérez, F. C. (2006). Trajectories associated to regional and extra-regional pollen transport in the southeast of Buenos Aires province, Mar del Plata (Argentina). *International Journal of Biometeorology*, 50, 280-291.

Geßler, A., Keitel, C., Kreuzwieser, J., Matyssek, R., Seiler, W., Rennenberg, H. (2007). Potential risks for European beech (*Fagus sylvatica* L.) in a changing climate. *Trees*, 21, 1–11.

González-Minero, F.J., Candau Fernández-Mensaque, P. (1996). Prediction of the beginning of the olive full pollen season in southwest Spain. *Aerobiologia*, 12, 91-96.

Hernández-Ceballos, M.A., García-Mozo, H, Adame, J.A., Domínguez-Vilches, E., De la Morena, B.A., Bolívar, J.P., Galán, C. (2011a). Synoptic and meteorological characterization of olive pollen transport in Cordoba province (South-western Spain). *International Journal of Biometeorology*, 55, 17-34.

Hernández-Ceballos, M.A., García-Mozo, H., Adame, J.A., Domínguez-Vilches, E., Bolívar, J.P., De la Morena, B.A., Pérez-Badía, R., Galán, C. (2011b). Determination of potential sources of *Quercus* airborne pollen in Córdoba city (southern Spain) using back-trajectory analysis. *Aerobiologia*. DOI: 10.1007/s10453-011-9195-1.

Hirst, J. (1952). An automatic volumetric spore-trap. Annal of Applied Biology, 36, 257-265.

Hondula, D.M., Sitka, L., Davis, R.E., Knight, D.B., Gawtry, S.D., Deaton, M.L., Lee, T.R., Normile, C., Stenger, P.J. (2010). A back-trajectory and air mass climatology for the Northern Shenandoah Valley, USA. *International Journal of Climatology. Published online (www.interscience.wiley.com)*. DOI: 10.1002/joc.1896.

Jorba, O., Pérez, C., Rocandenbosch, F., Baldasano, J. M. (2004). Cluster analysis of 4-day back trajectories arriving in the Barcelona area (Spain) from 1997 to 2002. *Journal of Applied Meteorology*, 43, 887-901.

Liccardi, G., D'Amato, M., D'Amato, G. (1996). Oleaceae pollinosis: a review. *International Archives of Allergy and Immunology*, 111, 210-217.

López Ontiveros, A. (coord). (2003). *Geografía de Andalucía*. Editorial Ariel Geografía.

Lozano, R.L., Hernández-Ceballos, M.A., Adame, J.A., Casas-Ruíz, M., Sorribas, M., San Miguel, E.G., Bolívar, J.P. (2011). Atmospheric routes involved in the radioactive impact of Fukushima accident on the Iberian Peninsula. *Environmental Internacional*, DOI: 10.1016/j.envint.2011.06.001.

Mahura, G. A., Korsholm, S. U., Baklanov, A. A., Rasmussen, A. (2007). Elevated birch pollen episodes in Denmark: Contributions from remote sources. *Aerobiologia*, 23, 171-179.

Maillard, R. (1975). *L'olivier*. INVUFLEC. Paris, France.

Marchuk, G. I. (1982). *Mathematical modeling in the environmental problems*. Moscow: ''Nauka'' publisher. (320 pp, in Russian).

Martínez Cañavate, A., Barbero, A., De Mayo, P., Sánchez Calderón, P. (1995). Estudio epidemiológico en la Unidad de alergia infantil en el área hospitalaria norte. – *In 12e Reun. Asoc. Pediatría Andalucía Occ. Extremadura and Andalucía Orient. Granada 1995. Actas (ed. Org. Comm.)*, 171- 179. APAOE, Sevilla.

Miller, J. (1981). A five-year climatology of five-day back-trajectories from Barrow, Alaska. *Atmospheric Environment*, 15, 1401-1405.

Orlandi, F., Garcia-Mozo, H., Galán, C., Romano, B., Diaz de la Guardia, C., Ruiz, L., Trigo, M.M., Dominguez-Vilches, E., Fornaciari, M. (2010). Olive flowering trends in a large Mediterranean area (Italy and Spain). *International Journal of Biometeorology*, 54, 151-163.

Pérez-Landa, G., Ciais, P., Gangoiti, G., Palau, J. L., Carrara, A., Gioli, B., et al. (2007b). Mesoscale circulations over complex terrain in the Valencia coastal region, Spain–Part 2: Modeling CO2 transport using idealized surface fluxes. *Atmospheric Chemistry and Physics*, 7, 1851-1868.

Pérez-Landa, G., Ciais, P., Sanz, M. J., Gioli, B., Miglietta, F., Palau, J. L., et al. (2007a). Mesoscale circulations over complex terrain in the Valencia coastal region, Spain–Part 1: Simulation of diurnal circulation regimes. *Atmospheric Chemistry and Physics*, 7, 1851-1868.

Petzold, A., Rasp, K., Weinzierl, B., Esselborn, M., Hamburger, T., Dornbrack, A., Kandler, K., Schutz, L., Knippertz, P., Fiebig, M., Virkkula, A. (2009). Saharan dust absorption and refractive indez from aircraft-based observation during SAMUM 2006. *Tellus*, 618, 118-130.

Recio, M., Cabezudo, B., Trigo, M,M., Toro, J. (1997). Accumulative air temperature as a predicting parameter for daily airborne olive pollen (*Olea* europaea L.) during the pre-peak period in Málaga (Western Mediterranean area). *Grana*, 36, 44-48.

Recio, M., Cabezudo, B., Trigo, M. M., Toro, F. J. (1996). *Olea* europaea L. pollen in the atmosphere of Málaga (S. Spain) and its relationship with meteorological parameters. *Grana,* 35, 307-312.

Sánchez-Mesa, J.A., Brandao, R., Lopes, L., Galan, C. (2005). Correlation between pollen counts and symptoms in two different areas of the Iberian Peninsula: Cordoba (Spain) and Evora (Portugal). *Journal of Investigational Allergology and Clinical Immunology*, 15, 112-116.

Sauliene, I., and Veriankaite, L. (2006). Application of backward air mass trajectory analysis in evaluating airborne pollen dispersion. *Journal of Environmental Engineering and Landscape Management*, XIV(3), 113-120.

Seinfeld, J. H., and Pandis, S. N. (2006). *Atmospheric Chemistry and Physics: From air pollution to climate change*. New York: John Wiley and Sons.

Siljamo, P., Sofiev, M., Severova, E., Ranta, H., Kukkonen, J., Polevova, S. (2008). Sources, impact and exchange of early-spring birch pollen in the Moscow region and Finland. *Aerobiologia*, doi:10.1007/s10453-008-9100-8.

SkjØth, C., Sommer, J., Brandt, J., Hvidberg, M., Geels, C., Hansen, K., et al. (2008). Copenhagen–a significant source of birch (*Betula*) pollen?. *International Journal of Biometeorology*, 52(6), 453-462.

Smith, M., Emberlin, J., Kress, A. (2005). Examining high magnitude grass pollen episodes at Worcester, United Kingdom, using backtrajectory analysis. *Aerobiología* , 21, 85-94.

Sofiev, M., Siljamo, P., Ranta, H., Rantio-Lehtimaki, A. (2006a). Towards numerical forecasting of long-range air transport of birch pollen: Theoretical considerations and a feasibility study. *International Journal of Biometeorology*, 50, 392-402.

Sofiev, M., Siljamo, P., Valkama, I., Ilvonen, M., and Kukkonen, J. (2006b). A dispersion modelling system SILAM and its evaluation against ETEX data. *Atmospheric Environment*, 40, 674-685.

Stach, A., Smith, M., SkjØth, C., Brandt, J. (2007). Examining Ambrosia pollen episodes at Poznan (Poland) using back-trajectory analysis. *International Journal of Biometeorology*, 51, 275-286.

Stohl, A., Hittenberger, M., Wotawa, G. (1998a). Validation of the Lagrangian particle dispersion model FLEXPART against large scale tracer experiments. *Atmospheric Environment*, 32, 4245-4264.

Stohl., A. (1998b). Computation, accuracy and applications of trajectories- A review and bibliography. *Atmospheric Environment*, 32, 947-966.

Toledano, C., Cachorro, V. E., de Frutos, A. M., Torres, B., Berjon, A., Sorribas, M., et al. (2009). Airmass classification and analysis of aerosols types at El Arenosillo. *Journal of Applied Meteorology and Climatology*, 48, 962-981.

Van de Water, K. P. and Levetin, E. (2001). Contribution of upwind pollen sources to the characterization of *Juniperus ashei* phenology. *Grana*, 40, 133-141.

Vázquez, L.M., Galán, C., Domínguez-Vilches, E. (2003). Influence of meteorological parameters on *Olea* pollen concentrations in Córdoba (South-western Spain). *International Journal of Biometeorology*, 48, 83-90.

Veriankaite, L., Siljamo, P., Sofiev, M., Sauliene, I., Kukkonen, J. (2010). Modelling analysis of source regions of long-range transported birch pollen that influences allergenic seasons in Lithuania. *Aerobiologia*, 26, 47-62.

Vogel, H., Pauling, A., Vogel, B. (2008). Numerical simulation of birch pollen dispersion with an operational weather forecast system. *International Journal of Biometeorology*, 52, 805-814.

In: Olive Consumption and Health
Editors: C. A. Savalas and S. M. Nicolau

ISBN: 978-1-62100-774-6

Chapter 7

FRYING WITH OLIVE OIL AND HEALTH

Sodeif Azadmard-Damirchi ***and Shiva Emami***
Department of Food Science and Technology,
Faculty of Agriculture, University of Tabriz, Tabriz, Iran

ABSTRACT

Frying is one of the most widely spread culinary methods in developed countries, whether in home, institutional, or industrial cooking. Frying is also a means of preserving food. Frying oils are subjected to various alterations such as hydrolysis and thermal oxidation during deep frying, which generate a large number of compounds due to high temperature. As frying oil becomes part of the food being fried, the quality of frying oil is of a great importance due to absorption of those compounds into the food during frying, thereby affecting the quality of the final products. Therefore, frying oil must have high oxidative stability during long-term use. Each vegetable oil has a characteristic stability against oxidation depending on the fatty acid composition and the content and composition of antioxidants and other minor components. Minor lipid components such as certain types of phytosterols, phenolic compounds and tocopherols play an important role in vegetable oil stability, both during frying operations and in the oxidative stability of the fried products. Substantial quantities of refined olive oil and refined olive-pomace oil are produced every year; therefore, they can be alternative frying oil for industrial applications. From a nutritional stand-point in particular, the low amount of saturated fatty acids and the high amount of oleic acid in olive oil are important advantages. Therefore, frying with olive oil can offer possibilities of lowering fat intake and improving the quality of fat actually consumed, which are important in preventing cardiovascular and other diseases.

Keywords: Antioxidant, frying, health, olive oil, oxidation

---

* Corresponding author:
Department of Food Science and Technology,
Faculty of Agriculture, University of Tabriz,
Tabriz 51664, Iran, Phone: + 98-411 3392032, Fax: + 98- 411 3345332
E-mail: s-azadmard@tabrizu.ac.ir, azadmardd@yahoo.com.

INTRODUCTION

Frying is one of the oldest food preparation processes that dates back as early as 1600 BC [Sahin and Gülüm Sumnu, 2009]. It is one of the most widely spread culinary methods in developed countries, whether in home, institutional, or industrial cooking, which palatability and short preparation time of fried foods contribute to its popularity [Varela and Ruiz-Roso, 2000].

During food frying, the hot frying fat penetrates into food and replaces part of the water, exerting a tenderizing effect on the crust, as well as a wetting effect on the food, and thus contributes for the popularity of deep fried foods, namely, their flavor, crispness and pleasant eating characteristics. The typical fried flavor is mainly due to lipid degradation products originating from frying oils. The volatile oxidation products of linoleic acid such as dienals, alcanals, lactones, hydrocarbons, and various cyclic compounds are the most important flavor compounds found in fried foods [Ghidurus *et al.*, 2010].

Frying is also a means of preserving food because in the process, heat destroys micro-organisms, inactives enzymes and reduces surface water activity [Quaglia and Bucarelli, 2001]. In addition, despite the common belief, frying process is considered to have almost the same or even less effect on nutrient losses compared to other cooking methods. However, the nutritive value of food may even increase due to the absorption of frying oils, which are rich in unsaturated fatty acids and vitamin E [Kalogeropoulos *et al.*, 2007]. Nevertheless, during the frying process, the oil or fat is exposed to high temperature in air and moisture. Under these conditions, a complex series of reactions takes place, resulting in the loss of quality of the frying oil and of the fried food [Velasco *et al.*, 2009]. In this chapter, different types of frying, using olive oil as frying oil, changes in olive oil composition during frying and health issues are discussed.

FRYING

There are two kinds of frying including deep frying: cooking of food submersed in hot fat or oil; shallow frying: cooking of food in shallow fat or oil in a pan [Quaglia and Bucarelli, 2001].

Of the mentioned methods, deep frying is the most often subject to technological study. This is because it is widely applied in industrial production and demands constant plant control. In deep frying, fat or oil is exposed for long periods to heat stress [Quaglia and Bucarelli, 2001]. During the deep fat frying process, oil is continuously or repeatedly subjected to high temperatures, 160–190°C, in the presence of air and moisture, which cause a variety of oil degradation reactions such as autoxidation, thermal polymerisation, thermal oxidation and hydrolysis. During frying, food can introduce various components in the oil, such as carbohydrates, phosphates, sulphur compounds, trace metals, etc., which many of them contribute to color formation and other changes, that can be deleterious, in the frying medium by reacting with the oil or its breakdown products [Kochhar, 2001]. The rate of fat degradation depends on many variables involved in the frying process, which some of them are linked to the process (e.g., temperature, length of heating, continuous or discontinuous heating, turnover rate), to the food (i.e., lipid composition, main and minor constituents) or to the oil or fat (e.g., degree of unsaturation, initial quality and additives) [Velasco *et al.*, 2009].

However, deep fat frying has significant advantages over other cooking methods: the temperature within the product (aside from the crust region) is below 100^0; the frying time is short and there is insolubility of water-soluble vitamins. Therefore, less deterioration is expected to heat-sensitive vitamins, in comparison with baking or boiling [Ghidurus *et al.*, 2010]. For example, deep frying is shown to retain the vitamins B_1, B_2, B_3 and C better than boiling, steaming and stewing in some foods. Also after frying of vegetable food, breaded meat, poultry and fish, the content of protein, carbohydrates and minerals is nearly fully retained while boiling and steaming can reduce the mineral content by 25-50% [Bognár, 1998].

During frying the frying oils decompose to form a variety of volatile compounds as well as monomeric and polymeric products. Several factors, such as contact with air, temperature and length of heating, type of frying vessel, degree of oil unsaturation, and presence of pro-oxidants or anti-oxidants, affect the overall performance of frying oils by diminishing their original characteristics. The most marked changes found in triglyceride fatty acids from frying oils during thermoxidation or frying are the decrease in unsaturated fatty acids, the increase of trans-isomers at high temperatures and the formation of short-chain fatty acid triglycerides, namely heptanoate and octanoate [Andrikopoulos *et al.*, 2002].

Interaction between food and the frying medium during deep-frying involves many physical and chemical modifications in both the oil and the food, among which physical changes stand out. Main physical changes include surface dehydration by continuous evaporation of food moisture, lipid exchanges in the two directions, i.e. used frying oil absorption by the food and migration of food lipids into the frying oil, and distillation of flavor compounds. These changes are the main contributors to the texture and odor of fried foods as well as to its caloric value. Chemical reactions between main food constituents and between oxidation compounds and proteins or amino acids seem to be the most important pathways for formation of compounds responsible for color and flavor [Dobarganes *et al.*, 2000].

The main reactions contributing to the golden color of fried products are considered to be produced by protein-carbohydrates reactions, i.e. the non-enzymatic browning (Maillard reaction); however, lipids can also play a role in Maillard reaction. Particularly, the reaction of lipid oxidation products with amines, aminoacids, and proteins has long been related to the browning observed in many foods during processing and storage. The intensity of browning has been primarily correlated with losses of lysine, histidine, and methionine while the main reactive compounds from lipids are aldehydes, epoxides, hydroxyketones, and dicarbonylic compounds [Dobarganes *et al.*, 2000]. The formation of acrylamide, which is a potential carcinogen, is also linked to Maillard reactions. Gelatinization of starch, denaturation of proteins, inactivation of enzymes, and destruction of microorganisms are also observed in the product being fried depending on its constituents, as in other food processes (e.g., drying, baking). However, various flavor components found in fried products are not developed during other cooking methods such as baking [Sahin and Gülüm Sumnu, 2009].

Water loss and oil absorption in a certain food are interrelated as the pressure inside the food is greater than that outside and limits penetration of the frying oil. Water loss and fat absorption clearly depend on both food and frying oil. With respect to the food, many variables affect the final composition of the finished fried product. Among them, food composition, in particular the surface structure and composition, moisture, lipid content, product shape, surface-to-weight ratio, porosity, and pre-frying treatment have been reported. As an example, even for a single non-lipid food, like potatoes, oil absorption and water loss strongly depend on the potato specific gravity – oil uptake being lower as the specific gravity increases – as well as on the surface-to-weight ratio exposed to the frying medium – the larger the ratio the higher the oil absorption. In the case of fatty foods, it has been shown that lipid exchanges as well as final lipid composition and quality might be very different in different types of fatty foods including: (i) natural fatty foods, i.e. fish or meat, which are normally coated by batter or bread and are characterised by a low content of lipids on their surface, and (ii) the increasing group of frozen pre-fried foods (potatoes, fish, vegetables, etc.) where the fat or oil is mainly located on the surface. [Dobarganes *et al.*, 2000].

With regard to the frying oil, as it becomes part of the food being fried, the quality of the frying oil is of great importance with regard to quality of the fried food [Rossi *et al.*, 2007]. Oil absorption depends on the frying oil quality more than on the oil or fat used for frying. Influence of oil quality is attributed to formation of degradation compounds which increases the polarity of the frying medium. On the one hand, the oil viscosity increases after several times of frying, which in turn could contribute to increase the amount of oil on the food surface and, on the other hand, the interfacial tension between the food and the oil would decrease, thus facilitating oil absorption [Dobarganes *et al.*, 2000].

Nevertheless, oil uptake can be modified by steam treatment to remove external oil or pre-drying. On the other hand, many foods are subjected to frying after modification of the surface by a cover of bread or batter which modify water loss and lipid interchange in fatty foods [Dobarganes *et al.*, 2000]. Coating of potatoes with hydrocolloids and/or modified starches is also an alternative way to reduce oil uptake during frying. Furthermore, incorporation of powdered cellulose or cellulose derivatives into batters or doughnut mixes reduces oil uptake due to their thermal gelation and film-forming properties. In addition, alternative frying technologies such as vacuum, pressure or microwave frying to reduce the oil content of these products appear promising [Sahin and Gülüm Sumnu, 2009].

There are many types of oils and fats available for frying. Generally, palm oil or slightly hydrogenated palm oil is used for producing pre-fried French fries, frozen chips and other convenience foods. Increasingly, palm olein because of its good performance due to natural high oxidative stability is becoming the oil of choice for the major snack food manufacturers in many EU countries, whilst the more unsaturated oil products or special long-life oils containing blends of hydrogenated oils are usually used by caterers and fast-food service industry [Kochhar, 2001].

Industrial frying oils should have high oxidative stability, high smoke point, low foaming, low melting point, bland flavor and nutritional value [Kochhar, 2001]. Crude vegetable oils contain a variety of minor components, such as hydrocarbons, sterols, tocopherols, polyphenols, color compounds and trace metals. Some of these components, e.g. tocopherols (particularly γ-tocopherol), phospholipids (at less than 100 mg/ kg), carotenoids (at low levels), squalene, and certain sterols, are beneficial to oil stability during frying [Rossi *et al.*, 2007]. It has been shown that olive oil has a remarkable stability during domestic deep frying or in other uses that require frying temperatures. Deep frying in olive oil offers a means to improve the profile of lipid intake [Varela, 1992], moreover, shallow frying of vegetables in virgin olive oil can be result in fried food enriched with α-tocopherol, terpenic acids and polyphenols, mainly tyrosol [Kalogeropoulos *et al.*, 2007]. Deep fat frying has both advantages and disadvantages related to olive oil degradation. The low oxygen exposure of the oil and a short cooking time reduce the potential for lipid peroxidation. However, because the oil is more likely to be re-used, accumulation of polymeric compounds occurs as the antioxidant capacity is being reduced. Compared to other oils, olive oil has a relatively long deep fat frying "shelf-life" and is comparatively more stable than other oils for repeated frying. Because exchange between lipids in the food and the oil occurs during cooking, the type of food fried also plays a role. For example, frying fish increases the oil's instability because the oil becomes enriched with polyunsaturated fatty acids, which are more susceptible to oxidative degradation than monounsaturated fatty acids (MUFA). Although frying foods with a high protein content such as meat, fish, and eggs can potentially produce carcinogenic heterocyclic amines (HCAs); however, the antioxidants present in olive oil limit the formation of HCAs [Waterman and Lockwood, 2007]. Also, when meat is cooked in olive oil there is a favorable change in saturated to polyunsaturated fatty acids ratio [Boskou, 2006].

Deep frying in olive oil also offers a means to improve the profile of lipid intake [Varela, 1992]. Table 1 shows changes in significant fatty acids after frying pre-fried potatoes, pre-fried hake, and sardines in olive oil to remark the differences between natural fatty foods and pre-fried foods. As it can be observed, the amounts of selected fatty acids in the fried potatoes and hake were very similar to those present in olive oil while in the case of sardines almost 50% of their characteristic fatty acids (C14:0 and C22:6) remained in the fried product. [Dobarganes *et al.*, 2000]. Because foods of plant origin absorb more than foods of animal origin, for example the highest fat uptake has been observed in fried vegetables, such as peeled eggplant, tomatoes, onion, mushrooms and flesh pineapple. The fat intake of peeled potatoes has been shown to be 19.4% after 70 seconds, which is higher than the fat intake of fried chicken, meat, fish or prawns. Low fat changes have also been determined in frying beef, pork, lamb or sausages [Ghidurus *et al.*, 2010].

Table 1. Quantitation of significant fatty acids before and after frying different fatty foods in olive oil

Sample	C14:0	C18:1	C18:2	C22:6
Before frying				
Olive oil	-	76.3	8.3	-
Potatoes	-	40.9	2.9	-
Hake	-	28.9	52.8	-
Sardines	6.6	13.2	1.2	11.5
After frying				
potatoes	-	73.4	7.9	-
Hake	-	72.3	11.2	-
Sardines	3.1	47.9	2.8	6.0

Dobarganes et al, 2000.

Frying with Olive Oil: Health Issues and Changes in Composition

Mediterranean diet's nutritional model of whole grains, vegetables, fruits, and olive oil is contribute to decreased rates of coronary heart disease. Because of olive oil's role as the primary source of fat intake, the Mediterranean diet is high in MUFA, specifically oleic acid, and low in saturated fatty acids (SFA). Studies affirm that dietary *cis*-MUFA have a great antiatherosclerotic effect and are comparable with the effects of polyunsaturated fatty acids (PUFA) on cardiovascular risk factors. Several components of olive oil have beneficial health effects on the atherosclerotic and thrombotic pathways, which include lipid oxidation, hemostasis, platelet aggregation, coagulation, and fibrinolysis. Oleic acid, a major fatty acid in olive oil, and polyphenols, tocopherol, hydroxytyrosol, and oleuropein exert the most substantial antiatherosclerotic effects [Huang *et al.*, 2008].

Olive oil has a remarkable oxidative stability. If properly stored, it can retain its characteristics for 18 months or even more. This resistance to the development of rancidity, combined with a variety of flavors and distinct features, offers the opportunity for many culinary applications, many of which demand no or very mild processing (addition to salads, marinades, sauces, dressings, dips). There are also many applications of the oil in the preparation of fried and baked or grilled foods. In comparison to other vegetable oils usually richer in polyunsaturated fatty acids, olive oil has a much lower rate of alteration during domestic frying or other uses that require high temperatures [Boskou, 2009]. It has been demonstrated that olive oil has a significantly lower rate of alteration in comparison to corn oil [Chatzilazarou *et al.*, 2006], cottonseed oil, Friol oil (commercial name of a blend of 75% sunflower oil, 25% palm oil and 5% peanut oil) [Aggelousis and Lalas, 1997], fresh commercial vegetable shortening [Andrikopoulos *et al.*, 2002], palm olein [Tabee *et al.*, 2009], sunflower oil [Quiles *et al.*, 2002] and soybean oil. The resistance of olive oil to rapid deterioration at elevated temperatures is attributed to its fatty acid composition and the presence of natural antioxidants such as squalene, α-tocopherol, and Δ5- avenasterol [Boskou, 2006]. Beneficial effects of olive oil compounds and also their changes during frying have been discussed as follow:

A) Fatty Acid Profile

Chemical composition of olive oil can be divided based on their content into major and minor components. Triacylglycerols (TAG) are the major components and represent about 98% of total olive oil weight [Aparicio and Aparicio-Ruiz, 2000; Azadmard-Damirchi, 2010]. The fatty acid composition of olive oil includes: myristic acid (C14:0): $\leq 0.05\%$, palmitic acid (C16:0): 7.5-20%, palmitoleic acid (C16:1): 0.3-3.5%, heptadecanoic acid (C17:0): $\leq 0.3\%$, stearic acid (C18:0): 0.5-5%, oleic acid (C18:1): 55-83%, linoleic acid (C18:2): 3.5-21%, linolenic acid (C18:3): 3.5-21%, eicosanoic acid (C20:0): $\leq 0.6\%$, gadoleic acid (C20:1): $\leq 0.4\%$, behenic acid (C22:0): $\leq 0.2\%$, lignoceric acid (C24:0): $\leq 0.2\%$ [IOOC, 2003].

The fatty acid composition of foods may change during frying, becoming similar to that of the oil used. For example, it has been shown that sardines fried in olive oil became greatly oleic acid-enriched, while their n-6:n-3 ratio varied moderately from that of their raw counterparts [Sanchez-Muniz and Bastida, 2006]. Capita *et al.* [2003] studied the changes produced by deep fat frying in the fatty acid composition of chicken meat and chicken-based products, found that frying with olive oil increased the percentage of oleic acid in chicken meat. Also Kalogeropoulos *et al.* [2004] showed that domestic pan frying of Mediterranean fish and molluscs in virgin olive oil modified the fatty acid profiles of fried seafood towards less SFA and more MUFA intake, while still provided significant n-3 PUFA amounts. However evaluation of fatty acid composition of oil extracted from French fries prepared in refined olive oil showed small changes for all fatty acids [Tabee *et al.*, 2009].

These findings are very important because lipoprotein metabolism, and therefore the cholesterol and low density lipoprotein (LDL) level, can be modulated by the type of fatty acid available in the liver, which in turn depends on the predominant dietary fatty acids [Dietschy, 1998]. LDL of individuals who consume olive oil appears to be oleic-acid enriched and are less susceptible to oxidation [Mata *et al.*, 2002]. These facts are important with regard to the prevention of cardiovascular disease [Sanchez-Muniz and Bastida, 2006]. Oleic acid also plays an important role in cancer prevention but it remains to be understood whether this is a secondary effect of the fatty acid on oil stability (preventing oxidative stress) or a direct anticancer effect [Bourre *et al.*, 2004; Gnoni *et al.*, 2010].

On the other hand, fatty acid composition of frying oil can change during frying. Chatzilazarou et al. [2006] reported an increase in the SFA content and a decrease in PUFA content of olive oil after 10 h of frying.

B) Phytosterols

Sterols are natural components present in many plants and animal species. They are also essential for human and animal health. The sterol fraction is specific from each oil and can be used to characterize oil [Chunhieng *et al.*, 2008]. Basic structure of sterols has been shown in Figure 1. Phytosterols (plant sterols) are similar in structure to cholesterol, having the same basic cyclopentanoperhydrophenanthrene ring structure but differing in the side chain at C24 and/ or the position and configuration of unsaturated double bonds and the optical rotation at chiral carbons. Phytosterols have been classified on the basis of the number of methyl groups at the C4 position [4-desmethyl-, 4-momomethyl-, and 4,4'-dimethylsterols] [Azadmard-Damirchi and Dutta, 2010].

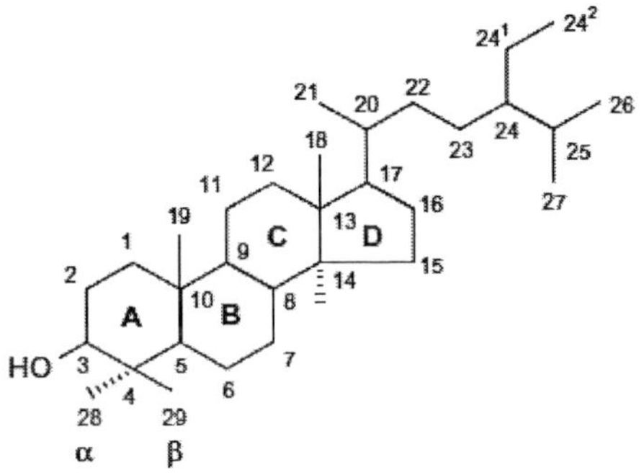

Figure 1. Basic structure of a sterol with standard carbon numbering according to the IUPAC system.

Phytosterols comprise a major proportion of the unsaponifiables in olive oil. Olive oils have the lowest amount of 4-monomethylsterols (9–11%) while 4-desmethyl and 4,4'-dimethylsterols constitute 51–57% and 32–40% of total sterols, respectively [Azadmard-Damirchi and Dutta, 2010]. Total sterol content of virgin olive oils varies mainly between 1000 mg/kg, which is the lower limit set by the European Union Commission [EC Regulation 2568, 1991], and 2000 mg/kg. Studies on olive oil sterol composition show that β-sitosterol makes up 75 to 90% of the total sterol fraction, while Δ5-avenasterol usually ranges between 5% and 20% [Boskou *et al.*, 2006].

Since the early 1950s, phytosterols have been indicated to lower cholesterol absorption in animals. The average daily intake of phytosterols is in the range 150–400 mg, while phytosterol intake from enriched foods needs to be between 1.5–2.0 g per day to be effective as a cholesterol-lowering agent [Normén *et al.*, 2004]. Epidemiological data suggest that the phytosterol content of the diet may be associated with a reduction in common cancers, including cancers of the colon, breast and prostate. In addition, phytosterols may directly inhibit tumor growth, including the slowing of cell cycle progression, the induction of apoptosis and the inhibition of tumor metastasis [Bradford and Awad, 2007].

Phytosterols, like unsaturated fatty acids, are prone to oxidation, especially when subjected to heat treatment or long-term storage. In general, sterol oxidation can proceed via nonenzymic or enzymic pathways. Nonenzymic pathways can further be divided into autoxidation, or photoxidation. Mechanisms in sterol autoxidation are similar to those in fatty acid oxidation [Soupas, 2006].

Formation of phytosterol oxidation products (POPs) and their distribution depends on the sterol structure, composition of the matrix and temperature and amounts of unoxidized sterols [Tabee *et al.*, 2008]. Soupas *et al.* [2004] showed that the interaction between lipid matrices and temperatures may have an effect on the stability of phytosterols in food. A study on the POPs contents of olive oil heated at 180 °C for 0–2 h reported an increase in total POPs content during heating for olive oil [Johnsson and Dutta, 2006]. Tabee *et al.* [2009] reported that the total POPs content in fresh refined olive oil was approximately 50% more than that in fresh palm olein, which this difference in POPs content between the two oils persisted in the oils extracted from the fifth batch of French fries, heated to 180 °C for 5 h in these frying oils. However, it should be noted that the lower content of POPs in palm olein compared with olive oil can be from low level of phytosterols in palm olein.

C) Tocopherols

Vitamin E is the collective term for a family of chemical substances that are structurally related to α-tocopherol. Vitamin E occurs naturally in eight different forms: four tocopherols, α-, β-, γ- and δ- tocopherol and four tocotrienols, α-, β-, γ- and δ-tocotrienol. All of these forms consist of a chromanol ring with a long aliphatic side chain, bound to the chromanol ring at the 2 position. Tocotrienols differ from their corresponding tocopherols in that the saturated phytyl side chain is replaced with an unsaturated isoprenoid side chain. The Greek characters refer to the number and position of the methyl groups at the 5, 7 and 8 positions [Amaral *et al.*, 2005]. Figure 2 gives a schematic presentation of the molecular structures of tocopherols and tocotrienols.

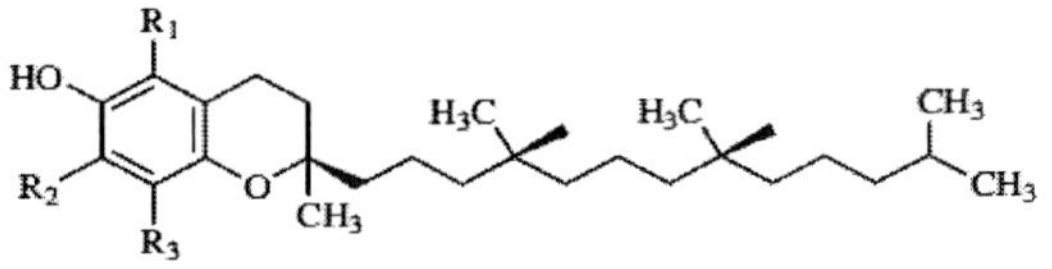

Tocopherol

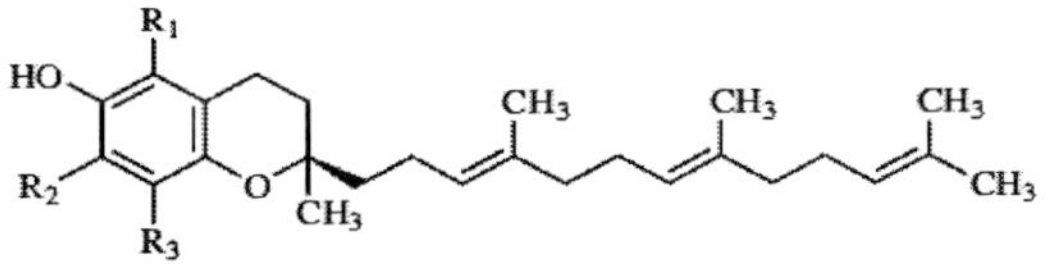

Tocotrienol

Tocopherol or Tocotrienol	R_1	R_2	R_3
α	CH_3	CH_3	CH_3
β	CH_3	H	CH_3
γ	H	CH_3	CH_3
δ	H	H	CH_3

Figure 2. Structures of tocopherols and tocotrienols.

From the nutritional point of view tocopherols has been shown to reduce the risk of coronary heart disease in high doses [Ryan *et al.*, 2006]. One of the most developed theories for their cardioprotective effect appears to be concerning tocopherols induced inhibition of LDL oxidation, which is proposed to be a key role in the atherogenic process [Kornsteiner *et al.*, 2006].

Tocopherols also have a fundamental role as lipid phase antioxidants, by scavenging radicals in membranes and lipoprotein particles [Kalogeropoulos and *et al.*, 2007]. The mode of action of tocopherols and tocotrienols as antioxidants at room and moderate temperatures can be explained by their role in free radical chain-breaking by donating hydrogen from their phenolic group to radicals to stabilise them. The resulting tocopheryl semiquinone radical-molecule, which does not have antioxidant properties, still shows possibilities of further different reactions at higher temperature. For instance, in the case of γ-tocopherol/ tocotrienol a reaction between the two such radicals can give rise to two tocopherol dimers, namely γ-tocopherol biphenyl-dimer and γ-tocopherol ether-dimer, both of which possess antioxidative properties. While α-tocopherol which degrades much faster in oils at frying temperature, produces four oxidation products which only one of these, α-tocopherol ethane-dimer, shows antioxidant activity. Therefore, γ-tocopherol is superior to α-tocopherol because it oxidises to more stable compounds which are still effective as antioxidants. Therefore, it improves frying oil stability more than α-tocopherol and thus can provide better protection to fried food in storage [Kochhar, 2001].

α-Tocopherol is traditionally considered to be the major antioxidant of olive oil and its concentration varies from a few ppm up to 300 ppm [Dionisi *et al.*, 1995; Blekas *et al.*, 2002]. The oxidative stability of olive oil can be related to some extent with the high amount of α-tocopherol that it contains [Chatzilazarou *et al.*, 2006]. β-, γ- and δ-tocopherols concentrations have also been reported to range from trace to 25 ppm [Dionisi *et al.*, 1995; Boskou *et al.*, 2006; Cunha *et al.*, 2006]. α-, β-, and γ-tocotrienols have also been reported in olive oils at concentrations from non-detectable to 3.1, 0.7 and 4.7 ppm, respectively [Benitez-Sanchez *et al.*, 2003; Azadmard-Damirchi, 2010].

Vitamin E is being used to protect the oils against the thermal damage [Quiles *et al.*, 2002].During frying tocopherols are often fully destroyed before the point at which the frying oil should be replaced, based on the contents of polymerized triacylglycerols (i.e. 12%) or polar compounds (i.e. 24%) [Normand *et al.*, 2001; Barrera-Arellano *et al.*, 2002; Réblova and Okrouhla, 2010]. The decrease in tocopherol content with the frying time is different, depending on the type of oil. Comparison of loss of tocopherols in olive oil with sunflower oil showed that in the case of virgin olive and olive oils, the loss of tocopherol started after 45 or 60 min of frying. While, sunflower oil lost tocopherol after 15 min and then the quantity of this antioxidant remained constant until the end. Sunflower lost tocopherol content, in absolute value, 201 mg kg^{-1}, followed by virgin olive oil (127 mg kg^{-1}) and olive oil (77.1 mg kg^{-1}).Therefore it seems that olive and virgin olive oils resist the frying procedure better [Quiles *et al.*, 2002]. However, the half-life of α-tocopherol (calculated as the time needed for the α-tocopherol content to decrease to 50% of the original value) is shown to be extended significantly by phenolic acids (gentisic, caffeic, and gallic acids) during the heating of sunflower oil at 180°C [Réblova and Okrouhla, 2010]. Pellegrini et al. [2001] suggested that polyphenols from extra virgin olive oil are effective stabilizers of α-tocopherol during olive oil heating, thus contributing to the nutritional value of cooked foods [Réblova and Okrouhla, 2010].

D) Polyphenols

During the last decades many studies have demonstrated that polyphenols, which are the most abundant natural antioxidants in our diet, prevent oxidative alterations due to free radicals and other reactive species and oxidation of LDL. The nutrition community has recognized the importance of dietary polyphenols as health-promoting agents. Polyphenol intake is associated with lower risk of coronary heart disease, some types of cancer, inflammation and inhibition of platelet-activating factor activity [Kalogeropoulos and *et al.*, 2007]. The reduction in the risk of several chronic diseases by consumption of plant phenols has been attributed to their array of bio-mechanisms, including antioxidation, anti-inflammation, carcinogen detoxification, and cholesterol reduction [Chen and Blumberg, 2008].

The total phenolic content of olive oil is in the range of 196-500 mg/kg. Although the reported levels of phenolic compounds in olive oil vary widely. Extra virgin olive oil has a higher phenolic content than other types of olive oils [Waterman and Lockwood, 2007]. The major phenolic compounds in olive oil are: (1) simple phenols (e.g., hydroxytyrosol, tyrosol, vanillic acid); (2) secoiridoids: oleuropein glucoside, and SIDs which are the dialdehydic form of oleuropein (SID-1) and ligstroside (SID-2) lacking a carboxymethyl group, and the aglycone form of oleuropein glucoside (SID-3) and ligstroside (SID- 4); and (3) polyphenols: lignans (e.g., (+)-pinoresinol and (+)-1-acetoxypinoresinol) and flavonols. Tyrosol, hydroxytyrosol, and their secoiridoid derivatives make up around 90% of the total phenolic content of a virgin olive oil [Covas *et al.*, 2010]. Figure 3 presents chemical structure of tyrosol and hydroxytyrosol.

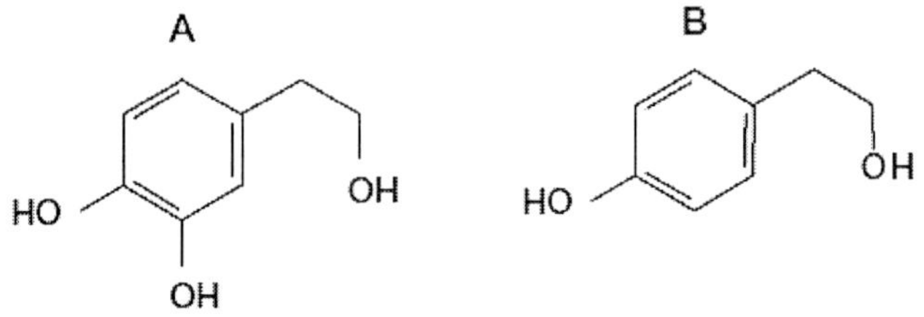

Figure 3. Structures of (A): hydroxytyrosol; (B): tyrosol.

Virgin olive oil also contains significant amounts of hydroxy pentacyclic triterpene acids (HPTAs), particularly oleanolic, maslinic and ursolic acids. Oleanolic and ursolic acids intake has been reported to have beneficial effects on human health, notably hepatoprotection, antiinflammation, antitumor promotion, and antihyperlipidemia while ursolic and maslinic acids have been reported to exhibit anti- HIV activity [Kalogeropoulos and *et al.*, 2007]. Data has demonstrated that the virgin olive oil having high concentrations of oleuropein derivatives efficiently inhibit acrylamide formation in crisps from mild to moderate frying conditions [Napolitano *et al.*, 2008]. In addition, it has been demonstrated a reduction of the formation of the different heterocyclic amines (HAs) which are mutagenic/carcinogenic compounds, in beefburgers fried in virgin olive oil that this reduction is probably linked to the high content of phenols in the virgin olive oil [Persson *et al.*, 2003].

During frying of virgin olive oil, all phenolic compounds concentration decreases with an increase in the number of frying operations, although the rate of loss depends on chemical structure and antioxidant activity, as the reduction in tyrosol and its derivatives is much smaller than that for hydroxytyrosol and its derivatives [Gomez-Alonso *et al.*, 2003]. The reduction of phenolic compounds during frying is probably as the result of thermal destruction of these molecules or because they are used in the protection of the oils against the oxidative insult. These compounds are also lost in the oil over time, as a consequence of hydrolytic or oxidative processes during storage [Quiles *et al.*, 2002; Cinquanta *et al.*, 1997].

Phenolic antioxidants are shown to be lost by steam distillation during frying of potatoes and other moisture containing foods [Fritsch, 1981] and consumed by reacting with lipid free radicals, originally formed by the action of oxygen on unsaturated fatty acids, to form relatively stable products which interrupt the propagation stage of oxidative chain reactions [Gordon & Kourimska, 1995; Andrikopoulos *et al.*, 2002]. Andrikopoulos *et al.* [2002] showed that pan-frying of potatoes in virgin olive oil caused more marked loss of phenols than deep-frying after 10 operations. This was because of higher surface/volume ratio, higher temperatures and contact with atmospheric oxygen, as the potatoes remain partly uncovered by oil.

E) Squalene

Squalene, a highly unsaturated hydrocarbon C30H50, that has been reported to possess moderate antioxidant activities, occurs about 10–1200 mg/100g in olive oil. The exact antioxidative mechanistic pathway of squalene at frying temperature is not clearly understood. It is, possibly, suggested that tocopherols and squalene act together in combination as chain-braking antioxidants. They scavenge the chain-carrying peroxy radicals, interrupt the chain propagation, but are themselves modified/oxidized during this reaction process. At first squalene is preferentially consumed, so its loss is greater than the tocopherol loss [Kochhar, 2001]. Squalene has been reported to have important beneficial effects on health, such as decreasing the risk for various cancers and reducing serum cholesterol levels. The protective effect of squalene may be attributed to its possible antioxidant functions. It has been demonstrated to be an efficient quencher of singlet oxygen [Kohno *et al.*, 1995] and protects against H_2O_2-induced sister chromatid exchange in Chinese hamster V79 cells [Ryan *et al.*, 2006].

Although squalene is widely distributed throughout the body, the majority is transported to the skin. Exposure to high levels of ultraviolet radiation causes the formation of carcinogenic singlet oxygen species within the skin, where a high concentration of squalene may provide a chemoprotective effect. Due to squalene's structure, it is more likely to scavenge singlet oxygen species than hydroxyl radicals. Squalene, found in high amounts in the Mediterranean diet, is believed to be responsible for the lower incidence of skin cancer seen in epidemiological studies of populations consuming this diet [Waterman and Lockwood, 2007]. Kalogeropoulos *et al.* [2004] evaluated the effect of domestic pan frying of Mediterranean fish and molluscs in virgin olive oil and showed a 20–78 times increase of squalene content.

REFERENCES

[1] Aggelousis, G. & Lalas, S. (1997). Quality changes of selected vegetable oils during frying of doughnuts. *La Rivista Italian Delle Sostanze Grasse*, Lxxiv, 559-565.

[2] Amaral, J. S., Casal, S., Torres, D., Seabra, R. M. & Oliveira, B. P. P. (2005). Simultaneous determination of tocopherols and tocotrienols in hazelnuts by a normal phase liquid chromatographic method. *J. Anal Sci*, 21, 1545-1548.

[3] Andrikopoulos, N. K., Kalogeropoulos, N., Falirea, A. & Barbagianni, M. N. (2002). Performance of virgin olive oil and vegetable shortening during domestic deep-frying and pan frying of potatoes. *International Journal of Food Science and Technology*, 37, 177-190.

[4] Aparicio, R. & Aparicio-Ruiz, R. (2000). Authentication of vegetable oils by chromatographic techniques. *Journal of Chromatography A,* 881, 93-104.

[5] Azadmard-Damirchi, S., & Dutta, P. C. (2010). Phytosterol Classes in Olive Oils and their Analysis by Common Chromatographic Methods. In: V. R. Preedy, & R. R. Watson (Eds.), Olives and Olive Oil in Health and Disease Prevention. (1st, pp. 249-257). San Diego, Elsevier Inc.

[6] Azadmard-damirchi, S. (2010). Minor compounds of olive oil: phytosterols and tocopherols. In: J. D. Corrigan (Ed.), Olive Oil and Health. Nova Science Publishers, USA.

[7] Barrera-Arellano, D., Ruiz-Mendez, V., Velasco, J., Marquez-Ruiz, G. & Dobarganes, C. (2002). Loss of tocopherols and formation of degradation compounds at frying temperatures in oils differing in degree of unsaturation and natural antioxidant content. Journal of the Science of Food and Agriculture, 82, 1696–1702.

[8] Benitez-Sanchez, P. L., Camacho, L. M. & Aparicio, R. (2003). A comprehensive study of hazelnut oil composition with comparisons to other vegetable oils, particularly olive oil, *European Food Research and Technology, 218,* 13-19.

[9] Blekas, G., Psomiadou, E., Tsimidou, M. & Boskou, D. (2002). On the importance of total polar phenols to monitor the stability of Greek virgin olive oil. *European Journal of Lipid Science and Technology,* 104, 340-346.

[10] Bognár, A. (1998). Comparative study of frying to other cooking techniques influence on the nutritive value. *Grasasy Aceites*, 49(3-4), 250-260.

[11] Boskou, D. (2006). Culinary Applications. In: D. Boskou (Ed), Olive Oil Chemistry and Technology. (2nd Ed, pp. 243-248). AOCS Press.

[12] Boskou, D. (2009). Culinary Applications of Olive Oil Minor Constituents and Cooking. In: D. Boskou (Ed), Olive Oil: Minor Constituents and Health. (pp. 1-6). Boca Raton, Taylor & Francis Group.

[13] Boskou, D., Blekas, G. & Tsimidou, M. (2006). Olive Oil Composition. In: D. Boskou (Ed), Olive Oil Chemistry and Technology. (2nd Ed, pp. 41-72). AOCS Press.

[14] Bourre, J. M., Dumont, O. & Durand, G., (2004). Dose-effect of dietary oleic acid: oleic acid is conditionally essential for some organs. Reprod. Nutr. Dev., 44, 371 – 380.

[15] Bradford, B. G. & Awad, A. B. (2007). Phytosterols as anticancer compounds. *Mol. Nutr. Food Res,* 51, 161 – 170.

[16] Capita, R., Garcia-Linares, M. C., Tome, M., Garcia-Fernandez, M. C., Garcia-Arias, M.T. & Sanchez-Muniz, F. J. (2003) Deep-frying of chicken meat and chicken-based product. Changes in the proximate and fatty acid compositions. *Italian Journal of Food Science,* 15, 225–240.

[17] Chatzilazarou, A., Lalas, O. G. S., Zoidis, E. & Tsaknis, J. (2006). Physicochemical changes of olive oil and selected vegetable oils during frying. *Journal of Food Lipids*, 13, 27–35.

[18] Chen, C-Y. O. & Blumberg, J. B. (2008). Phytochemical composition of nuts. *Asian Pac J Clin Nutr*, 17, 329-332.

[19] Chunhieng, T., Hafidi, A., Pioch, D., Brochier, J. & Montet, D. (2008). Detailed study of Brazil nut (*Bretholletia excelsa*) oil micro-compounds: phospholipids, tocopherols and sterols, *J. Braz. Chem. Soc*, 19(7), 1374-1380.

[20] Cinquanta, L., Esti, M. & La Notte, E. (1997). Evolution of phenolic compounds in virgin olive oil during storage. *Journal of the American Oil Chemists Society*, 74, 1259–1264.

[21] Covas, M. I., Fito, M., Khymenets, O. & de la Torre, R. (2010). The Bioavailability of Olive Oil Phenolic Compounds. In: V. R. Preedy, & R. R. Watson (Eds.), Olives and Olive Oil in Health and Disease Prevention. (1st Ed, pp. 699-703). San Diego, Elsevier Inc.

[22] Cunha, S. C., Amaral, J. S., Fernandes, J. O. & Oliveira, M. B. P. P. (2006). Quantification of tocopherols and tocotrienols in Portuguese olive oils using HPLC with three different detection systems. *Journal of Agriculture and Food Chemistry*, 54, 3351- 3356.

[23] Dietschy, J.M. (1998) Dietary fatty acids and the regulation of plasma low density lipoprotein cholesterol concentrations. *Journal of Nutrition,* 128, 444S–448S.

[24] Dionisi, F., Prodolliet, J. & Tagliaferri, E. (1995). Assessment of olive oil adulteration by reversed-phase high-performance liquid chromatography/ amperometric

determination of tocopherols and tocotrienols. *Journal of the American Oil Chemist's Society, 72,* 1505-1511.

[25] Dobarganes, C., Márquez-Ruiz, G. & Velasco, J. (2000). Interactions between fat and food during deep-frying. *Eur. J. Lipid Sci. Technol,* 102, 521–528.

[26] Fritsch, C.W. (1981). Measurement of frying fat deterioration: a brief review. *Journal of the American Oil Chemists Society*, 58, 272-274.

[27] Ghidurus, M., Turtoi, M., Boskou, G., Niculita, P. & Stan, V. (2010). Nutritional and health aspects related to frying (I). *Romanian Biotechnological Letter*, 15(6), 5675-5682.

[28] Gnoni, G. V., Natali, F., Geelen, M. J. H. & Siculella, L. (2010). Oleic Acid as an Inhibitor of Fatty Acid and Cholesterol Synthesis. In: V. R. Preedy, & R. R. Watson (Eds.), Olives and Olive Oil in Health and Disease Prevention: (1st Ed, pp. 1365-1373). San Diego, Elsevier Inc.

[29] Gomez-Alonso, S., Fregapane, G., Desamparados Salvador, M. & Gordon, M. H. (2003). Changes in phenolic composition and antioxidant activity of virgin olive oil during frying. *J. Agric Food Chem*, 51, 667-672.

[30] Gordon, H.M. & Kourimska, L. (1995). Effects of antioxidants on losses of tocopherols during deep-fat frying. *Food Chemistry*, 52, 175-177.

[31] Huang, Ch. L. & Sumpio, B. E. (2008). Olive Oil, the Mediterranean Diet, and Cardiovascular Health. *J Am Coll Surg*, 207(3), 407-416.

[32] IOOC. (2003). *International Olive Oil Council activities: World Olive Oil Consumption.* Available from: <www.internationaloliveoil.org/>.

[33] Johnsson, L. & Dutta, P. C. (2006). Determination of phytosterol oxides in some food products by using an optimized transesterification method. *Food Chem*, 97, 606–613.

[34] Kalogeropoulos, N., Andrikopoulos, N. K. & Hassapidou, M. (2004). Dietary evaluation of Mediterranean fish and molluscs pan-fried in virgin olive oil. *Journal of the Science of Food and Agriculture,* 84, 1750–1758.

[35] Kalogeropoulos, N., Chiou, A., Mylona, A., Ioannou, M. S. & Andrikopoulos, N. K. (2007). Recovery and distribution of natural antioxidants (a-tocopherol, polyphenols and terpenic acids) after pan-frying of Mediterranean finfish in virgin olive oil. *Food Chemistry*, 100, 509–517.

[36] Kochhar, S. P. (2001). The composition of frying oils. In: J. B. Rossell (Ed), Frying Improving quality. (pp. 87-114).Cambridge, Woodhead Publishing Limited.

[37] Kohno, Y., Egawa, Y., Itoh, S., Nagaoka, S., Takahashi, M. & Mukai, K. (1995). Kinetic study of quenching reaction of singlet oxygen and scavenging reaction of free radical by squalene in n-butanol. *Biochim. Biophys. Acta*, 1256, 52-56.

[38] Kornsteiner, M., Wanger, K. H. & Elmadfa, I. (2006). Tocopherols and total phenolics in 10 different nut types, *J. Food Chem,* 98, 381-387.

[39] Mata, P., Alonso, R. & Mata, N. (2002) Los omega-3 y omega-9 en la enfermedad cardiovascular. In: Mataix, J. and Gil, A. (eds) *Libro blanco de los omega-3. Los acidos grasos poliinsaturados omega 3 y monoinsaturados tipo oleico y su papel en la salud.* Instituto Omega 3, Puleva Food, Madrid, pp. 50–63.

[40] Napolitano, A., Morales, F., Sacchi, R. & Fogliano, V. (2008). Relationship between Virgin Olive Oil Phenolic Compounds and Acrylamide Formation in Fried Crisps. *J. Agric. Food Chem*, 56, 2034–2040.

[41] Normand, L., Eskin, N.A.M. & Przybylski, R. (2001). Effect of tocopherols on the frying stability of regular and modified canola oils. Journal of the American Oil Chemists' Society, 78, 369–373.

[42] Normén, L., Frohlich, J. & Trautwein, E. (2004). Role of plant sterols in cholesterol lowering. In: P. C. Dutta (Ed), Phytosterols as Functional Food Components and Nutraceuticals. (pp. 243-315). NewYork, Marcel Dekker Inc.

[43] Pellegrini N., Visioli F., Buratti S. & Brighenti F. (2001). Direct analysis of total antioxidant activity of olive oil and studies on the influence of heating. *Journal of Agricultural and Food Chemistry*, 49, 2532–2538.

[44] Persson, E., Graziani, G., Ferracane, R., Fogliano, V. & Skog, K. (2003). Influence of antioxidants in virgin olive oil on the formation of heterocyclic amines in fried beefburgers. *Food and Chemical Toxicology*, 41, 1587-1597.

[45] Quaglia, G. B. & Bucarelli, F. M. (2001). Effective process control in frying. In: J. B. Rossell (Ed), Frying Improving quality. (pp. 236-265).Cambridge, Woodhead Publishing Limited.

[46] Quiles, J. L., Ramı´rez-Tortosa, M. C., Gomez, J. A., Huertas, J. R. & Mataix, J. (2002). Role of vitamin E and phenolic compounds in the antioxidant capacity, measured by ESR, of virgin olive, olive and sunflower oils after frying. *Food Chemistry*, 76, 461–468.

[47] Réblova, Z. & Okrouhla, P. (2010). Ability of Phenolic Acids to Protect α-Tocopherol. *Czech J. Food Sci*, 28(4), 290–297.

[48] Rossi, M., Alamprese, C. & Ratti, S. (2007). Tocopherols and tocotrienols as free radical-scavengers in refined vegetable oils and their stability during deep-fat frying. *Food Chemistry*, 102, 812–817.

[49] Ryan, E., Galvin, K., O'Connor, T. P., Maguire, A. R. & O'Brien, N. M. (2006). Fatty acid profile, squalene and phytosterol content of brazil, pecan, pine, pistachio and cashew nuts. *Int. J. Food Sci Nutr*, 57(3/4), 219-228.

[50] Sahin, S. & Gülüm Sumnu, S. (2009). Introduction. In: S. Sahin, & S. Gülüm Sumnu, (Eds.), Advances in deep-fat frying of foods: (pp. 1-4). Boca Raton, Taylor & Francis Group.

[51] Sanchez-Muniz, F. J. & Bastida, S. (2006). Effect of Frying and Thermal Oxidation on Olive Oil and Food Quality. In: J. L. Quiles, M. C. Ramirez-Tortosa, & P. Yaqoob (Eds.), Olive oil and health: (pp. 74-108). Trowbridge, Columns Design Ltd.

[52] Soupas, L. 2006. Oxidative stability of phytosterols in food models and foods. PhD thesis. University of Helsinki

[53] Soupas, L., Juntunen, L., Lampi, A. M. & Piironen, V. (2004). Effects of sterol structure, temperature, and lipid medium on phytosterol oxidation. *J. Agric. Food Chem*, 52, 6485-6491.

[54] Tabee, E., Azadmard-Damirchi, S., Ja¨gerstad, M. & Dutta, P. C. (2008). Effects of *a*-Tocopherol on Oxidative Stability and Phytosterol Oxidation during Heating in Some Regular and High-Oleic Vegetable Oils. J Am Oil Chem Soc (2008) 85:857–867.

[55] Tabee, E., Jagerstad, M. & Dutta, P. C. (2009). Frying Quality Characteristics of French Fries Prepared in Refined Olive Oil and Palm Olein. *J Am Oil Chem Soc*, 86, 885–893.

[56] Varela G. (1992). Some Effects of Deep Frying on Dietary Fat Intake, *Nutrition Reviews*, 50, 256-262.

[57] Varela, G. & Ruiz-Roso, B. (2000). Some nutritional aspects of olive oil. In: J. Harwood, & R. Aparicio (Eds.), Hand book of olive oil analysis and properties. (pp. 565-582). Maryland, Aspen publishers Inc.

[58] Velasco, J., Marmesat, S. & Dobarganes, M. C. (2009). Chemistry of Frying. In: S. Sahin, & S. Gülüm Sumnu, (Eds.), Advances in deep-fat frying of foods: (pp. 33-56). Boca Raton, Taylor & Francis Group.

[59] Waterman, E. & Lockwood, B. (2007). Active Components and Clinical Applications of Olive Oil. *Alternative Medicine Review*, 12(4), 331-342.

In: Olive Consumption and Health
Editors: C. A. Savalas and S. M. Nicolau
ISBN: 978-1-62100-774-6

Chapter 8

OLIVE OIL PHENOLICS AND OXIDATIVE STRESS

Verónica Leticia Colin*
PROIMI-CONICET. Av. Belgrano y Pasaje Caseros,
T4001 MVB, Tucumán, Argentina

ABSTRACT

Olive oil, which has been part of the human diet for more than 5000 years, is almost unique among oils in that it can be consumed in the crude form without refining. This has the effect of conserving all its vitamins, essential fatty acids, and other nutrients. In addition to the fatty acid profile of olive oil, which is high in the monounsaturated oleic acid and appears to be beneficial in reducing several risk factors for coronary heart disease and certain cancers, extra virgin olive oil contains powerful antioxidants. In this connection, the incidence of degenerative pathologies, including those in which the excessive free radical formation has been suggested, is very low in the Mediterranean area, where the diet is rich in antioxidant compounds. Among such antioxidants, the contribution of olive oil phenolics is currently under active investigation, since they affords considerable protection against cancer (colon, breast, and skin), coronary heart disease, and ageing by inhibiting oxidative stress. This chapter focuses on antioxidant role and additional biological actions of olive oil phenolics.

1. INTRODUCTION

The olive, native to Asia Minor, spread from Iran, Syria and Palestine to the rest of the Mediterranean basin 6000 years ago. Interesting epidemiologic studies have demonstrated that a Mediterranean diet rich in olive oil is associated with decrease in risk for cardiovascular disease, certain types of cancers and other chronic diseases [1–6]. Traditionally, the beneficial health effects of virgin olive oil intake were attributed to unsaturated fatty acid components,

* Corresponding author. Tel: +54 381 4344888; fax: +54 381 4344887. E-mail address: veronicacollin@yahoo. com.ar.

particularly oleic acid [7]. However, several seed oils including sunflower, soybean and rapeseed, which containing high quantities of this acids, are ineffective in beneficially altering chronic diseases risk factors [8, 9].

Reactive oxygen species (ROS), considered as a by-product of aerobic metabolism, have been implicated in the natural cellular aging process as well as in cardiovascular disease (atherosclerosis), disease states neoplastic (hematological and solid tumor), metabolic (obesity and diabetes) and neurological (Alzheimer's and Parkinson's diseases) [10, 11]. Oxidative stress caused by the presence of ROS, which the cell is unable to counterbalance, could result in damage to one or more biomolecules including DNA, RNA, proteins and lipids. A substantial number of researches have focused on the biologically active phenolic compounds naturally present in virgin olive oil to aid in explaining reduced mortality and morbidity experienced by people consuming a traditional Mediterranean diet. Olive oil phenolic compounds have been shown to scavenge ROS under natural and chemically simulated oxidative stress conditions [12–14]. Both *in vivo* and *in vitro* studies have demonstrated that these compounds have positive effects on certain physiological parameters such as plasma lipoproteins, inflammatory markers, oxidative damage, etc.

This chapter focuses on antioxidant role and other biological actions of olive oil phenolics.

2. Olive Oil Composition

2.1. Triacylglycerols and Fatty Acids

Olive oil is composed mainly of triacylglycerols (TGs) and contains small quantities of free fatty acids (FFAs), glycerol, phosphatides, pigments, flavor compounds, sterols and microscopic bits of olive. From a chemical point of view, TGs are molecules derived from the natural esterification of three fatty acid molecules, which varying (in the case of olive oil) from about 14 to 24 carbon atoms in length with a glycerol molecule. The fatty acids composition that forming part of the TG molecule of olive oil varies widely depending on the cultivar, maturity of the fruit, altitude, climate and other factors. The primary fatty acids in olive oil are all long chain fatty acids. Very long-chain fatty acids have greater than 20 carbon atoms. These tend to be more solid at room temperature, such as waxes. There are no appreciable amounts of these acids in olive oil. The major fatty acids in olive oil are showed in Table 1.

Regarding the polyunsaturated fatty acids, there is a wide range acceptable for extra virgin olive oil. However, the linolenic acid has to be less than 0.9% per the International Olive Oil Council (IOOC) guidelines. Higher levels, e.g. 1.5%, do not present a nutritional problem, but the IOOC uses the linolenic acid level to establish the authenticity of the olive oil. Seed oils like canola oil have higher levels of linolenic acid.

Triacylglycerols are normally composed of a mixture of three fatty acids. Most prevalent in olive oil is the oleic-oleic-oleic triacylglycerol, followed, in order of incidence by palmitic-oleic-oleic, oleic-oleic-linoleic, palmitic-oleic-linoleic, stearic-oleic-oleic, and so on. Concerning to essential fatty acids, from a medical point of view, these are the ones that the human body cannot make. There are only two, which are the building blocks from which many of the other omega-3 and omega-6 fatty acids are made in a healthy body: linoleic acid and alpha-linolenic acid.

Table 1. Chemical structure and percentage of the most common fatty acids in the olive oil [15]

Name of fatty acids	Structure (xx:y)	Formula	Contain in olive oil (%)
Palmitic	16:0	$C_{16}H_{32}O_2$	11.2 to 20.7
Palmitoleic	16:1	$C_{16}H_{30}O_2$	0.67 to 2.9
Stearic	18:0	$C_{18}H_{36}O_2$	1.7 to 4.3
Oleic	18:1	$C_{18}H_{34}O_2$	47.1 to 78.0
Linoleic	18:2	$C_{18}H_{32}O_2$	3.6 to 27.5
Linolenic	18:3	$C_{18}H_{30}O_2$	6.7 to 1.5
Arachidic	20:0	$C_{20}H_{40}O_2$	0.0 to 0.84

(xx:y) carbon chain length: number of unsaturated bonds.

2.2. Free Fatty Acids and Acidity

The 'acidity' in olive oil is the result of the degree of breakdown of the TGs, due to a chemical reaction called hydrolysis or lipolysis, in which FFAs are formed. In exceptional circumstances, even oils made from fresh, healthy olives can have significant amounts of acidity, caused by anomalies during the actual biosynthesis of the oil in the olive fruit. Oil extracted carelessly and/or from poor quality fruit suffers from a very significant breakdown of the TGs into fatty acids. These 'broken off fatty acids' are called FFAs. The free fatty acidity is thus a direct measure of the quality of the oil, and reflects the care taken right from blossoming and fruit set to the eventual sale and consumption of the oil.

2.3. Peroxides

Fats and oils such as olive oil are oxidized when they come in contact with oxygen. In this connection, peroxides are the primary products of oxidation of olive oil. The oxidation products have an unpleasant flavor and odor and may adversely affect the nutritional value of the oil. Essential fatty acids such as linoleic and linolenic are destroyed, and certain fat soluble vitamins disappear. Fatty acids can be oxidized either 1) auto-oxidation, which occurs in the absence of air by reactive oxygen species or 'free radicals' or, 2) photo-oxidation, which occurs when the oil is exposed to natural and/or artificial light sources. It causes serious deterioration of olive oil, as it can occur up to 30,000 times faster than auto-oxidation.

2.4. Pigments

The unique color of olive oil is due to pigments like chlorophyll, pheophytin and carotenoids. The presence of various pigments depends on factors such as the fruit ripeness, the olive cultivar, the soil and climatic conditions, the extraction and processing procedures. According to Apostolos Kiritsakis [16], one of the premier researchers on olive oil components, fresh olive oil contains between 1 and 10 parts per million chlorophyll, which is miniscule compared for example to a portion of spinach. In the light, chlorophyll and pheophytin will promote formation of oxygen radicals and speed up oxidation, but in the dark chlorophyll acts as an antioxidant.

2.5. Vitamins

Vitamins can be divided into the fat soluble and water soluble varieties. Fat soluble vitamins, such as the ones found in olive oil, are stored in the liver and body fat for long periods so it is not essential to eat them with every meal.

Vitamin E is a natural antioxidant present in olive oil. Vitamin K, on the other hand, is found in green, leafy vegetables. Seems that, vegetable oils such as olive oil are one of best source of vitamine K. Olive oil is also rich in vitamins A, B-1, B-2, C, D and in iron.

2.6. Polycyclic Aromatic Hydrocarbons

Many foods naturally contain small quantities of polycyclic aromatic hydrocarbons (PAHs). Olive oil, like other vegetable cooking oils, has been found to contain minute amounts of up to 17 PAHs such as benzanthracene and chrysene. Burning any cooking oil can increase the amounts of PAHs. This is not considered a major risk source in the diet and the oil would have to be heated repeatedly and for extended periods to the smoking point. It is unlikely that, in home use, olive oil or other cooking oils would be a significant source of PAHs.

2.7. Polyphenols

The polyphenols in olive oil are natural antioxidants that contribute to a bitter taste, astringency and resistance to oxidation. They have been shown to have a host of beneficial effects from healing sunburn to lowering cholesterol, blood pressure, risk of coronary disease, etc. Olive oil is a source of at least 30 phenolic compounds. Oleuropein, hydroxytyrosol and tyrosol are some of the most common phenolic compounds of olive oil, which are related structurally (Figure 1). Oleuropein is the major phenolic compound in olive fruit, which can be as much as 14% in dried fruit. Hydroxytyrosol is the major phenolic component in olive oil [17]. The polyphenol content is determined by many factors including olive varietal, time of picking, environmental factors such as altitude, cultivation practices and the amount of irrigation, extraction conditions, and storage conditions and refining. Concerning to this last, refined oils are low in tyrosol and other phenols.

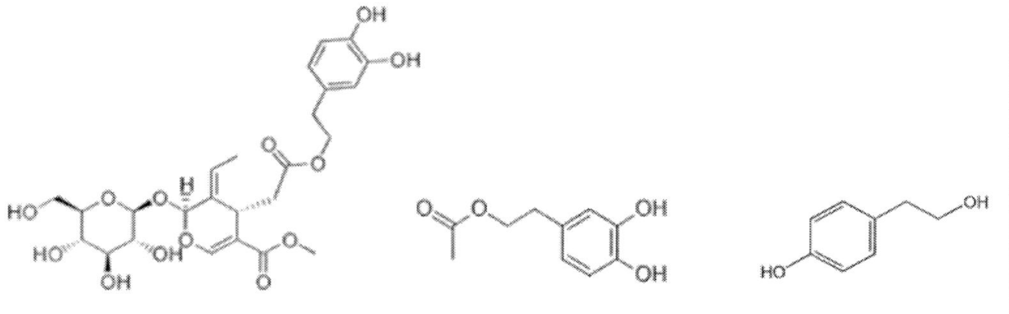

Figure 1. Chemical structure of major phenol compounds of olive oil.

3. Bioavailability of Olive Oil Phenolic Compounds

Much research has focused on the biologically active phenolic compounds naturally present in virgin olive oils, since diverse studies (human, animal, *in vivo* and *in vitro*) have demonstrated that they have positive effects on certain physiological parameters, such as plasma lipoproteins, oxidative damage, inflammatory markers, etc. The majority of research regarding the bioavailability of olive oil phenolic compounds has focused on three major phenolics: hydroxytyrosol, tyrosol and oleuropein. Many studies demonstrated the dose-dependent absorption of olive oil phenolics in humans and their urinary excretion as glucuronide conjugates [18–26]. In general, phenolics from virgin olive oil have been demonstrated to be readily bioavailable. In this connection, Tuck et al. [18] demonstrated increased bioavailability of hydroxytyrosol and tyrosol when administered as an olive oil solution compared to an aqueous solution. A further study found that absorption of administered ligstroside-aglycone, hydroxytyrosol, tyrosol and oleuropein-aglycone was as high as 55–66% in humans [19].

The mechanism by which absorption occurs with regards to olive oil phenolic compounds remains unclear. However, the different polarities of the various phenolics have been postulated to play a role in the absorption of these compounds [19].

Studies examining the quantity of phenolics excreted have also been carried out. A low quantity of phenolics present in urine after ingestion would indicate that these compounds are readily absorbed. Excreted phenolics, mainly in the form of hydroxytyrosol and tyrosol, were determined to be 5–16% of the total ingested [19]. Excretion of approximately 24% of administered tyrosol was demonstrated in a study by Miro-Cases et al. [20]. Visioli et al. [21] reported the excretion of administered hydroxytyrosol and tyrosol to be between 30–60% and 20–22% respectively, of the total ingested by human subjects. Another interesting finding of that study was that increasing amounts of phenolics administered with olive oil stimulated the rate of conjugation with glucuronide [19–23]. It is also important considering the metabolism of olive oil phenolic compounds since it may affect their availability. In this connection, it was reported that phenolic compounds oleuropein-glycoside, oleuropein and ligstroside-aglycones are converted to hydroxytyrosol or tyrosol [19]. As mentioned above, hydroxytyrosol and tyrosol themselves are generally conjugated to glucuronic acid and excreted in urine as glucuronides [19, 24–26].

4. Antioxidant Role and other Biological Actions of Phenolic Compounds

In addition of ROS, oxidative stress can be indicated by the presence of markers such as F2-isoprostanes, lipid peroxides (LPO), oxidized gluthathione (GSSG) and reduced gluthathione (GSH), and glutathione peroxidase (GSH-Px). F2-isoprostanes are a result of the free radical induced peroxidation of arachidonic acid. LPO is more than likely a by-product of the oxidation of fatty acids [27] and depletion of the protective GSH precedes lipid oxidation and atherogenesis *in vivo* [28].

As mentioned before, human and animal research have shown that olive oil phenolic compounds possess important biological activities that may exert a preventative effect in regards to the development of chronic degenerative diseases. Total plasma antioxidant activity has been reported to increase in humans after the ingestion of olive oil phenolic compounds [29–31]. However, interesting aspects of olive oil phenolics, in many cases, are unrelated to their antioxidant potential (Figure 2). The main biological activities of olive oil phenolics are described next:

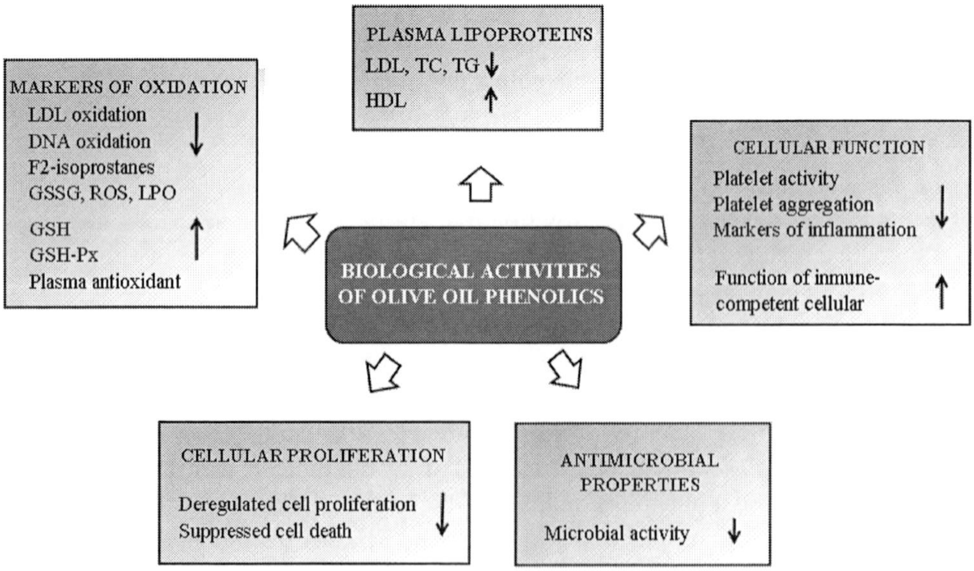

Figure 2. Biological activities of olive oil phenolic compounds. LDL: low density lipoprotein. HDL: high density lipoprotein. TC: total cholesterol. TG: triglyceride. GSSG: oxidized gluthathione. ROS: reactive oxygen species. LPO: lipid peroxides. GSH: reduced gluthathione. GSH-Px: glutathione peroxidase.

4.1. Effect of Olive Oil Phenolic Compounds on Plasma Lipoproteins

Elevated levels of total cholesterol (TC) and low density lipoprotein (LDL) have been established as risk factors for atherosclerosis, which is the primary cause of cardiovascular disease (CVD). Oxidation of LDL causes damage to the vascular wall, stimulating macrophage uptake and formation of foam cells, which in turn result in the formation of plaque within the arterial wall [32–34] (Figure 3). Contrarily, elevated levels of high density lipoprotein (HDL) are believed to have protective and anti-inflammatory properties [35].

A series of *in vitro* experiments aimed at investigating the antioxidant activities of virgin olive oil phenolics on parameters that are considered relevant to human health were initiated in 1994. The first paper reported inhibition of LDL oxidation by oleuropein glycoside, which was, to our knowledge, the only phenol typical of olive oil that was commercially available (Extrasynthese, France). Oleuropein was found to potently and dose-dependently inhibit LDL oxidation induced by copper sulphate [36]. This study was subsequently expanded to include hydroxytyrosol, which wasn't commercially available but was isolated from olive oil and other catechols [37]. Subsequent experiments showed that both oleuropein and hydroxytyrosol effectively scavenge superoxide anion generated by either human polymorphonuclear cells or by the xantine/xantine oxidase system [38]. It is noteworthy that, in these experimental setups, both vitamin E and butylated hydroxytoluene were found to be inactive. A scavenging effect of oleuropein and hydroxytyrosol was also demonstrated with respect to hypochlorous acid [38], a potent and dangerous oxidant species produced *in vivo* by activated neutrophils at the site of inflammation [39].

Both human and animal *in vivo* studies have also shown that the level at which LDL oxidizes, decreases linearly with increasing phenolic concentration [32, 40–49]. Fitó et al. [32] examined the antioxidant and anti-hypertensive effect of two similar olive oils, but with differences in their phenolic compounds content (refined: 14.7 mg/kg *versus* virgin: 161.0 mg/kg), in 40 males with coronary heart disease. Lower plasma oxidized LDL and LPO levels, together with higher activities of GSH-Px, were observed after virgin olive oil intervention. Data from a controlled human study containing 200 healthy male subjects, found a decrease in TC to HDL ratio with increasing phenolic content of the virgin olive oil consumed. An increase in HDL was also noted with increasing phenolic concentration of the oil [40]. On the other hand, Covas et al. [41] examined the role of phenolic compounds from olive oil on postprandial oxidative stress and LDL antioxidant content. According to this study, olive oil phenolic content seems to modulate the LDL phenolic content and the postprandial oxidative stress promoted by olive oil ingestion in humans. Furthermore, has been reported that the consumption of virgin olive oils have resulted in increases in circulating HDL ranging between 5.1–6.7% in two further human studies [42, 43]. Gimeno et al. [44] reported on an increase in the incorporation of oleic acid and antioxidants (phenols and vitamin E) to LDL after acute and short-term ingestion of virgin olive oil. An improvement of LDL resistance to oxidation was also observed.

Ocho et al. [45] provided evidence *in vivo* of the considerable antioxidant capacity of the phenolic fraction of virgin olive oil in rabbit LDL and the important role that this fraction can play in the overall antioxidant benefit attributed to this oil. Interestingly, two further mechanistic studies, demonstrated that phenolic compounds are able to bind to LDL, which could account for the increase in LDL resistance to oxidation [46, 47]. Also, studies involving animals have demonstrated that ingestion of phenol rich virgin olive oil led to improvements in blood lipid profile. A study involving rabbits demonstrated a reduction in circulating TC and an increase in HDL upon virgin olive oil consumption. Studies in rats have found that the intake of phenol rich virgin olive oil decreases TC, LDL and TG levels [48] and substantially increases HDL concentrations [49].

4.2. Effect of Olive oil Phenolic Compounds on Oxidative DNA Damage

Oxidative damage to DNA is a precursor for human carcinogenesis [50] and it is well known that oxygen radicals continually attack human cells [51]. Unless damage to these cells is counteracted, DNA damage may result, and such damage can lead to cancer development [51].

The activities of hydroxytyrosol toward chemically-induced DNA and aminoacid modification have been investigated [52, 53] and it was found that low concentrations of hydroxytyrosol, are able to scavenge peroxynitrite and therefore, to prevent of peroxynitrite-dependent DNA damage and tyrosine nitration. A randomized cross-over intervention trial has shown that intake of phenol rich virgin olive oil decreases oxidative DNA damage by up to 30% compared to a low phenol virgin olive oil [51]. An additional research demonstrated that after consumption of phenol rich virgin olive oil there was decreased urinary excretion of 8-oxo-deoxygyuanosine, a systemic marker of DNA oxidation [50, 54]. In support of these findings, animal studies have reported that a diet enriched with olive oil phenolic compounds has a protective effect against DNA damage [55, 56]. In agreement with these researches, an *in vitro* study reported that olive oil phenolic compounds showed DNA oxidation preventative activity [57].

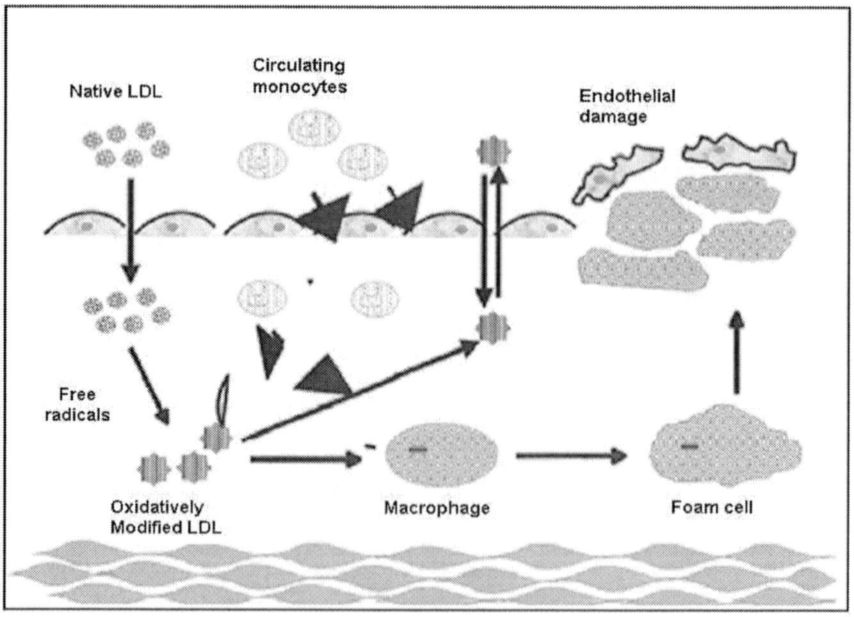

Figure 3. Flow-chart showing mechanism by which the oxidation of LDL may contribute to atherosclerosis.

4.3. Effect of Olive Oil Phenolic Compounds on Diverse Cellular Functions

Blood platelets have been demonstrated to play a role in CVD and atherosclerosis development. Continual damage to the vascular epithelium results in the development of lesions and these lesions stimulate endothelial adhesion molecule expression, platelet activity and aggregation [58, 59]. Circulating monocytes are attracted by these particular molecules and adhere to the endothelium and differentiate into macrophages, which in turn scavenge LDL and TG rich lipoproteins, becoming foam cells and forming fatty streaks [60]. Olive oil phenolic compounds have been demonstrated to inhibit human platelet activity in vitro [61, 62]. They inhibit also endothelial adhesion molecule expression upon incubation with human umbilical vein endothelial cells [63]. Virgin olive oil containing a high content (400 mg/kg) of phenolic compounds has been demonstrated to also decrease plasminogen activator inhibitor-1 (PAI-1) and factor VII (FVII). Both PAI-1 and FVII are pro-coagulant factors that have been linked to the development of coronary heart disease (CHD) [64]. Furthermore, olive oil phenolics have been shown to decrease homocysteine, which has been linked to increased adhesiveness of the endothelium [65].

One of the most interesting aspects of olive oil phenolics biochemistry is the discovery of their enzyme-modulating properties, which in many cases, are unrelated to their antioxidant potential. Olive oil phenolics such as oleuropein might be able to interact with enzymes relevant to human pathology such as atherosclerosis. *In vitro* studies on murine macrophages revealed that oleuropein increases the functional response of immune-competent cells when they are stimulated with bacterial polysaccharide [66]. This increase is due to a direct effect of oleuropein, which increases both the activity and the expression of the inducible form of the enzyme nitric oxide synthase. As relevant to atherosclerosis, it should be noted that during acute sepsis and inflammation that take place in the arterial wall, macrophages react to the endotoxin challenge by increasing the production of nitric oxide, which inhibits platelet aggregation and adherence and maintains a proper end-organ perfusion rate through increased vase-relaxation. In agreement with this finding, inhibition of nitric oxide synthesis during sepsis increases cellular damage and animal mortality [67]. Finally, macrophagic nitric oxide exerts antioxidant activities that play a protective role in preventing oxidative LDL modification that occur at the site of inflammation during enhanced ROS production [68].

4.4. Effect of Olive oil Phenolic Compounds on Cellular Proliferation

Cell proliferation and suppressed cell death are underlying factors for tumor formation and progression [69]. Research to date has shown that the olive oil phenolic inhibits cell proliferation in human promyelocytic HL60 leukemia cells and in human colon cancer lines [70–72]. Hashim et al. [73] demonstrated a dose-related inhibition of colon cancer cell invasion by olive oil phenolic compounds. Also, hydroxytyrosol has been found to exert strong anti-proliferative effects against human colon adenocarcinoma cells [74]. On the other hand, research using MCF-7 and SKBR3 breast cancer cells showed that phenolic compounds inhibit growth in these cell lines in a dose dependent manner and reduce expression of the HER2 oncogene, which plays a integral role in malignant transformation, tumorigenesis and metastasis [75–77]. Han et al. [78] studied the effects of oleuropein and hydroxytyrosol on growth in MCF-7 human breast cancer cells using assays for proliferation, cell viability, cell apoptosis and cellcycle. These phenolic compounds decreased cell viability, inhibited cell proliferation and induced cell apoptosis in MCF-7 cells. Result of proliferation assay showed that 200 μg/mL of oleuropein or 50 μg/mL of hydroxytyrosol remarkably reduced cell viability of MCF-7 cells. Oleuropein or hydroxytyrosol decrease of the number of MCF-7 cells by inhibiting the rate of cell proliferation and inducing cell apoptosis.

4.5. Antimicrobial Properties of Olive Oil Phenolic Compounds

The antimicrobial properties of plant molecules have been known for a long time and the commercial potential for their use was discussed by Wilkins and Board [79]. The olive leaf is known among other things to be resistant in nature to microbe and insect attack and much research has been focused on the antimicrobial activity of compounds contained in olives, olive oil and vegetation extracts [80–83]. *In vitro* research has shown that olive oil phenolic compounds have antimicrobial properties. Particularly, the phenolic compounds oleuropein, hydroxytyrosol and tyrosol have demonstrated potent antimicrobial activity against several strains of bacteria responsible for intestinal and respiratory infections [80]. Romero et al. [81] found that the dialdehydic form of decarboxymethyl ligstroside is not hydrolyzed in the stomach and therefore aids in inhibiting the growth of *Helicobacter pylori* bacteria. Interestingly, *Helicobacter pylori* are linked to the development of peptic ulcers and some types of gastric cancer. Hydroxytyrosol and oleuropein have also been shown to be cytotoxic to a large number of bacterial strains [82]. Interestingly, it was demonstrated the antimicrobial activities some phenolic components against fungal strains such as *Alternaria alternata, Aspergillus chevalieri, A. chrysogenum, A. elegans, A. flavus, A. fumigatus, A. nidulans, A. niger, A. oryzae, A. parasiticus, A. tamari, P. verrucosum, A. versicolor, A. wentii, Fusarium oxysporum, F. semitectum, Mucor racemosus, Neurospora crassa, Penicillium citrinum, P. echinulatum, P. griseofulvum, P. italicum, P. roqueforti* and *Rhizopus oligosporus* [83].

Conclusion and Future Perspectives

As noted throughout this chapter, free radicals have been implicated in the etiology of large number of chronic pathology. They can adversely alter many crucial biological molecules leading to loss of form and function. Such undesirable changes can lead to diseased conditions. Antioxidants can protect against the damage induced by free radicals acting at various levels. In this connection, the relation between free radicals, antioxidants and functioning of various organs and organ systems is highly complex; and many novel approaches are made and significant findings have come to light in the last few years.

As mentioned before, the amount of olive oil phenolics is a very important parameter when evaluating the quality of virgin olive oil. Diverse studies have shown that the amount of phenols, together with a favourable monounsaturated to polyunsaturated fatty acid ratio, is related to several healthy attributes. However, if the literature is analyzed in detail, it is evident that phenolic compounds of virgin olive oil have not been completely studied, because of the complexity of their chemical nature and the complexity of the matrix in which they are found. Therefore, it is expected that the use of potent techniques coupled with rapid, reliable and sophisticated detectors will become more common in the near future.

REFERENCES

[1] Stark, A.H.; Madar, Z. Olive oil as a functional food: epidemiology and nutritional approaches. *Nutr. Rev.* 2002, *60*, 170–176.

[2] Fortes, C.; Forastiere, F.; Farchi, S.; Mallone, S.; Trequattrinni, T.; Anatra, F.; Schmid, G.; Perucci, C.A. The protective effect of the Mediterranean diet on lung cancer. *Nutr. Cancer* 2003, *46*, 30–37.

[3] Herrera, M.D.; Perez-Guerrero, C.; Marhuenda, E.; Ruiz-Gutierrez, V. Effects of dietary oleic- rich oils (virgin olive and high-oleic-acid sunflower) on vascular reactivity in Wistar-Kyoto and spontaneously hypertensive rats. *Br. J. Nutr.* 2001, *86*, 349–357.

[4] Grasso, S.; Siracusa, L.; Spatafora, C.; Renis, M.; Tringali, C. Hydroxytyrosol lipophilic analogues: Enzymatic synthesis, radical scavenging activity and DNA oxidative damage protection. *Bioorg. Med. Chem.* 2006, *35*, 137–152.

[5] Trichopoulou, A.; Costacou, T.; Bamia, C.; Trichopoulos, D. Adherence to a Mediterranean diet and survival in a Greek population. *N. Engl. J. Med.* 2003, *348*, 2599–2608.

[6] Singh, R.B.; Dubnov, G.; Niaz, M.A.; Ghosh, S.; Singh, R.; Rastogi, S.S.; Manor, O.; Pella, D.; Berry, E.M. Effect of an Indo-Mediterranean diet on progression of coronary artery disease in high risk patients (Indo-Mediterranean Diet Heart Study): A randomised single-blind trial. *Lancet* 2002, *360*, 1455–1461.

[7] Tripoli, E.; Giammanco, M.; Tabacchi, G.; Di Majo, D.; Giammanco, S.; La Guardia, M. The phenolic compounds of olive oil: structure, biological activity and beneficial effects on human health. *Nutr. Res. Rev.* 2005, *18*, 98–112.

[8] Aguilera, C.M.; Mesa, M.D.; Ramirez-Tortosa, M.C.; Nestares, M.T.; Ros, E.; Gil, A. Sunflower oil does not protect against LDL oxidation as virgin olive oil does in patients with peripheral vascular disease. *Clin. Nutr.* 2004, *23*, 673–681

[9] Harper, C.R.; Edwards, M.C.; Jacobson, T.A. Flaxseed oil supplementation does not affect plasma lipoprotein concentration or particle size in human subjects. *J. Nutr.* 2006, *136*, 2844–2848.

[10] Witztum, J.L. The oxidation hypothesis of atherosclerosis. *Lancet.* 1994, *344*, 793–795.

[11] Reinisch, N.; Kiechl, S.; Mayr, C.; Schratzberger, P.; Dunzendorfer, S.; Kahler, C.M.; Buratti, T.; Willeit, J.; Wiedermann, C.J. Association of high plasma antioxidant capacity with new lesion formation in carotid atherosclerosis: a prospective study. *Eur. J. Clin. Invest.* 1998, *28*, 787–792.

[12] De la Puerta, R.; Martinez Domínguez, M.E.; Ruiz-Gutierrez, V.; Flavill, J.A.; Hoult, J.R. Effects of virgin olive oil phenolics on scavenging of reactive nitrogen species and upon nitrergic neurotransmission. *Life Sci.* 2001, *69*, 1213–1222.

[13] Owen, R.W.; Giacosa, A.; Hull, W.E.; Haubner, R.; Spiegelhalder, B.; Bartsch, H. The antioxidant/anticancer potential of phenolic compounds isolated from olive oil. *Eur. J. Cancer.* 2000, *36*, 1235–1247.

[14] Paiva-Martins, F.; Fernandes, J.; Rocha, S.; Nascimento, H.; Vitorino, R.; Amado, F.; Borges, F.; Belo, L.; Santos-Silva, A. Effects of olive oil polyphenols on erythrocyte oxidative damage. *Mol. Nutr. Food Res.* 2009, *53*, 609–616.

[15] Zarrouk, W.; Baccouri, B.; Taamalli, W.; Trigui, A.; Daouda, D.; Zarrouka, M. Oil fatty acid composition of eighteen Mediterranean olive varieties cultivated under the arid conditions of Boughrara (southern Tunisia). *Grasas y Aceites* 2009, *60*, 498–506.

[16] Kiritsakis, A.K. Composition of olive oil and its nutritional and health effect. *In* 10th International Rapeseed Congress, Canberra, Australia, 1999.

[17] Amiot, M.J.; Fleuriet, A.; Macheix, J.J. Importance and evolution of phenolic compounds in olive during growth and maturation. *J. Agric. Food Chem.* 1996, *34*, 823–826.

[18] Tuck, K.L.; Freeman, M.P.; Hayball, P.J.; Stretch, G.L.; Stupans, I. The in vivo fate of hydroxytyrosol and tyrosol, antioxidant phenolic constituents of olive oil, after intravenous and oral dosing of labeled compounds to rats. *J. Nutr.* 2001, *131*, 1993–1996.

[19] Vissers, M.N.; Zock, P.L.; Roodenburg, A.J.; Leenen, R.; Katan, M.B. Olive oil phenols are absorbed in humans. *J. Nutr.* 2002, *132*, 409–417.

[20] Miro Casas, E.; Albadalejo, M. F.; Covas Planells, M. I.; Colomer, F. M.; Lamuela Raventos, R. M.; de la Torre Fornell, R. Tyrosol bioavailability in humans after ingestion of virgin olive oil. *Clin. Chem.* 2001, *47*, 341–343.

[21] Visioli, F., Caruso, D., Galli, C., Viappiani, S., Galli, G., Sala, A. Olive oils rich in natural catecholic phenols decrease isoprostane excretion in humans. *Biochem. Biophys. Res. Commun.*2000, *278*, 797–799.

[22] Miro-Casas, E.; Covas, M.I.; Farre, M.; Fito, M.; Ortuno, J.; Weinbrenner, T.; Roset, P.; De la Torre, R. Hydroxytyrosol disposition in humans. *Clin. Chem.* 2003, *49*, 945–952.

[23] Miro-Casas, E.; Covas, M.I.; Fito, M.; Farre-Albadalejo, M.; Marrugat, J.; De la Torre, R. Tyrosol and hydroxytyrosol are absorbed from moderate and sustained doses of virgin olive oil in humans. *Eur. J. Clin. Nutr.* 2003, *57*, 186–190.

[24] Visioli, F.; Galli, C.; Plasmati, E.; Viappiani, S.; Hernandez, A.; Colombo, C.; Sala, A. Olive phenol hydroxytyrosol prevents passive smoking-induced oxidative stress. *Circulation* 2000, *102*, 2169–2171.

[25] Caruso, D.; Visioli, F.; Patelli, R.; Galli, C.; Galli, G. Urinary excretion of olive oil phenols and their metabolites in humans. *Metabolism* 2001, *50*, 1426–1428.

[26] Visioli, F.; Caruso, D.; Plasmati, E.; Patelli, R.; Mulinacci, N.; Romani, A.; Galli, G.; Galli, C. Hydroxytyrosol, as a component of olive mill waste water, is dose-dependently absorbed and increases the antioxidant capacity of rat plasma. *Free Rad. Res.* 2001, *34*, 301–305.

[27] Ruano, J.; Lopez-Miranda, J.; Fuentes, F.; Moreno, J.A.; Bellido, C.; Perez-Martinez, P.; Lozano, A.; Gomez, P.; Jimenez, Y.; Perez Jimenez, F. Phenolic content of virgin olive oil improves ischemic reactive hyperemia in hypercholesterolemic patients. *J. Am. Coll. Cardiol.* 2005, *46*, 1864–1868.

[28] Biswas, S.K.; Newby, D.E.; Rahman, I.; Megson, I.L. Depressed glutathione synthesis precedes oxidative stress and atherogenesis in Apo-E(-/-) mice. *Biochem. Biophys. Res. Comm.* 2005, *338*, 1368–1373.

[29] Bogani, P.; Galli, C.; Villa, M.; Visioli, F. Postprandial anti-inflammatory and antioxidant effects of extra virgin olive oil. *Atherosclerosis* 2007, *190*, 181–186.

[30] Salvini, S.; Sera, F.; Caruso, D.; Giovannelli, L.; Visioli, F.; Saieva, C.; Masala, G.; Ceroti, M.; Giovacchini, V.; Pitozzi, V.; Galli, C.; Romani, A.; Mulinacci, N.; Bortolomeazzi, R.; Dolara, P.; Palli, D. Daily consumption of a high-phenol extra-virgin olive oil reduces oxidative DNA damage in postmenopausal women. *Br. J. Nutr.* 2006, *95*, 742–751.

[31] Visioli, F.; Caruso, D.; Grande, S.; Bosisio, R.; Villa, M.; Galli, G.; Sirtori, C.; Galli, C. Virgin Olive Oil Study (VOLOS): Vasoprotective potential of extra virgin olive oil in mildly dyslipidemic patients. *Eur. J. Nutr.* 2005, *44*, 121–127.

[32] Fitó, M.; Cladellas, M.; de la Torre, R.; Marti, J.; Alcantara, M.; Pujadas-Bastardes, M.; Marrugat, J.; Bruguera, J.; Lopez-Sabater, M.C.; Vila, J.; Covas, M.I. Antioxidant effect of virgin olive oil in patients with stable coronary heart disease: a randomized, crossover, controlled, clinical trial. *Atherosclerosis* 2005, *181*, 149–158.

[33] Vissers, M.N.; Zock, P.L.; Wiseman, S.A.; Meyboom, S.; Katan, M B. Effect of phenol-rich extra virgin olive oil on markers of oxidation in healthy volunteers. *Eur. J. Clin. Nutr. 2001*, 55, 334–341.

[34] Patrick, L.; Uzick, M. Cardiovascular disease: C-reactive protein and the inflammatory disease paradigm: HMG-CoA reductase inhibitors, alpha-tocopherol, red yeast rice, and olive oil polyphenols. A review of the literature. *Altern. Med. Rev.* 2001, *6*, 248–271.

[35] Chrysohoou, C.; Pitsavos, C.; Skoumas, J.; Masoura, C.; Katinioti, A.; Panagiotakos, D.;Stefanadis, C. The emerging anti-inflammatory role of HDL-cholesterol, illustrated in cardiovascular disease free population; the ATTICA study. *Int. J. Cardio.* 2006, *122*, 29–33.

[36] Visioli, F., Galli, C. Oleuropein protects low density lipoprotein from oxidation. *Life Sci.*1994, *55*, 1965–1971.

[37] Visioli, F.; Bellomo, G.; Montedoro, G.; Galli, C. Low density lipoprotein oxidation is inhibited in vitro by olive oil constituents. *Atherosclerosis* 1995, *117*, 25–32.

[38] Visioli, F.; Bellomo, G.; Galli, C. Free radical-scavenging properties of olive oil polyphenols. *Biochem. Biophys. Res. Commun.*1998, *247*, 60–64.

[39] Aruoma, O.I.; Halliwell, B. Action of hypochlorous acid on the antioxidant protective enzymes superoxide dismutase, catalase and glutathione peroxidase. *Biochem. J.* 1987, *248*, 973–976.

[40] Covas, M.I.; Nyyssonen, K.; Poulsen, H.E.; Kaikkonen, J.; Zunft, H.J.; Kiesewetter, H.; Gaddi, A.; de la Torre, R.; Mursu, J.; Baumler, H.; Nascetti, S.; Salonen, J.T.; Fito, M.; Virtanen, J.; Marrugat, J.; Group, E.S. The effect of polyphenols in olive oil on heart disease risk factors: a randomized trial. *Ann. Int. Med.* 2006, 145, 333–341.

[41] Covas, M.I.; de la Torre, K.; Farre-Albaladejo, M.; Kaikkonen, J.; Fito, M.; Lopez-Sabater, C.; Pujadas-Bastardes, M.A.; Joglar, J.; Weinbrenner, T.; Lamuela-Raventos, R.M.; de la Torre, R. Postprandial LDL phenolic content and LDL oxidation are modulated by olive oil phenolic compounds in humans. *Free Rad. Biol. Med.* 2006, *40*, 608–616.

[42] Marrugat, J.; Covas, M.I.; Fito, M.; Schroder, H.; Miro-Casas, E.; Gimeno, E.; Lopez-Sabater, M.C.; de la Torre, R.; Farre, M. Effects of differing phenolic content in dietary

olive oils on lipids and LDL oxidation--a randomized controlled trial. *Eur. J. Nutr.* 2004, *43*, 140–147.

[43] Weinbrenner, T.; Fito, M.; de la Torre, R.; Saez, G.T.; Rijken, P.; Tormos, C.; Coolen, S.; Albaladejo, M.F.; Abanades, S.; Schroder, H.; Marrugat, J.; Covas, M.I. Olive oils high in phenolic compounds modulate oxidative/anti oxidative status in men. *J. Nutr.* 2004, *134*, 2314–2321.

[44] Gimeno, E.; Fito, M.; Lamuela-Raventos, R.M.; Castellote, A.I.; Covas, M.; Farre, M.; de La Torre-Boronat, M.C.; Lopez-Sabater, M.C. Effect of ingestion of virgin olive oil on human low- density lipoprotein composition. *Eur. J. Clin. Nutr.* 2002, *56*, 114–120.

[45] Ochoa, J.J.; Quiles, J.L.; Ramirez-Tortosa, C.; Mataix, J.; Huertas, J.R. Dietary oil high in oleic acid but with different unsaponifiable fraction contents have different effects in fatty acid composition and peroxidation in rabit LDL. *Nutrition* 2002, *18*, 60–65.

[46] Gimeno, E.; de la Torre-Carbot, K.; Lamuela-Raventos, R.M.; Castellote, A.I.; Fito, M.; de la Torre, R.; Covas, M.I.; Carmen Lopez-Sabater, M. Changes in the phenolic content of low density lipoprotein after olive oil consumption in men. A randomized crossover controlled trial. *Br. J. Nutr.* 2007, 1–8.

[47] De la Torre-Carbot, K.; Chavez-Servin, J.L.; Jauregui, O.; Castellote, A.I.; Lamuela-Raventos, R.M.; Fito, M.; Covas, M.I.; Munoz-Aguayo, D.; Lopez-Sabater, M.C. Presence of virgin olive oil phenolic metabolites in human low density lipoprotein fraction: determination by high-performance liquid chromatography-electrospray ionization tandem mass spectrometry. *Analyt. Chim. Acta* 2007, *583*, 402–410.

[48] Gorinstein, S.; Leontowicz, H.; Lojek, A.; Leontowicz, M.; Ciz, M.; Krzeminski, R.; Gralak, M.; Czerwinski, J.; Jastrzebski, Z.; Trakhtenberg, S.; Grigelmo-Miguel, N.; Soliva-Fortuny, R.; Martin-Belloso, O. Olive oils improve lipid metabolism and increase antioxidant potential in rats fed diets containing cholesterol. *J. Agric. Food Chem.* 2002, *50*, 6102–6108.

[49] Mangas-Cruz, M.A.; Fernandez-Moyano, A.; Albi, T.; Guinda, A.; Relimpio, F.; Lanzon, A.; Pereira, J.L.; Serrera, J.L.; Montilla, C.; Astorga, R.; Garcia-Luna, P.P. Effects of minor constituents (non-glyceride compounds) of virgin olive oil on plasma lipid concentrations in male Wistar rats. *Clin. Nutr.* 2001, *20*, 211–215.

[50] Cooke, M.S.; Evans, M.D.; Dizdaroglu, M.; Lunec, J. Oxidative DNA damage: mechanisms, mutation, and disease. *Fed. Am. Soc. Exp. Biol. J.* 2003, *17*, 1195–1214.

[51] Salvini, S.; Sera, F.; Caruso, D.; Giovannelli, L.; Visioli, F.; Saieva, C.; Masala, G.; Ceroti, M.; Giovacchini, V.; Pitozzi, V.; Galli, C.; Romani, A.; Mulinacci, N.; Bortolomeazzi, R.; Dolara, P.; Palli, D. Daily consumption of a high-phenol extra-virgin olive oil reduces oxidative DNA damage in postmenopausal women. *Br. J. Nutr.* 2006, *95*, 742–751.

[52] Deiana, M.; Aruoma, O.I.; Bianchi, M.L.; Spencer, J.P.; Kaur, H.; Halliwell, B.; Aeschbach, R.; Banni, S.; Dessi, M.A.; Corongiu, F.P. Inhibition of peroxynitrite dependent DNA base modification and tyrosine nitration by the extra virgin olive oil-derived antioxidant hydroxytyrosol. *Free Radic. Biol. Med.*1999, 26, 762–769.

[53] de la Puerta, R.; Martinez, D.M.; Ruiz-Gutierrez, V.; Flavill, J.A.; Hoult, J.R. Effects of virgin olive oil phenolics on scavenging of reactive nitrogen species and upon nitrergic neurotransmission. *Life Sci.* 2001, 69, 1213–1222.

[54] Machowetz, A.; Poulsen, H.E.; Gruendel, S.; Weimann, A.; Fito, M.; Marrugat, J.; de la Torre, R.; Salonen, J.T.; Nyyssonen, K.; Mursu, J.; Nascetti, S.; Gaddi, A.;

Kiesewetter, H.; Baumler, H.; Selmi, H.; Kaikkonen, J.; Zunft, H.J.; Covas, M.I.; Koebnick, C. Effect of olive oils on biomarkers of oxidative DNA stress in Northern and Southern Europeans. *FASEB J.* 2007, *21*, 45–52.
[55] Jacomelli, M.; Pitozzi, V.; Zaid, M.; Larrosa, M.; Tonini, G.; Martini, A.; Urbani, S.; Taticchi, A.; Servili, M.; Dolara, P.; Giovannelli, L. Dietary extra-virgin olive oil rich in phenolic antioxidants and the aging process: long-term effects in the rat. *J. Nutr. Biochem.* doi:10.1016/j.jnutbio.2008.12.014.
[56] Quiles, J.L.; Farquharson, A.J.; Simpson, D.K.; Grant, I.; Wahle, K.W. Olive oil phenolics: effects on DNA oxidation and redox enzyme mRNA in prostate cells. *Br. J. Nutr.* 2002, *88*, 225–234.
[57] Fabiani, R.; Rosignoli, P.; De Bartolomeo, A.; Fuccelli, R.; Servili, M.; Montedoro, G.F.; Morozzi, G. Oxidative DNA damage is prevented by extracts of olive oil, hydroxytyrosol, and other olive phenolic compounds in human blood mononuclear cells and HL60 cells. *J. Nutr.* 2008, *138*, 1411–1416.
[58] White, J.G. Platelets and atherosclerosis. *Eur. J. Clin. Invest.* 1994, *24*, 25–29.
[59] De La Cruz, J.P.; Villalobos, M.A.; Carmona, J.A.; Martin-Romero, M.; Smith-Agreda, J.M.; de la Cuesta, F.S. Antithrombotic potential of olive oil administration in rabbits with elevated cholesterol. *Thromb. Res.* 2000, *100*, 305–315.
[60] Perona, J.S.; Cabello-Moruno, R.; Ruiz-Gutierrez, V. The role of virgin olive oil components in the modulation of endothelial function. *J. Nutr. Biochem.* 2006, *17*, 429–445.
[61] Togna, G.I.; Togna, A.R.; Franconi, M.; Marra, C.; Guiso, M. Olive oil isochromans inhibit human platelet reactivity. *J. Nutr.* 2003, *133*, 2532–2536.
[62] Dell' Agli, M.; Maschi, O.; Galli, G. V.; Fagnani, R.; Dal Cero, E.; Caruso, D.; Bosisio, E. Inhibition of platelet aggregation by olive oil phenols via cAMP-phosphodiesterase. *Br. J. Nutr.* 2008, *99*, 945–951.
[63] Petroni, A.; Blasevich, M.; Salami, M.; Papini, N.; Montedoro, G.; Galli, C. Inhibition of platelet aggregation and eicosanoid production by phenolic components of olive oil. *Thromb. Res.* 1995, *78*, 151–160.
[64] Ruano, J.; Lopez-Miranda, J.; de la Torre, R.; Delgado-Lista, J.; Fernandez, J.; Caballero, J.; Covas, M.I.; Jimenez, Y.; Perez-Martinez, P.; Marin, C.; Fuentes, F.; Perez-Jimenez, F. Intake of phenol-rich virgin olive oil improves the postprandial prothrombotic profile in hypercholesterolemic patients. *Am. J. Clin. Nutr.* 2007, *86*, 341–346.
[65] Manna, C.; Napoli, D.; Cacciapuoti, G.; Porcelli, M.; Zappia, V. Olive oil phenolic compounds inhibit homocysteine-induced endothelial cell adhesion regardless of their different antioxidant activity. *J. Agric. Food Chem.* 2009, *57*, 3478–3482.
[66] Visioli, F.; Bellosta, S.; Galli, C. Oleuropein, the bitter principle of olives, enhances nitric oxide production by mouse macrophages. *Life Sci.* 1998, *62*, 541–546.
[67] Lowenstein, C.J.; Hill, S.L.; Lafond-Walker, A.; Wu, J., Allen; G., Landavere, M.; Rose, N.R.; Herskowitz, A. Nitric oxide inhibits viral replication in murine myocarditis. *J. Clin. Invest.* 1996, *97*, 1837–1843.
[68] Jessup, W.; Mohr, D.; Gieseg, S.P.; Dean, R.T.; Stocker, R. The participation of nitric oxide in cell free- and its restriction of macrophage-mediated oxidation of low-density lipoprotein. *Biochim. Biophys. Acta* 1999, *1180*, 73–82.

[69] Evan, G.I.; Vousden, K.H. Proliferation, cell cycle and apoptosis in cancer. *Nature* 2001, *411*, 342–348.

[70] Fabiani, R.; De Bartolomeo, A.; Rosignoli, P.; Servili, M.; Selvaggini, R.; Montedoro, G.F.; Di Saverio, C.; Morozzi, G. Virgin olive oil phenols inhibit proliferation of human promyelocytic leukemia cells (HL60) by inducing apoptosis and differentiation. *J. Nutr.* 2006, *136*, 614–619.

[71] Gill, C.I.; Boyd, A.; McDermott, E.; McCann, M.; Servili, M.; Selvaggini, R.; Taticchi, A.; Esposto, S.; Montedoro, G.; McGlynn, H.; Rowland, I. Potential anti-cancer effects of virgin olive oil phenols on colorectal carcinogenesis models in vitro. *Int. J. Cancer* 2005, *117*, 1–7.

[72] Fini, L.; Hotchkiss, E.; Fogliano, V.; Graziani, G.; Romano, M.; De Vol, E.B.; Qin, H.; Selgrad, M.; Boland, C.R.; Ricciardiello, L. Chemopreventive properties of pinoresinol-rich olive oil involve a selective activation of the ATM-p53 cascade in colon cancer cell lines. *Carcinogenesis* 2008, *29*, 139–146.

[73] Hashim, Y.Z.; Rowland, I.R.; McGlynn, H.; Servili, M.; Selvaggini, R.; Taticchi, A.; Esposto, S.; Montedoro, G.; Kaisalo, L.; Wahala, K.; Gill, C.I. Inhibitory effects of olive oil phenolics on invasion in human colon adenocarcinoma cells in vitro. *Int. J. Cancer* 2008, *122*, 495–500.

[74] Corona, G.; Deiana, M.; Incani, A.; Vauzour, D.; Dessi, M.A.; Spencer, J.P.E. Hydroxytyrosol inhibits the proliferation of human colon adeocarcinoma cells through ihibition of ERK1/2 ad cyclin D1. *Mol. Nutr. Food Res.* 2009, *53*, 897–903.

[75] Menendez, J.A.; Vazquez-Martin, A.; Colomer, R.; Brunet, J.; Carrasco-Pancorbo, A.; Garcia- Villalba, R.; Fernandez-Gutierrez, A.; Segura-Carretero, A. Olive oil's bitter principle reverses acquired autoresistance to trastuzumab (Herceptin) in HER2-overexpressing breast cancer cells. *BMC Cancer* 2007, *7*, 80–99.

[76] Menendez, J.A.; Vazquez-Martin, A.; Oliveras-Ferraros, C.; Garcia-Villalba, R.; Carrasco Pancorbo, A.; Fernandez-Gutierez, A.; Segura-Carretero, A. Analysing effects of extra-virgin olive oil polyphenols on breast cancer-associated fatty acid synthase protein expression using reverse-phase protein microarrays. *Int. J. Mol. Med.* 2008, *22*, 433–439.

[77] Menendez, J.A.; Vazquez-Martin, A.; Oliveras-Ferraros, C.; Garcia-Villalba, R.; Carrasco Pancorbo, A.; Fernandez-Gutierrez, A.; Segura-Carretero, A. Extra-virgin olive oil polyphenolics inhibit HER2 (erbB-2)-induced malignant transformation in human breast epithelial cells: Relationship between the chemical structures of extra-virgin olive oil secoiridoids and lignans and their inhibitory activities on the tyrosine kinase activity of HER2. *Int. J. Oncol.* 2009, *34*, 43–51.

[78] Han, J.; Talorete, T.P.N.; Yamada, P.; Isoda, H. Anti-proliferative and apototic effects of oleuropein and hydroxytyrosol on human breast cancer MCF-7 cells. *Cytotechnology* 2009, *59*, 45–53.

[79] Wilkins, K.M.; Board, R.G. Natural antimicrobial systems. In: G.W. Gould, Editor, *Mechanisms of action of food preservation procedures*, Elsevier Applied Sciences, London, 1989.

[80] Medina, E.; de Castro, A.; Romero, C.; Brenes, M. Comparison of the concentrations of phenolic compounds in olive oils and other plant oils: correlation with antimicrobial activity. *J. Agric. Food Chem.* 2006, *54*, 4954–4961.

[81] Romero, C.; Medina, E.; Vargas, J.; Brenes, M.; De Castro, A. In vitro activity of olive oil polyphenols against Helicobacter pylori. *J. Agric. Food Chem.* 2007, *55*, 680–686.
[82] Bisignano, G.; Tomaino, A.; Lo Cascio, R.; Crisafi, G.; Uccella, N.; Saija, A. On the in-vitro antimicrobial activity of oleuropein and hydroxytyrosol. *J. Pharma. Pharmacol.* 1999, *51*, 971–974.
[83] Korukluoglu, M.; Sahan, Y.; Yigit, A. Antifungal properties of olive leaf extracts and their phenolic compounds. *J. Food Saf.* 2008, *28*, 76–87.

In: Olive Consumption and Health
Editors: C. A. Savalas and S. M. Nicolau

ISBN: 978-1-62100-774-6

Chapter 9

OLIVE OIL TRACEABILITY THROUGH DNA MARKERS

P. Martins-Lopes* and S. Gomes†
Institute of Biotechnology and Bioengineering,
Centre of Genomics and Biotechnology,
University of Trás-os-Montes and Alto Douro
(IBB/CGB-UTAD), Portugal

ABSTRACT

Traceability/product tracing has been defined by the *Codex Alimentarius Commission* as the ability to follow the movement of a food through specified stage(s) of its production, processing, and distribution [CODEX, 2006]. The development of food traceability systems is becoming more demanding once consumers and producers are seeking for more notable foods with high quality guarantee. Consumers are interested in choosing what they are eating based on nutrition value, food safety and products' origin guarantee. As a consequence, food traceability is required by consumers and government organizations because it is a significant component of food and human safety. The European Union regulation allows the application of the following geographical indications to a food product: protected designation of origin (PDO), protected geographical indication (PGI), and traditional specialities guaranteed (TSG). An olive oil with a PDO designation demands precise definitions of several parameters such as the olive cultivar used for the oil production, cultivar geographical origin, olive orchards agronomic practice, technology used for olive oil production, and oil organoleptic characteristics. Nowadays, these parameters are defined by legislation, and are considered for olive oil certification purposes.

Because chemical analyses *per se* are not sufficient to verify olive oil authenticity, DNA markers, which have already been used for olive cultivars fingerprinting, are increasingly being applied to solve food traceability and provenance issues. Nowadays, DNA analysis with molecular markers has opened way to understand complex organism's genome. Nevertheless, it is presently being applied in a vast number of areas,

* E-mail: plopes@utad.pt.
† E-mail: sgomes@utad.pt.

where food traceability is going to have a preeminent positioning. This chapter addresses recent advances concerning traceability of olive oils, aspects related to the DNA fingerprinting application in the olive oil production chain, and problems related to the DNA extraction methods and molecular marker choices.

1. Introduction

Many consumers identify olive oil as a food product that perfectly combines nutritional and sensory values. Apart from these values olive oil consumption has been largely associated as beneficial for human health, so oil quality became more appreciated [Willett, 2006].

Traceability or product tracing has been defined by the *Codex Alimentarius Commission* as "the ability to follow the movement of a food product through specified stage(s) of its production, processing and distribution" [CODEX, 2006], and the same definition is adopted by European Union Regulation 178/2002 including besides food, "feed, food-producing animal or substance intended to be, or expected to be, incorporated into a food or feed". For food producing companies' food traceability legislation may be considered an additional production cost, but it could as well play an interesting commercial role to consumers' attention if directed to specific market niches linked to food safety and high quality products with certified origin. As a matter of fact, besides consumer's growing interest in these issues, each country is also interested in protecting their own quality products, increasing the regulation on certified products worldwide. The legislation although tight is still able to be overcome, since most of the control measures used is sometimes ambiguous in the correct determination of the controlled parameters. Thus, the European Union has recognized and supported the potential of differentiating quality products on a regional basis [Dimara and Skuras, 2003]. In 1992, European Union regulation 2081/92 and 2082/92 introduced an integrated framework for the protection of geographical indications and designations of origin for agricultural products and foodstuffs. Recently, these last regulations have been replaced by regulation 510/2006 and 509/2006, respectively, and European Union regulation 1898/2006 was added. The European Union regulation allows the application of the following geographical indications to a food product: protected designation of origin (PDO), protected geographical indication (PGI) and traditional specialities guaranteed (TSG). The protected designation of origin (PDO) is the term used to describe foodstuffs that are produced, processed and prepared in a specific geographical area using recognized and certified methods.

Several protected denomination of origin (PDO) for olive oil regions have been established by legislation in order to: (i) enhance the quality of certified product, and (ii) ensure both consumers' expectations and producers' profits. Virgin olive oils command a premium in the market, leading to a great temptation to adulterate them with vegetable seed oils [Cercaci et al., 2003]. Several techniques based on olive oil composition (e.g., gas chromatography and silica gel column chromatography) have been applied to detect adulterations [Pasqualone and Catalano, 2000; Damirchi et al., 2005; Flores et al., 2006; Mariani et al., 2006]. However, some difficulties have been found in distinguishing among different olive cultivars [De la Torre et al., 2004]. Nevertheless, several problems concerning *Olea europaea* L. cultivars homonymous and synonymous have been pointed out in the literature in terms of olive germplasm [Gemas et al., 2004; Martins-Lopes et al., 2007], which may compromise a correct cultivar identification, and consequently influence the development of a reliable traceability system in the olive sector. A part from this, intra-varietal genetic variation has also been detected among olive clones [Gemas et al., 2004; Gomes et al., 2008; Martins-Lopes et al., 2009], which can complicate even more this DNA approach. Thus, it is urgent that a dependable olive database can be generated, containing all available data, in order to have a better prospect of the work that is needed in terms of olive germplasm evaluation. Moreover, this database may define a set of molecular markers that are discriminatory for traceability purposes.

In order to fulfil all the purposes mentioned above, the analysis methods applied to detect the presence of a particular component in food must be sensitive and accurate. When compared to other molecules, DNA is more stable (e.g., proteins) to a physical and chemical actions during food processing. Therefore, DNA is an interesting target for food control, in what concerns traceability purposes. The DNA-based methods that have been more widely used in authenticity of species, used in foodstuffs production, have been realtime (RTi) and other techniques based on polymerase chain reaction (PCR). One of the reasons for the success in their application is due to the fact that PCR based methods require very small amount of starting sample, which can sometimes be a problem when using other detection methods. With the large genome sequencing programmes and the development of chips with wider information, we foresee that a system with multi-genes will exist and will be able to trace all these occurrences in one single reaction.

2. Olive Oil DNA Extraction Protocols

One of the principal constrains when applying molecular marker technology to the olive oil traceability is related to obtaining DNA samples suitable for PCR amplification procedures. In order to extract and purify olive oil a series of procedures are undertaken (centrifugation, filtration and decantation), which have a direct influence on the amount of DNA that will remain with the oil [Busconi et al., 2003; Consolandi et al., 2008], due to the shear forces and further mechanical stress [Adam and Zimm, 1977]. However, the quantity of DNA available in the olive oil is normally sufficient to be suitable for molecular marker application [Montemurro et al., 2008]. The problem that remains is normally associated to the presence of PCR inhibitors that constrains further analysis. The compounds that can interfere with the DNA polymerase activity are mainly, in this matrix, the phenolic compounds [Muzzalupo et al., 2007, Agrimonti et al., 2011], polysaccharides [Muzzalupo et al., 2007] and the fat presence [Agrimonti et al., 2011]. The DNA extraction buffer most widely used in food products is based on hexadecyltrimethylammonium bromide (CTAB). However, each method has to be adapted according to the specificity of each matrix. Nowadays, there are several DNA extracting kits available in the market that have demonstrated to be appropriate for traceability of processed food [Doveri and Lee, 2007; Brezná and Kuchta, 2008]. However, some of them are not always suitable for all food matrices, having to be adapted to each one in particular.

Table 1. Olive oil DNA extraction methods

Method	Starting material	Previous amplification	Yield	Molecular Marker	Reference
Gene Elute Plant kit (Sigma)	200 mL	NA	ND	AFLP	Montemurro et al. [2008]
	250 mL	NA	ND	SSR	Alba et al. [2009]
QIAamp DNA Stool (Qiagen) following Testolin and Lain [2005]	100- 300 μL	GenomePlex Whole Genome Amplification (WGA) kit (Sigma Chemical Company)	73-300 ng (QIAamp DNA) 17-22 fold higher (WGA)	SSR	Muzzalupo et al. [2007]
CTAB method adapted from Doyle and Doyle [1987]	100 mL	NA	ND	RAPD	Muzzalupo and Perri [2002]
	6 mL	NA	387 ng		Martins-Lopes et al. [2008]
CTAB based method	1 mL	NA	ND	qRT-PCR	Gimenez et al. [2010]
CTAB method adapted from Murray and Thompson [1980]	50-100 mL	NA	ND	chloroplast DNA markers SCAR and AFLP	Busconi et al. [2003]
Qiagen Plant	1 mL	NA	87 ng		Martins-Lopes et al. [2008]
NucleoSpin Plant	1 mL	NA	1320 ng		Martins-Lopes et al. [2008]
	1 mL	NA	40 ng mL^{-1}	SSR	Vietina et al. [2011]
NucleoSpin Food	4.2 mL	NA	2300 ng		Martins-Lopes et al. [2008]
Hexane method	1.0 mL	NA	500-750 ng	LDR-UA SNP	Conslandi et al. [2008]
	2.0 mL	NA	3520 ng	RAPD, ISSR, SSR	Martins-Lopes et al. [2008]
	1.0 mL	NA	ND	qRT-PCR	Gimenez et al. [2010]
CTAB–hexane method	1.0 mL	NA	ND	qRT-PCR	Gimenez et al. [2010]
CTAB–hexane–chloroform method	0.5 mL	NA	ND	qRT-PCR	Gimenez et al. [2010]
Wizard Magnetic DNA Purification System for Food (Promega)	40 mL	NA	Not detectable	SSR	Breton et al. [2004]

NA- Not applicable; ND- Not determined.

Although DNA is present in the olive oil samples, the yields obtained are normally very low and highly dependent on the applied DNA extraction method. An overview of the DNA extraction methods and DNA yields obtained in the several protocols are reported in table 1.

Apart from the low yields, DNA extracted from virgin olive oils appeared to be highly degraded due to the mechanical stress connected with olive processing [Muzzalupo and Perri, 2002; Breton et al., 2004; De la Torre et al., 2004; Pasqualone et al., 2004; Pafundo et al., 2005; Testolin and Lain, 2005; Muzzalupo et al., 2007]. Muzzalupo et al. [2007] referred a DNA size range between 100 to 1500 bp, which was detectable on an agarose gel electrophoresis using ethidium bromide as detection method, once it had been previously amplified using the GenomePlex Whole Genome Amplification (WGA) kit. In a previous work, Muzzalupo and Perri [2002] reported high molecular weight DNA extracted from olive oil samples prepared with the resource to malaxation with proteinase K prior to centrifugation in laboratory conditions. However, in the same work no DNA was visible from the other lab controlled and commercial samples, fact that is coincident with the majority of the reports [Breton et al., 2004; Doveri et al., 2006; Martins-Lopes et al., 2008].

3. DNA Based Methods

Recently, DNA-based markers, which are independent from environmental conditions, have been successfully applied to the olive oil matrices evaluation. Following we will describe the most applied techniques used in olive oil traceability as well as the limitations that have been found when applying them. Busconi et al. [2003] refer that an important aspect, in terms of reproducibility of the fingerprinting technique, is the length and quantity of the recovered DNA.

3.1. Random Amplified Polymorphic DNA (RAPD)

RAPD markers were developed by Williams et al. [1990] that relies on the differential enzymatic amplification of small DNA fragments using arbitrary primers, normally 10-mers long. This technique requires low amounts of DNA and no previous knowledge of the genome sequence is required [Fabbri et al., 1995]. The principle constrains reported are related to the low hybridization temperature used in the PCR cycle and the low data reproducibility observed.

When Muzzalupo and Perri [2002] performed RAPD-PCR amplification of DNA extracted from olive leaves and olive oil sediments, from the same tree, the RAPD patterns were similar. One of the explanations advanced for this occurrence was attributable to the presence of seed DNA characteristic of cross-pollination crops, such as *Olea europaea* L.

Even so an attempt was made to use this technique for olive oil traceability system [Martins-Lopes et al., 2008]. When comparing the DNA profiles obtained from olive oil and leaf samples, it was clear that the there was coincidence of the low molecular weight fragments, but the high molecular weight ones were absent in all the olive oil DNA samples. This result is related to the DNA fragmentation observed in the olive oil samples [Muzzalupo and Perri, 2002; Breton et al., 2004; De la Torre et al., 2004; Pasqualone et al., 2004; Pafundo et al., 2005; Testolin and Lain, 2005; Muzzalupo et al., 2007]. Another interesting observation is that although some RAPD primers were suitable in the DNA leaf samples they were not successful when applied to DNA extracted from olive oil [Martins-Lopes et al., 2008]. In order to overcome the problems related to this type of markers, more reproducible markers are developed from the sequencing information of the markers that may differentiate between olive cultivars such as, sequence characterized amplified region (SCAR) which are further applied in olive oil traceability.

3.2. Sequence Characterized Amplified Region (SCAR)

The sequence characterized amplified region (SCAR) markers are developed with a pair of longer primers (usually the extended sequence of a RAPD primer) that has a specific sequence of approximately 20 nucleotides. Compared with universal primers, specific primers for special genome regions prevent site-competition among primers, and make the results less sensitive to PCR reaction and more reproducible by increasing the specificity [Hernández et al., 1999]. Busconi et al. [2003] used cultivar nonspecific sequence and developed a sequence characterized amplified region (SCAR) primer in order to prove that this primer combination, nuclear origin, could amplify DNA extracted from olive oil samples. Pafundo et al. [2007] used specific bands obtained through amplified fragment length polymorphism (AFLP) to develop several sequence characterized amplified region (SCAR) markers in order to obtain more reproducible DNA profiles in olive oil samples. The results pointed out that this technique is able to be used for olive oil traceability and food authenticity.

3.3. Microsatellites or Single Sequence Repeats (SSRs)

Microsatellites are the class of repetitive DNA sequences present in all organisms, both Eukaryotes and Prokaryotes. They consist of tandemly arranged repeats of several nucleotides, usually 2-6, in tracts up to 10^2 bp that are distributed through the whole genome (although their distribution depends on the species and chromosome), and are flanked by highly conserved sequences [Chambers and MacAvoy, 2000]. By using SSR markers it is possible to detect several alleles at a high frequency, therefore, SSRs turned out to be an ideal tool for identifying individuals. Breton et al. [2004] used twelve SSR markers in several type of olive oils, differing in terms of cultivar composition (Monovarietal and Mulivarietal), and on controlled and commercial blends. The authors verified that in the controlled olive oil blends only alleles from some major cultivars were detectable, limiting the use of SSRs for traceability purposes at that time. Muzzalupo et al. [2007] used six SSR markers to compare between monovarietal oils from the single, self-sterile cultivar, and the corresponding leaf sample, and the authors proved that DNA purified from oil and from the leaves, of the same cultivar presented the same microsatellite profile. They were therefore able to prove that there is no contamination of seed embryo DNA in a monovarietal olive oil. Alba et al. [2009] referred that olive oil DNA is not always suitable for SSR amplification. In seventy PCR experiments they only produced reliable results in 85.7% of the cases. However, the successful amplifications led to a 90% of identical patterns between leaf and olive oil samples. Moreover, the authors reported a single microsatellite, UDO43, able to distinguish seven types of olive oils, demonstrating the potential use of this type of markers in traceability systems. Vietina et al. [2011] accessed 21 monovarietal olive oils produced from 16 olive cultivars with nine nuclear, and two shortened nuclear microsatellite markers. Vietina et al. [2011] referred that the size of SSR amplicons may interfere in the success of amplification due to a low amount of degraded DNA. Therefore, the authors suggested that smaller size amplicons produced better amplification efficiency and higher allele correspondence between leaf and olive oil samples.

3.4. Intermicrosatellites (ISSRs)

In order to resolve some of the inconveniences associated with RAPDs molecular markers (low reproducibility), the high cost of AFLP technique, and the need to know the flanking sequences in order to developed primers for SSR polymorphism, the intermicrosatellites (ISSR) markers were developed [Zietkiewicz et al., 1994; Terzopoulos et al., 2005]. The intermicrosatellites approach is based on the amplification of regions (200-2000 bp) between inversely oriented closely spaced microsatellites. This marker system was used in olive oil traceability by Martins-Lopes et al. [2008], and in a total of eight primers tested, three revealed to be highly polymorphic. The molecular weights of amplicons ranged between 100-2000 bp, although they did not always correspond with the leaf DNA profile.

3.5. Single Nucleotide Polymorphisms (SNPs)

Single nucleotide polymorphisms (SNPs) are the smallest unit of genetic variation and represent the most common type of sequence polymorphism in plant and animal genomes. The single nucleotide polymorphisms (SNPs) can be discovered on preexisting datasets as are genomic sequences or expressed sequence tags (ESTs) [Kota et al., 2003; Rostoks et al., 2005] or through sequencing of candidate genes or PCR products [Ponting et al., 2007]. When compared with other types of markers they offer higher levels of genotyping throughput [Rafalski, 2002]. This marker system is biallelic (in diploids) providing an specific allele information. The application of single nucleotide polymorphisms (SNPs) for food traceability may offer several advantages, being the most attractive one the fact that they can be detected on a very small portion of DNA, which in case of having fragmented DNA may constitute an advantage. This molecular technology has been applied for food traceability purposes in olive oil context [Doveri et al., 2006]. The development of microarrays based on SNP sequences maybe in the near future a main application for food traceability purposes. In a preliminary study, Consolandi et al. [2008] used seventeen olive single nucleotide polymorphisms (SNP) and tested them by ligation detection reaction on an universal array (LDR-UA) platform, developed for olive cultivar identification [Consolandi et al., 2007]. In this assay SNPs were previously amplified using a multiplex PCR and subsequently were used in ligation detection reactions to genotype. Thirteen of the seventeen investigated SNPs were sufficient to unequivocally discriminate the forty-nine olive cultivars and consequently used in monovarietal identification [Consolandi et al., 2008].

3.6. Amplified Fragment Length Polymorphism (AFLP)

The amplified fragment length polymorphism (AFLP) markers are one of the most efficient markers, once they are capable of revealing many polymorphic bands in a single assay [Vos et al., 1995]. Furthermore, AFLP require very low amounts of starting DNA, which makes them interesting when dealing with samples that are difficult to extract and therefore produce low yields. Associated to this advantage, AFLPs enables the analysis of samples without requiring any previous genome sequencing information, making AFLPs very useful in species where little genetic information is available, as in *Olea europaea* L. species. Busconi et al. [2003] were able to demonstrate that the DNA extracted from olive oil could be applied in AFLP analysis, and that the profile obtained for a monovarietal olive oil was highly correspondent to the profile generated by DNA from leaf samples of the same cultivar. Pafundo et al. [2005] were able to obtain an AFLP profile of olive oil with a similarity of about 70% of the corresponding cultivar leaf AFLP profile. Although, some of the AFLP bands were highly conserved, the profiles obtained from the same olive oil with different extractions were considered the limiting step. Montemurro et al. [2008] referred that the AFLP profiles of olive oil samples were less intense than those obtained from leaf samples, and the coincident bands were restricted to fragments under 350 bp. The olive oil storage-time (one and three weeks, one, three, six and nine months, and one and two years) and its effect on DNA quality were studied by Pafundo et al. [2010] using AFLP analysis. The authors reported that there is progressive loss of information by the stored oil DNA, with the reduction of correspondence between DNA fingerprinting of long stored oil (more than one month) and of plant leaves.

3.7. Chloroplast DNA

The resource to chloroplast DNA polymorphism for traceability purposes has been proposed by Intrieri et al. [2007]. Chloroplast polymorphism using microsatellites and restriction fragment length polymorphism (PCR–RFLP) has been reported [Besnard and Berville, 2000; Intrieri et al., 2007]. However, the level of polymorphism may not be enough to be used for unique cultivar identification. Recently, Mariotti et al. [2010] have completed the sequence of olive cultivar 'Frantoio', and they have identified mutations that may represent a valuable tool to assess the level of olive intercultivar plastome variation for use in DNA food tracking. Giménez et al. [2010] used chloroplast DNA (cpDNA) to check their application for olive oil traceability purposes and verified that the potential of using chloroplast DNA (cpDNA) for olive oil authentication needs to be further explored. One of the reasons pointed out is the fact that the quantity of chloroplastic DNA was higher than that of nuclear DNA, which makes it more accessible when applying DNA based methods. Another fact is related to the avoidance of the effect of the pollen donor on traceability cytoplasmic DNA authentication.

4. Limitation of Olive Oil DNA for Traceability

Problems associated with alogamic polinization and their effect on traceability issues were advanced by several authors [Muzzalupo and Perri, 2002; Doveri et al., 2006]. This is purposed due to the fact that most olive cultivars are considered self-incompatible, being that the flowers are wind pollinated. The presence of pollinators DNA is considered one of the limitations for olive oil authentication based on DNA. Once olive oil is produced by crushing whole fruits, paternal DNA may hamper the traceability when using markers based on nuclear DNA [Doveri et al., 2006]. Doveri et al. [2006] reported that the profiles obtained from olive oil were composed of maternal and paternal alleles, suggesting that cultivar identification cannot be based on the match of reference leaf samples profiles, and olive oil profiles. However, Muzzalupo et al. [2007] when studying oil extracted from olives with and/or without pits found a similar electrophoretic pattern, and in the case of SSR marker GAPU59 the exact same sequence was found among different source samples (leaf, drupe, and olive oil). Muzzalupo et al. [2007] demonstrated that on a monovarietal oil, obtained from the self-sterile cultivar 'Ogliarola salentina', there is no contamination of DNA from the pollinators present in the genome of the seed embryo, once no differences in the DNA fingerprinting extracted from oils with or without pits was observed.

The olive oil extraction may largely influence the DNA extraction efficiency and may limit the application of olive oil authentication using DNA-based markers. Therefore, the marker choice for the amplification of DNA extracted from olive oil is an important issue. Doveri et al. [2006], Pafundo et al. [2005] and Testolin and Lain [2005] reported that DNA fragments longer than 300 bp could not be amplified. Microsatellite markers have been suggested for DNA tracking in olive oil samples due to their small size (200–300 bp) [Pasqualone et al., 2004]. Thus, this marker is widely used in food traceability. Recently, Giménez et al. [2010] have suggested that the quantity of templates for the amplification of PCR products around 80 bp is much higher than that of 200 bp, independently of the DNA extraction protocol used. Similar results were obtained by Vietina et al. [2011] when reducing amplicon SSR size. Thus, molecular marker systems that comprehend smaller targets are more likely to succeed when aiming olive oil traceability.

Another issue that is not all the times taken into account is the wide genetic variability present in the *Olea europaea* L. species. This feature may affect the reliability of the traceability procedure, mainly when cultivars used in certain olive protected designation of origin (PDO) regions are not genetically uniform, as has been proved when intra-varietal assessment has been looked into [Belaj et al., 2004; Gemas et al., 2004; Gomes et al., 2008; Martins-Lopes et al., 2009].

Conclusion

Interest in food traceability has been increasing with consumers' demand and concern in controlling what they are eating. New DNA based diagnostic methodologies are being developed in order to increase consumer's confidence and to guarantee producer's profit in high quality food as are protected designation of origin (PDO) olive oils. The main advantage of DNA based technology is that it is not dependent on environmental conditions, which makes it reliable. However, there are still some bottlenecks in what olive oil traceability is concerned, that need to be improved in order for it to be widely applied, being the first the DNA recovery from olive oil. Pafundo et al. [2010] advanced several guidelines that may help in the preservation of DNA quality for reliable DNA fingerprinting. Those are related to storage conditions (dark, temperature, and avoidance of oxidation reactions) and with time between production and DNA extraction (one-month). Although these are valuable guidelines they are not always possible to fulfill and control. The use of smaller polymorphisms, possibly associated to SNP markers, and the resource to more sensitive detection systems, as microchips, may increase the overall application of more accurate and quicker traceability platforms.

Acknowledgment

This research was funded by Fundação para a Ciência e Tecnologia, Portugal through SFRH/BPD/70378/2010 grant.

References

Adam, R. E. and Zimm, B. H. (1977). Shear degradation of DNA. *Nucleic Acids Research*, Vol.4, No.5, pp. 1513-1537.

Agrimonti, C., Vietina, M., Pafundo, S. and Marmiroli, N. (2011). The use of food genomics to ensure the traceability of olive oil. *Trends in Food Science and Technology*, Vol.22, pp. 237-244.

Alba, A., Sabetta, W., Blanco, A., Pasqualone, A. and Montemurro, C. (2009). Microsatellite markers to identify specific alleles in DNA extracted from monovarietal virgin olive oils. *European Food Research and Technology,* Vol.229, pp. 375–382.

Belaj, A., Rallo, L., Trujillo, I. and Baldoni, L. (2004). Using RAPD and AFLP markers to distinguish individuals obtained by clonal selection of 'Arbequina' and 'Manzanila de Sevilla' olive. *Hortscience*, Vol.39, pp. 1566–1570.

Besnard, G. and Bervillé, A. (2000). Multiple origins of the Mediterranean olive (*Olea europaea* L. ssp. *europaea*) based upon mitochondrial DNA polymorphisms. *Comptes rendus de l'Académie des Sciences,* Vol.323, pp. 173–181.

Breton, C., Claux, D., Metton, I., Skorski, G. and Berville, A. (2004). Comparative study of methods for DNA preparation from olive oil samples to identify cultivar SSR alleles in commercial oil samples: possible forensic applications. *Journal of Agricultural and Food Chemistry,* Vol.52, pp. 531-537.

Brezná, B. and Kuchta, T. (2008). A novel real-time polymerase chain reaction method for the detection of pecan nuts in food. *European Food Research and Technology*, Vol.226, pp. 1113–1118.

Busconi, M., Foronib, C., Corradib, M., Bongiornia, C., Cattapanc, F., Foghera, C. (2003). DNA extraction from olive oil and its use in the identification of the production cultivar. *Food Chemistry*, Vol.83, pp. 127–134.

Cercaci, L., Rodriguez-Estrada, M. T. and Lercker, G (2003). Solid-phase extraction-thin-layer chromatography-gas chromatography method for the detection of hazelnut oil in olive oils by determination of esterified sterols. *Journal of Chromatography*, Vol.24, pp. 211–20.

Chambers, G. K. and MacAvoy, E. S. (2000). Microsatellites: consensus and controversy. *Comparative Biochemistry and Physiology*, Vol.126, pp. 455-476.

CODEX. (2006) Principles for traceability/product tracing as a tool within a food inspection and certification system. http://www.codexalimentarius.net/web/standard_list.do?lang=en.

Consolandi, C., Palmieri, L., Doveri, S., Maestri, E., Marmiroli, N., Reale, S., Lee, D., Baldoni, L., Tosti, N., Severgnini, M., De Bellis, G. and Castiglioni, B. (2007). Olive variety identification by ligation detection reaction in a universal array format. *Journal of Biotechnology,* Vol.129, No.3, pp. 565–574.

Consolandi, C., Palmieri, L., Severgnini, M., Maestri, E., Marmiroli, N., Agrimonti, C., Baldoni, L., Donini, P., De Bellis, G. and Castiglioni, G. (2008). A procedure for olive oil traceability and authenticity: DNA extraction, multiplex PCR and LDR-universal array analysis. *European Food Research and Technology*, Vol.227, No.5, pp. 1429-1438.

Damirchi, S., Savage, G, and Dutta, P. (2005). Sterol fractions in hazelnut and virgin olive oils and 4,4′-dimethylsterols as possible markers for detection of adulteration of virgin olive oil. *Journal of the American Oil Chemists' Society,* Vol.82, pp. 717–725.

De la Torre, F., Bautista, R., Cánovas, F. and Claros, G. (2004). Isolation of DNA from olive oil and oil sediments: Application in oil fingerprinting. *Journal of Food Agriculture and Environment*, Vol.2, pp. 84-89.

Dimara, E. and Skuras, D. (2003). Consumer evaluations of product certification, geographic association and traceability in Greece. *European Journal of Marketing*, Vol.37, No.5-6, pp. 690–705.

Doveri, S. and Lee, D. (2007). Development of sensitive crop-specific polymerase chain reaction assays using 5S DNA: applications in food traceability. *Journal of Agricultural and Food Chemistry*, Vol.55, pp. 4640–4644.

Doveri, S., O'Sullivan, D. and Lee, D. (2006). Non-concordance between genetic profiles of olive oil and fruit: a cautionary note to the use of DNA markers for provenance testing. *Journal of Agricultural and Food Chemistry*, Vol.54, pp. 9221–9226.

Fabbri, A., Hormaza, J. I. and Polito, V. S. (1995). Random Amplified Polymorphic DNA analysis of olive (*Olea europaea* L.) cultivars. *Journal of the American Society for Horticultural Science*, Vol.120, No.3, pp. 538–542.

Flores, G., Castillo, M., Blanch, G. and Herraiz, M. (2006). Detection of the adulteration of olive oils by solid phase microextraction and multidimensional gas chromatography. *Food Chemistry*, Vol.97, pp. 336– 342.

Gemas, V. J. V., Almadanim, M. C., Tenreiro, R., Martins, A. and Fevereiro, P. (2004). Genetic diversity in the Olive tree (*Olea europaea* L. subsp. *europaea*) cultivated in Portugal revealed by RAPD and ISSR markers. *Genetic Resources and Crop Evolution*, Vol.51, pp. 501–511.

Giménez, M. J., Pistón, F., Martín, A. and Atienza, S. G. (2010). Application of real-time PCR on the development of molecular markers and to evaluate critical aspects for olive oil authentication. *Food Chemistry*, Vol.118, pp. 482–487.

Gomes, S., Martins-Lopes, P., Lima-Brito, J., Meirinhos, J., Lopes, J., Martins, A. and Guedes-Pinto, H. (2008). Evidence for clonal variation in 'Verdeal-Transmontana' olive using RAPD, ISSR and SSR markers. *The Journal of Horticultural Science and Biotechnology*, Vol.83, pp. 395–400.

Hernández, P., Martin, A. and Dorado, G. (1999). Development of SCARs by direct sequencing of RAPD products: a practical tool for the introgression and marker-assisted selection of wheat. *Molecular Breeding, Vol.***5, No.**3, pp. 245–253.

Intrieri, M. C., M. R., Buiatti, M. (2007). Chloroplast DNA polymorphisms as molecular markers to identify cultivars of *Olea europaea* L. *Journal of Horticultural Science and Biotechnology*, Vol.82, No.1, pp. 109-113.

Kota, R., Rudd, S., Facius, A., Kolesov, G., Thiel, T., Zhang, H., Stein, N., Mayer, K. and Graner, A. (2003). Snipping polymorphisms from large EST collections in barley (*Hordeum vulgare* L.). *Molecular Genetics and Genomics*, Vol.270, pp. 24–33.

Mariani, C., Bellan, G., Lestini, E. and Aparicio, R. (2006). The detection of the presence of hazelnut oil in olive oil by free and esterified sterols. *European Food Research and Technology*, Vol.223, pp. 655–661.

Mariotti, R., Cultrera, N., Muñoz Díez, C., Baldoni, L and, Rubini, A. (2010). Identification of new polymorphic regions and differentiation of cultivated olives (*Olea europaea* L.) through plastome sequence comparison. *BMC Plant Biology*, Vol.10, No.211, pp. 2-13.

Martins-Lopes, P., Gomes, S., Lima-Brito, J., Lopes, J. and Guedes-Pinto, H. (2009). Assessment of clonal genetic variability in *Olea europaea* L. 'Cobrançosa' by molecular markers. *Scientia Horticulturae*, Vol.123, No.1, pp. 82-89.

Martins-Lopes, P., Gomes, S., Santos, E. and Guedes-Pinto, H. (2008). DNA markers for Portuguese olive oil fingerprinting. *Journal of Agricultural and Food Chemistry*, Vol.*56, No.*24, pp. 11786–11791.

Martins-Lopes, P., Lima-Brito, J., Gomes, S., Meirinhos, J., Santos, L. and Guedes-Pinto, H. (2007). RAPD and ISSR molecular markers in *Olea europaea* L.: Genetic variability and cultivar identification. *Genetic Resources and Crop Evolution*, Vol.54, pp. 117-128.

Montemurro, C., Pasqualone, A., Simeone, R., Sabetta, W. and Blanco A. (2008). AFLP molecular markers to identify virgin olive oils from single Italian cultivars. *European Food Research and Technology*, Vol.226, pp. 1439–1444.

Muzzalupo, I. and Perri, E. (2002). Recovery and characterisation of DNA from virgin olive oil. *European Food Research and Technology*, Vol.214, pp. 528–531.

Muzzalupo, I., Pellegrino, M. and Perri, E. (2007). Detection of DNA in virgin olive oils extracted from destoned fruits. *European Food Research and Technology*, Vol.224, pp. 469–475.

Pafundo, S., Agrimonti, C. and Marmiroli, N. (2005). Traceability of plant contribution in olive oil by AFLPs. *Journal of Agricultural and Food Chemistry*, Vol.53, pp. 6995–7002.

Pafundo, S., Agrimonti, C., Maestri, E. and Marmiroli, N. (2007). Applicability of SCAR markers to food genomics: olive oil traceability. *Journal of Agricultural and Food Chemistry*, Vol.55, pp. 6052–6059.

Pafundo, S., Busconi, M., Agrimonti, C., Fogher, C., Marmiroli, N. (2010). Storage-time effects on olive oil DNA assessed by amplified fragments length polymorphisms. *Food Chemistry*, Vol.123, pp. 787–793.

Pasqualone, A. and Catalano, M. (2000). Free and total sterols in olive oils. Effects of neutralization. *Grasas Aceites*, Vol.51, pp. 177–182.

Pasqualone, A., Montemurro, C., Caponio, F. and Blanco, A. (2004). Identification of virgin olive oil from different cultivars by analysis of DNA microsatellites. *Journal of Agricultural and Food Chemistry*, vol.52, pp. 1068–1071.

Ponting, R. C., Drayton, M.C., Cogan, N. I. O., Dobrowolski, M. P., Spangenberg, G. C., Smith, K. F., Forster, J. W. (2007). SNP discovery, validation, haplotype structure and linkage disequilibrium in full-length herbage nutritive quality genes of perennial Ryegrass (*Lolium perenne* L.). *Molecular Genetics and Genomics*, Vol.278, pp. 585–597.

Rafalski, A. (2002). Applications of single nucleotide polymorphisms in crop genetics. *Current Opinion in Plant Biology*, Vol.5, pp. 94–100.

Rostoks, N., Mudie, S., Cardle, L., Russell, J., Ramsay, L., Booth, A., Svensson, J. T., Wanamaker, S. I., Walia, H., Rodriguez, E. M., Hedley, P. E., Liu, H., Morris, J., Close, T.J., Marshall, D. F and Waugh, R. (2005). Genome-wide SNP discovery and linkage analysis in barley based on genes responsive to abiotic stress. *Molecular Genetics and Genomics*, Vol.274, pp. 515–527.

Terzopoulos, P. J., Kolano, B. and Bebeli, P.J. (2005). Identification of *Olea europaea* L. cultivars using inter-simple sequence repeat markers. *Scientia Horticulturae,* Vol.105, pp. 45–51.

Testolin, R. and Lain, O. (2005). DNA extraction from olive oil and PCR amplification of microsatellite markers. *Journal of Food Science*, Vol.70, pp. 108-112.

Vietina, M., Agrimonti, C., Marmiroli, M., Bonas, U. and Marmiroli, N. (2011). Applicability of SSR markers to the traceability of monovarietal olive oils. *Journal of the Science of Food and Agriculture*, Vol.91, pp. 1381–1391.

Vos, P., Hogers, R., Bleeker, M., Reijans, M. Van De Lee, T., Hornes, M., Frijters, A., Pot, J., Peleman, J. and Kuiper, M. (1995). AFLP: a new technique for DNA fingerprinting. *Nucleic Acids Research,* Vol.21, pp. 4407-4414.

Willett, W. C. (2006). The Mediterranean diet: science and practice. *Public Health Nutrition*, Vol.9, No.1A, pp. 105–110.

Williams, J. G. K., Kubelik, A. R., Livak, K. J., Rafalski, J.A. and Tingey, S.V. (1990). DNA polymorphisms amplified by arbitrary primers are useful as genetic markers. *Nucleic Acids Research*, Vol.18, pp. 6531-6535.

Zietkiewicz, E., Rafalski, A., Labuda, D. (1994). Genome fingerprinting and simple sequence repeat (SSR)- anchored polymerase chain reaction amplification. *Genomics*, Vol.20, pp. 176-183.

In: Olive Consumption and Health
Editors: C. A. Savalas and S. M. Nicolau
ISBN: 978-1-62100-774-6

Chapter 10

Is Region of Origin a Valuable Cue for the Consumer? The Case of Olive Oil Sector

Sihem Dekhili *
HuManiS (EA 1347), EM Strasbourg Business School, University of Strasbourg, Strasbourg Cedex, France

Abstract

In the marketing literature, authors have favored the study of "country of origin" concept, and less attention was given to the "region of origin", and the question of the combined use of the two concepts was neglected. The general goal of this research is to investigate whether the two concepts are distinct or in interaction.

The results of an empirical study involving French consumers of olive oil show that the indication of the name of the "region", in addition to that of the "country", has a positive effect on the consumer choice.

Keywords: Country of origin, region of origin, perceived quality, olive oil, choice modelling

An extensive marketing literature adresses the question of the "country of origin" and in particular the "*made in*", suggesting that it is used as a quality cue (Han, 1990; Schooler and Wildt, 1968; Verlegh and Steenkamp, 1999).

Studying the "region of origin", on the other hand, has interested fewer researchers in the field of management. The scarce research (Van der Lans et al. 2001; Van Ittersum, 2001) that does explore the concept of "region of origin" looks almost exclusively at examples of food products, and has shown that the region is indeed also a quality cue, with comparable effects to those of the country.

Yet the "region of origin" concept has several specific features which differentiate it from the "country". The region might benefit from a more coherent and homogeneous image than

* Telephone number: (+33) 6 09 49 42 63; Fax number: (+33) 3 90 41 42 70; Email address: sihem.dekhili@em-strasbourg.eu.

that of the country, which would make it more effective when used in a brand strategy, because it provides a higher diagnostic value when choosing a product. Thus using the “region” name to enhance the value of food products would seem in certain cases to be more relevant than a strategy based on the name of the “country”, and especially for food products (Stefani et al. 2006).

Besides, when the marketing research explore the region of origin, authors do not consider the question of a possible link between country and region, and therefore have not explored the effects of a combined use of the two concepts (country and region) and rather considered them as alternatives.

Our research context is the olive oil markets, particularly in France. From a managerial point of view, the raised question is twofolds. Is it relevant to promote production regions as quality cues, in the same way this is successfully done for wine or cheese for instance? If yes, at what conditions such policies would be efficient ? Is it interesting to use the region names when they are less known by the consumers ?

The main objective of this paper is to explore the benefits of the combined use of the two concepts (country and region) on the national and international market. In a first part, we review the marketing literature on the geographic origin, which allows us to suppose a possible link between the two concepts and derive our research hypothesis. In a second part, we describe the research design and the results obtained from a protocol study which has been carried out on French olive oil consumers (n=123). Lastly, we discuss the results from both a theoretical and managerial point of view, in the light of the limitations to the research.

THEORETICAL CONSIDERATIONS

The Concept of Country of Origin and its Limitations

A large Marketing literature has extensively studied the country of origin effects on product evaluation. According to Usunier (2006), over four hundred academic articles have been produced in the last forty years, with a wide diversity in product categories, countries of origin and consumer nationalities. In these researches, the country of origin is often considered as an essential extrinsic attribute to indicate quality (Agrawal and Kamakura, 1999; Ahmed and d’Astous, 1993; Hong and Wyer, 1989; Steenkamp and Van Trijp, 1996; Verlegh and Steenkamp, 1999).

Dichter (1962) was among the first to demonstrate that country of origin can have a major influence on whether products are accepted or are successful. Later, Schooler and Wildt (1968) carried out an empirical test using glassware identical in every respect, except for their country of origin, and concluded that there were evaluated differently. The researches which followed often assimilate the notion of “country of origin” with the *made in* mention.

Usunier (2002) rises however the exaggeration of the country of origin effects on consumer behavior. Using the case of household electrical goods and stereo systems, he showed that 35% of consumers knew the country of origin of their latest purchase, and that only 25% considered that the country of origin label had been “important” or “very important” in their purchases.

Moreover, this *made in* expression is ambiguous, if only from a legal point of view; it can mean in certain countries "produced in", "assembled in", "designed in", "invented in" or "assembled by a producer whose headquarters are in ..." (Papadopoulos, 1993; Peterson and Jolibert, 1995). Interpreting how consumers use this cue in a given situation is difficult.

Some authors (Chao, 1993; Han and Terpstra, 1988; Li et al. 2000; Tse and Lee, 1993) have therefore proposed the decomposition of the "country of origin" construct into several dimensions (country of product design, country of assembly, country of manufacture, etc.). Whereas Li et al. (2000) find this decomposition approach rather deficient, their research showed that only the country of design is relevant in the product evaluation.

The "country image" concept was suggested as another way to try to enrich the "country of origin" concept and the decomposition approach. Several researchers explored the cognitive processes that create a country image, like political and economic informations (Nagashima, 1970; Han, 1989) or the perception of the design quality, of workers' manufacturing skill, of innovative ability (Roth and Romeo, 1992). As a result, the "country image" cannot be generalised to all products. Roth and Romeo (1992) indicate that is more interesting to examine country of origin in terms of the fit between countries and product categories. So the matches between product category dimensions with the perceived image of the country of origin can be captured.

The literature cited above raises the limits of the country of origin concept. The *made in* approach is too reductive to reflect all the matches between a country and a product. The "product-specific country image" concept was suggested to cover this limit. A large part of the research on the "made in" is based on industrial examples with an overrepresentation of involving products for the consumer, such as electronic goods, cars, clothes or a few generic agricultural products such as "Columbian coffee" (Usunier, 2006; 2002).

A few studies on food products (Carter et al. 2006; Kleppe et al. 2002; Loureiro and Umberger, 2005) have begun to appear in the literature about country of origin. According to Kleppe et al. (2002), the product-specific country image has gained importance in the marketing of food products, with examples like French wine and cheese, German beer and Swiss chocolate. In these examples, the origin is used as the most important heuristic evaluation. A country-product marketing strategy, suggesting better quality and enabling a better differentiation of food products, facilitates the evaluation process for consumers. But how relevant are these historic and factual references for decision making ? Papadopoulos (2004) suggested that French wine, for example, has a strong image but that this image has evolved through the product itself rather than through systematic promotion. We need deeper insigths into the cognitive processes by which this "country of origin cues" do function.

Is the Region of Origin Concept Different from Country of Origin?

A region is defined according to Van Ittersum (2001) as "an area, situated within one or more countries, which forms an entity based on local characteristics such as traditions, culture, and scenery"

Like the country of origin, the region is also used as a quality cue (Van der Lans et al. 2001). Lagrange and Trognon (1995) state that there are specific associations to certain *terroirs,* and a certain specialization of geographical areas in the consumers' minds (Auvergne-cheese, Bordeaux-wine, etc.). In this case, the region draws benefit from a reputation around the production of a particular product. This suggests that the region or the *terroir* constitutes a cognitive category with which consumers associate specific products and that certain products appear to be more typical than others.

The "region of origin" cue evokes general regional beliefs (traditions, inhabitants, culture). Consumers' general beliefs about a product's region of origin are proposed to be an important source for their affective feelings related to the regional product (Obermiller and Spangenberg, 1989; Van Ittersum, 2001; Verlegh and Steenkamp, 1999).

Thus the "region of origin" indication, like the "country", influences perceived quality through a cognitive process. Although region of origin effects are expected to operate through similar processes as country of origin effects, the region of origin has some specific aspects which we will try to investigate, by raising two questions: a) is region of origin a relevant attribute in consumer decision making ? and b) are there any differences between regions depending on their reputation as a production locations ?

a) The Region as an Attribute for Differentiation

Several studies (Aaker, 1991; Keller, 1998; Samiee, 1994) indicate that the use of the region of origin image to differentiate products can be compared with the application of a brand strategy.

The image consistence (Kapferer, 1992) is an important success determinant of a brand strategy. From this point of view, regions are more homogeneous in terms of human and natural environment dimensions than countries. They can be better demarcated by natural characteristics than countries, which are more demarcated by their national borders (Cordell, 1992).

On the other hand, the use of a regional cue, comparing to the "country of origin" label, makes it possible to differentiate products both from foreign and domestic competitors. French wine is a good example of a product that is well differentiated according to regions (Van Ittersum et al. 2003).

The emotional value of the region of origin associated with other specific values is particularly linked with food products, since by nature their geographic origins are rooted in the land in, and on, which they are produced (Sheth et al. 1999). Delamont (1995) referred to the strong historical and symbolic links between regions and foods, due to the interactions between natural resources and people's lifestyles.

b) Should the Region Be Known in Order to Constitute an Effective Cue ?

For the success of the marketing of products on the basis of their region of origin, two conditions are necessary, according to Keller (1998). First, a significant proportion of the target market should be aware of the region. Second, consumers' regional associations should be favourable and relevant. In the same way, Van der Lans et al. (2001) indicate that the capacity of a regional indication to influence the performance of regional products requires that consumers should not only be aware of the region and have favourable associations with it (Kapferer, 1992), but they should also be familiar with this region.

Other studies (Aaker, 1991; Van der Lans et al. 2001), however, note that the promotion of regional products based on the regional characteristics and the product dimensions may be efficient on foreign markets in the same way as the development of a new unknown brand name.

Hence we can ask the following question: is knowledge of a region's reputation for the product production a necessary condition for the success of a strategy based on the regional indication? Obviously, some regional products have successfully entered foreign markets and contribute to the success of French agro-food exports, and this in spite of the recurring criticism carried to the lack of visibility of the products and regional specialities which are candidates for export. Well known or not, it would seem that the region of origin is a geographical level of definition that is suitable for getting the best value from food products.

The next question is the following: is it the country or the region of origin that is more relevant when identifying a food product?

Country and/or Region: Which Level Is More Relevant ?

In a recent empirical study concerning Italian consumers, Stefani et al. (2006) looked at the size effect of a place of origin on consumer preference in the case of spelt from Garfagnana, a food speciality with a strong regional identity, and they found that more the area is small and well defined, better the consumers value the products.

This interesting study presents however some limitations; first, the notions of "terroir", "region" and "country" were considered as being alternatives. But is it relevant to dissociate these concepts? A product marketed "Garfagnana" or "Tuscany" includes implicitly the "Italy" origin. The methodology used in the study does not enable us to determine whether there are any interactions' effects between these concepts. Next, because of the Italian sample, we may have a familiarity bias with the product and the region.

As a conclusion of these discussions, we underline that the literature suggests that "country of origin" and "region of origin" may be conceptually different and do not provide to consumers the same informations and images. We propose then to study the combined effect of these two different concepts and to check whether mentioning the region of origin (associated with the country of origin) influences consumer choice behaviour, in particular when he does not know that this region is related to the quality of a particular product.

Method and Results

123 French consumers were questioned. Participants were recruited from people who consumed and purchased olive oil. The surveys took place in Paris, city that is not situated in olive oil production area. Ten sessions were organized, with an average duration of one hour. Each participant received a twenty euros fee and a bottle of olive oil. Table 1 summarizes the characteristics of respondents.

Experimental Design

In order to test our hypotheses (the mention of the region of origin, added to the country of origin, influences consumer choice positively), we used the discrete choice method (Hair et al. 1998) to measure the perceived value of the olive oil attributes. The choice experimental design enabled us to measure the utility of three attributes: country of origin, region of origin and price.

For the "country of origin" attribute, we selected five olive oil producing countries: Spain, Italy, France, Tunisia and Morocco. For the "regions of origin", we chose to consider both a region that is known and one that is less known for production in each of the five selected countries, relying on the opinions of experts. With the help of professionals from AFIDOL (French association of olive oil), we were able to draw up a list of countries and production regions (See table 2). A last option was the absence of the name of the region of origin. In this case, only information on the country was displayed.

We decided to retain in this research three price ranges which are representative of the French market, and which include both French oils and oils from abroad, expressed on the basis of 0.5 litre containers, which seems to be a familiar reference for purchasers in France.

The attributes of the experiment were manipulated according to the procedure of the individualised experimental design and each of the 123 respondents had to carry out 12 choice tasks. Each task contained three alternatives plus a "non-choice" option. Each alternative was described according to country of origin, absence or presence of the name of the region of origin and price level. No particular context of oil consumption was suggested to the respondents. Only the place of purchase was specified: the subject is asked to represent himself standing in front of an olive oil shelf in a supermarket (See figure 1).

Table 1. Characteristics of participants

Variables		Sample
Number of participants		123
Sex	Men	41
	Women	82
Age	From18 to 44 years	49
	45 years and more	74
Education level	Secondary	56
	University	67
Income level	Low and average*	85
	High*	38
Consumption level	Big consumers**	18
	Average consumers**	62
	Small consumers **	43
Usual purchase price of olive oil (1Liter)		
	Less than 6.1 TD/ 6 €	8
	From 6.1 to 6.8 TD/ From 6 to 8 €	46
	From 6.9 to 7.9 TD/ From 8.7 to 13.5€	53
	8 TD and more /From 13.6 to 19.4 €	13
	19.5€ and more	3

* Low and average income: $<$ 3693 Euros.

* High income: $\geq$ 3693 Euros.

** Big consumers: 1 liter and more/week (Krystallis et Ness, 2005).

** Average consumers: 1-2 litrers/month.

** Small consumers: 1-2 liters/quarter or more rarely.

Table 2. List of known and less known regions for producing olive oil

Country	**Known region**	**Less known region**
Spain	Andalusia	Bajo Aragon
Italy	Tuscany	Calabre
France	Nyons	Nîmes
Tunisia	Sfax	Nabeul
Marocco	Meknès	Azilal

Aggregate Results

In the Logit model with main effects, the estimated value of $\chi2$ (415.45) exceeded the critical value of the $\chi2$ test (16.92) by a large margin with a confidence level of $\alpha=5\%$. The model is therefore reliable, and we can conclude that the respondents' choices were influenced by the variations in the attributes' modalities that were presented in the choice alternatives.

In Table 3 we show the individual utility values, and the Student's t test for the three different modalities of the "region" attribute.

As expected, the name of a known region for production was favourably perceived by consumers, the effect of this attribute was significant (t = +3.42) and its utility value was of the order of +0.1523. In contrast, the absence of the name of the production region had a significant negative effect on the consumers' choice (t = -3.80), its utility value was negative at -0.1805. In the case of a less known region for production, no significant effect was found (t = +0.61; the utility value = +0.0282).

None of the interactions between the attributes proved to be significant, which means that there is no discernible synergy between region names and country names, and that only the main effects are detectable.

You are in front of an olive oil shelf in a supermarket. Which of these three bottles do you choose?

Spain Region Bajo Aragon 9.55 € 1	France 3.40 € 2	Tunisia Region Sfax 6.95 € 3	I will not buy any one 4

The bottles each are containing 0.5 litre of extra virgin olive oil.

Please circle the number of the bottle you've chosen (or the option "I will not buy any one").

Figure 1. Example of a task choice.

Table 3. Effects and t Ratio of the region of origin attribute levels

Region of origin attribute level	Effect	t Ratio
Known region	+0.1523	+ 3.42
Less known region	+0.0282	+0.61
Absence of the region name	-0.1805	-3.80

We conclude that mentioning the region of origin has a positive influence on consumer choice, at least when this name is known to the respondents, which supports our hypothesis.

The question rises as to the effect of the initial knowledge of the respondents on the regions and their associations with oil production.

Effect of Consumers Knowledge about the Regions' Reputation as Producer of Olive Oil

In order to draw up a list of regions that are known for olive oil production and others that are less known in relation to the five countries selected for the survey, we relied on the experts' opinion, then verified whether the consumers' perceptions regarding these regions matched those of the experts.

The study controls the degree to which the respondents associated the regions with olive oil production by measuring on a 5-point scale the degree of agreement with the proposals: "*Region X, Y, Z...is known for the production of olive oil*" and we carried out a t-test on paired samples (See table 4).

Results show that only for three countries (Spain, Italy and Morocco), respondents make distinctions between known and less known regions (significant t-test). So a gap between the consumers' perception and experts' point of view exist. We propose to take into account this gap of perception which can bias our conclusions.

We divided the sample on two groups on the basis of the consumers' knowledge. The differences between the two groups were significant. The group of consumers whose perceptions are coherent with those of professionals in terms of regions' reputation knowledge are more familiar with the tested regions than the less knowledgeable group (familiarity mean score for the first group = 3.87 against 3.08 for the second group on a 7-point scale), and has a higher level of expertise with the product (expertise mean for the first group = 4.37 versus 3.54 for the other group on a 7-point scale).

Table 4. Distinction between the known and the less known regions from consumers (t-test paired samples)

		t	D.F	Sig. (two-tailed test)
Pair 1	Andalusia (KR) - Bajo Aragon (LKR)	8,205	1 21	**,000**
Pair 2	Calabre (LKR) - Tuscany (KR)	-4,776	1 22	**,000**
Pair 3	Azilal (LKR) - Meknès (KR)	-2,887	1 21	**,005**
Pair 4	Nyons (KR) - Nîmes (LKR)	-,118	1 18	,906
Pair 5	Sfax (KR) - Nabeul (LKR)	-,883	1 18	,379

KR: Known Region according to experts ; LKR: Less known Region according to experts.

Table 5. Importance of "country of origin", "region of origin" and "price" attributes for the two groups of respondents (experts and non-experts)

Attributes		Country of origin	Region of origin	Price
Importance percentage	Expert group	61.79	16.84	21.38
	Non-expert group	50.36	7.01	42.63

We established two separate Logit models: the first included subjects belonging to the first group (the more knowledgeable respondents n = 66), the second included subjects from the second group (the less knowledgeable respondents n = 57). Both models are significant (1st model: maximum likelihood = -1005.57, $\chi 2 = 184.74$; 2nd model: maximum likelihood = -813.93, $\chi 2 = 268.58$).

The percentages of importance for the three considered attributes: "country of origin", "region of origin" and "price" for the two groups of respondents are summarised in the table 5.

Results show that knowledgeable consumers give more attention to origin cues (country and region) than the non-knowledgeable consumers (importance percentage of country of origin attribute are 61.79 and 50.36 respectively; importance percentage of region of origin attribute are 16.84 and 7.01 respectively). The importance of the price as a choice criteria is different between the two groups, less knowledgeable respondents give more attention to this attribute (importance percentage = 42.63 versus 21.38 for the more knowledgeable consumers).

Figure 2 illustrates the utility values for three modalities of the "region of origin" attribute for the two groups of consumers.

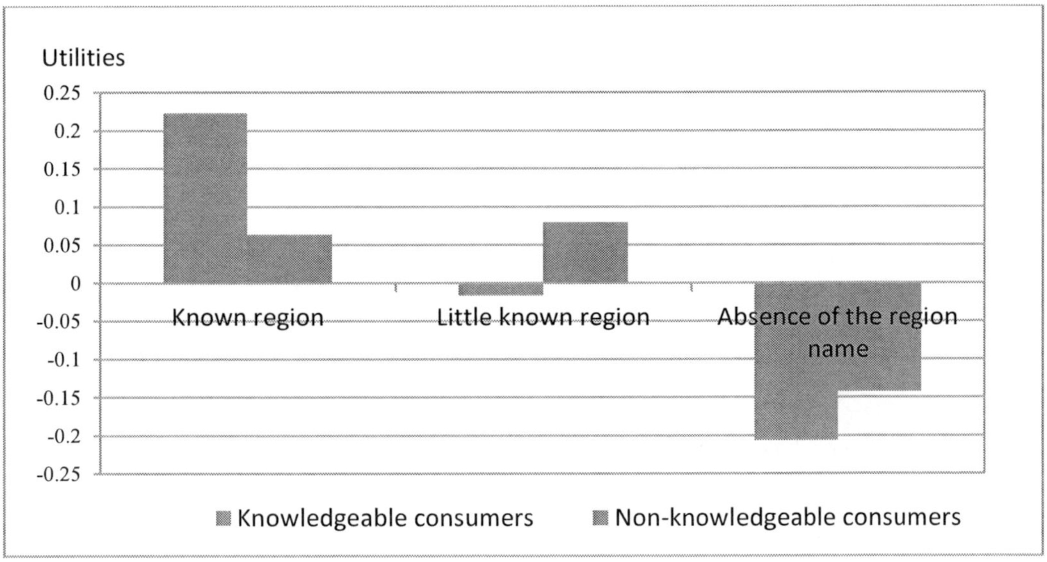

Figure 2. Utility values of the "region of origin" attribute levels according to the degree of knowledge of the producing reputation of the regions.

The segmentation suggests that knowledgeable consumers are, with a significant degree, favourably influenced by the known regions (Student t = +3.76). The absence of information about the regions of production, on the other hand, has a significant negative effect (Student t = -3.23). In the case of the less known regions, no significant effect was found (Student t = -0.26; utility value = -0.0163).

For the non-knowledgeable consumers, the effects of the different modalities of the "region of origin" attribute proved to be non-significant (Student t = +0.92 for the "known region" modality, +1.15 for the "less known region" modality and -1.98 in the absence of information about the region of production). Even though the trend is the same as for the first group (positive effects for a known region and negative in the absence of information about the region of production), it is interesting to highlight that the utility value of the known region is similar to that for the less known region (+0.0634 and +0.0793 respectively), which confirms the fact that the non-knowledgeable consumers did not differentiate between the two types of regions. On the other hand, even though the effects are not significant, the non-experts seem to distinguish only two cases: indication of the name of the region of production (whether the region is known or not) which is perceived positively. The second case is the absence of information about the region (only the name of the country is displayed) which is perceived negatively.

DISCUSSION

The results from the aggregated discrete choice model show that giving the name of a region can have contrasting effects, depending first on whether the regions are well known or not and second on the level of consumers own knowledge.

For all of our respondents, when the region is known for its olive oil production, mention of the name has a significant positive effect on their choice, when the region is less known for olive oil production the effect tended to be neutral (not significant). On the other hand, we noted that the absence of any indication as to region of origin had a significant negative effect.

However, these observations were more contrasted for the "knowledgeable" than for the "non-knowledgeable" consumers. For the latter, the trends were the same but the results were not significant. On first analysis, these results confirm Keller's thesis (1998) which postulates that one of the conditions of success of the region of origin cue on the international market is that the consumer should be aware and informed about the region.

For non-knowledgeable consumers, the absence of a regional name could also have an unfavourable effect even if this effect does not emerge as significant. Thus, even if the consumers are not aware of the region's production potential, they perceive more favourably the display of extra information (region of origin) when they are in a comparative choice situation with products that mention an unknown region and products with no mention of a region of origin. So these results would tend to support Aaker's position (1991) when he suggests that the promotion of regional products could be successful in foreign markets, in the same way as a brand strategy and therefore it is not a precondition that the foreign consumer has to be familiar with the region in order for the cue to be effective.

However in general, everything happens as though the aware or non-aware consumer spontaneously credits a smaller geographical area with a higher level of performance in terms of know-how or *terroir*, whatever its reputation.

CONTRIBUTIONS, LIMITATIONS AND LINES FOR FURTHER RESEARCH

Our contribution is to shed light on the function of region of origin used as a brand, namely whether knowledge of the name of the region on the part of the consumer is a precondition to his experiencing the full impact of the brand's effects. Our results clearly confirm the positive link that exists between the reputation of the region and consumer preference, and they also show that the more expert the consumers, the more value they place on the region being mentioned. Obviously, these consumers use the reputation of a known region in the same way they would consider brand reputation.

However, our results also show that consumers to whom the name of a region means nothing still place more value on the fact that the name of a less known region is mentioned than on the absence of a name altogether. We may hypothesise that this positive effect is not necessarily associated with representations of regions or with emotional ties between the consumer and a given region, but perhaps with the simple fact that the region provides extra and more specific information. It would therefore be interesting to explore the determinants that account for this positive effect.

These findings have to be considered in the light of some of the study's limitations. Results will be probably different if we had a sample of consumers who are not familiar at all with olive oil or with the notion of *terroir*. Geographic and cultural distance could modify our conclusions. We assume that it would be interesting in future research to explore the perceptions of non-European consumers (for example, Canadian or Japanese consumers).

We are aware about the limitations related to the external validity of the results which affect research on "made in", nor the contradictions in the conclusions which are attributable to the different contexts of the study and in particular to the product categories tested. It would be useful to carry out similar experiments on other food products.

From a managerial point of view, there are in our opinion two recommendations that can be drawn from these results.

The first recommendation is that such a policy can be effective even if initially the consumers do not know the region. In other words, the process to favour does not follows necessarily a logical route in the style of: "first to make known the country, then the regions, then possibly zones even more specified", but it could be efficient to consider thse components in a different order.

The second one is that if the products are to be marketed to knowledgeable consumers, the mention of a known region will be very highly appreciated, whereas the mention of a less known region will provide little benefit and may even be detrimental.

REFERENCES

Aaker DA. 1991. *Managing brand equity: capitalizing on the value of a brand name.* Free Press, New York.

Agrawal J, Kamakura W-A. 1999. Country of origin: A competitive advantage? International *Journal of Research in Marketing* 16: 255-267.

Ahmed S-A, d'Astous A. 1993. Cross-national evaluation of made-in concept using multiple cues. *European Journal of Marketing* 27, 7: 39-52.

Carter C, Krissoff B, Zwane AP. 2006. Can country-of-origin labelling succeed as a marketing tool for produce? Lessons from three case studies. *Canadian Journal of Agricultural Economics* 54, 4: 513-530.

Chao P. 1993. Partitioning country of origin effects: Consumer evaluations of a hybrid product. *Journal of International Business Studies* 24, 2: 291-306.

Cordell VV. 1992. Effects of consumer preferences for foreign sourced products. *Journal of International Business Studies* 23: 251-296.

Delamont S. 1995. *Appetites and identies: an introduction to the social anthropology of Western Europe.* Routledge edition: London.

Dichter E. 1962. *The World Customer.* Harvard Business Revue 40, 4: 113-122.

Hair JF, Anderson RE, Tatham RL, Black WC. 1998. *Multivariate Data Analysis.* USA.

Han C-M, Terpstra V. 1988. Country-of-origin effects for Uni-National and Bi-National products. *Journal of International Business Studies* 19, 2: 235-255.

Han CM. 1989. Country image: Halo or summary construct. *Journal of Marketing Research* 26: 222-229.

Han C-M. 1990. Testing the role of country image in consumer choice behaviour. *European Journal of Marketing* 24, 6: 24-40.

Hong ST, Wyer RS. 1989. Effects of Country-of-origin and product attribute information on product evaluation: an information processing perspective. *Journal of Consumer Research* 16: 175-187.

Kapferer JN. 1992. *Strategic brand management, new approaches to creating and evaluating brand equity.* Les Editions d'Organisation: London.

Keller KL. 1998; In: Van der Lans I-A, Van Ittersum K, De Cicco A et al. 2001. The role of the region of origin and EU certificates of origin in consumer evaluation of food products. *European Review of Agricultural Economics* 28, 4: 451-477.

Kleppe IA, Iversen NM, Stensaker IG. 2002. Country images in marketing strategies: Conceptual issues and an empirical Asian illustration. *Journal of Brand Management* 10, 1: 61-74.

Lagrange L, Trognon L. 1995. Produits alimentaires des terroirs du Massif Central. *Collection «Etudes».* ENITAC 1: 80 p.

Li ZG, Murray L-W, Scott D. 2000. Global sourcing, multiple country-of-origin facets, and consumer reactions. *Journal of Business Research* 47: 121-133.

Loureiro ML, Umberger WJ. 2005. Assessing consumer preferences for country-of-origin labelling. *Journal of Agricultural and Applied Economics* 37, 1: 49-63.

Nagashima A. A. 1970. Comparison of Japanese and U.S. Attitudes Toward Foreign Products. *Journal of Marketing* 34: 68-74.

Obermiller C, Spangenberg E. 1989. Exploring the effects of country of origin labels: an information processing framework. *Advances in Consumer Research* 16, 1: 454-459.

Papadopoulos N. 2004. Place branding: Evolution, meaning and implications. *Place Branding* 1, 1: 36-49.

Peterson RA, Jolibert AJP. 1995. A meta-analysis of country-of-origin effects. *Journal of international business studies* 26, 4: 883-900.

Roth M-S, Romeo J-B. 1992. Matching product category and country image perceptions: a framework for managing country-of-origin effects. *Journal of international business studies* 477-497.

Samiee S. 1994. Customer evaluation of products in a global market. *Journal of international business studies* 25, 3: 579-604.

Schooler RD, Wildt AR. 1968. Elasticity of product bias. *Journal of Marketing Research* 5, 1: 78-81.

Sheth JN, Mittal B, Newman BI. 1999. *Customer behavior: consumer behavior and beyond.* Dryden Press, London.

Steenkamp J-B, Van Trijp H. 1996. Quality guidance: A consumer-based approach to food quality improvement using partial least squares. *European Review of Agricultural Economics* 23: 195-215.

Stefani G, Romano D, Cavicchi A. 2006. Consumer expectations, liking and willingness to pay for speciality foods: Do sensory characteristics tell the whole story? *Food Quality and Preference* 17: 53-62.

Tse DK, Lee WN. 1993. Removing negative country images: effects of decomposition, branding, and product experience. *Journal of International Marketing* 1, 4: 25-48.

Usunier J-C. 2002. Le pays d'origine du bien influence-t-il encore les évaluations des consommateurs? *Revue Française du Marketing* 189/190: 49-65.

Usunier J-C. 2006. Relevance in business research: the case of country-of-origin research in marketing. *European Management Review* 3: 60-73.

Van der Lans I-A, Van Ittersum K, De Cicco Aea. 2001. The role of the region of origin and EU certificates of origin in consumer evaluation of food products. *European Review of Agricultural Economics* 28, 4: 451-477.

Van Ittersum K, Candel M-J-M, Meulenberg MT-G. 2003. The influence of the image of a product's region of origin on product evaluation. *Elsevier* 56: 215-226.

Van Ittersum K. 2001. *The Role of Region of Origin in Consumer Decision-Making and Choice*, PhD thesis, Social Sciences, Mansholt Graduate School of Social Sciences: Wageningen: 85p.

Verlegh PW-J, Steenkamp J-BEM. 1999. A review and meta-analysis of country-of-origin research. *Journal of Economic Psychology* 20: 521-546.

In: Olive Consumption and Health
Editors: C. A. Savalas and S. M. Nicolau
ISBN: 978-1-62100-774-6

Chapter 11

ANTIOXIDANT COMPOUNDS OF OLIVE PRODUCTS AND HUMAN HEALTH

T. Chatzistathis* and I. Therios
Laboratory of Pomology, School of Agriculture,
Aristotle University, 54124, Thessaloniki, Greece

ABSTRACT

During the last decades there is an increasing interest of people for the benefits of the Mediterranean diet, since, from many years ago, it was known that citizens from the Mediterranean countries suffered less from cardiovascular diseases, compared to others from Northern European countries and USA. Since olive oil has a dominant role in the Mediterranean diet, most of the papers during the last years were focused on the beneficial compounds of olive oil for health, as well as on their protective properties for heart and other human organs. Throughout the history, olive leaves have been exploited for the prevention, or the treatment, of hypertension, carcinogenesis, diabetes, atherosclerosis and many other traditional therapeutic uses.

The most 'famous' and abundant component of olive oil is oleuropein, which is the bitter substance that has antioxidant and anti-inflammatory properties. Apart from these beneficial properties of oleuropein, other very important effects for human organism are the increase of high density lipoprotein (HDL) (good cholesterol), as well as the decrease of bad cholesterol (LDL) and blood pressure. Other very important compounds of olive oil are those of oleic acid, linoleic acid, elenolic acid, hydroxytyrosol, tyrosol, caffeic acid, ferulic acid, o-coumaric acid, gallic acid, benzoic acid e.t.c. For example, oleic acid has been associated with a reduced risk of human cancer and cardiovascular diseases. However, the benefits of olive oil consumption on human health can be ascribed not only to the elevated oleic acid content, but also to the antioxidant, antidiabetic and other properties of its minor components, such as polyphenols, and especially hydroxytyrosol, which is present in high concentrations in the extra virgin olive oil. The concentration of polyphenols in the extra virgin olive oil depends on genotype, location, latitude, climate, ripening stage, irrigation, density of planting, storage conditions of olive oil, and other

* Corresponding author. Tel.: +30-2310-991391. Fax: +30-2310995292. E-mail address: ChChatzi@in.gr (T. Chatzistathis).

agronomic and technological factors. Therefore, with the correct management of the previous factors it can be achieved the maximum concentration of polyphenols, leading to the best quality of the extra virgin olive oil, and of course, to the maximum benefit for human health. The beneficial properties for human health of the most important olive oil compounds, as well as of the compounds found in olive leaves, are presented and discussed under the most recent research findings.

INTRODUCTION

In the Mediterranean diet olive oil has a dominant place. Virgin olive oil is well known for its high content of phenolic substances, amount of oleic acid and tocopherols, that are thought to have health promoting properties (Owen et al., 2000). Historically, olive leaves were used by old civilizations for the treatment of many illnesses. In the middle of the previous century, olive leaves extract was found to be positively acting on hypertension. Recently, olive leaves are used not only in medicine, but also in cosmetics and pharmaceutical products, while they have a high potential for industrial exploitation in the food industry (Erbay and Icier, 2010). During the last decades, the scientific research concerning the benefits of olive trees' products (and especially those of virgin olive oil) on human health has been dramatically increased. For example, the incidence of cancer overall in the Mediterranean basin has been thought to be the lowest, compared to the other parts of the world. This is mostly accounted for the incidence of cancer of the breast, endometrium, prostate, colon and leukaemia (Trichopoulou et al., 2000; La Vecchia, 2004). Almost all of the 16 countries bordering the Mediterranean Sea are sharing a common Mediterranean dietary pattern, characterized by a high consumption of fruit and vegetables, bread, wheat and other cereals, fish and of course olive oil (Bouallagui et al., 2011). After that, a strong association between the Mediterranean diet, and especially between the olive oil diet, and lower incidence of cancer, cardiovascular and neurodegenerative diseases, has been established (La Vecchia and Bosetti, 2006; Sotiroudis and Kyrtopoulos, 2008).

The most 'famous' and abundant phenolic component of olive oil is oleuropein, which gives to it the bitter substance, that has, apart from anticancer, antioxidant, anti-inflammatory, antiproliferative, pharmacological, antimicrobial and antiviral properties (Fabiani et al., 2006; Lee-Huang et al., 2007; Fabiani et al., 2008; Therios, 2009; Omar, 2010; Bulotta et al., 2011). Apart from all these beneficial properties of oleuropein, other very important effects for human organism are the increase of high density lipoprotein (HDL) (good cholesterol), as well as the decrease of bad cholesterol (LDL) and blood pressure (Therios, 2009). From the other compounds of olive oil, those of hydroxytyrosol, tyrosol, oleic, linoleic, palmitic, elenolic, syringic, caffeic, ferulic, o-coumaric, gallic and benzoic acid should be distinguished (Therios, 2009; Allalout et al., 2010; Cioffi et al., 2010). Hydroxytyrosol, for example, (one of the polyphenols), which is present in high concentrations in the extra virgin olive oil, has antidiabetic and anti-tumoral properties and activities, which have been investigated by many researchers (Bouallagui et al., 2011). Tyrosol is the third main olive compound present in the olive tree, which has important antioxidant properties (Ortega-Garcia and Peragon, 2010). Generally, the higher polyphenols' concentration of virgin olive oil, the better quality it has, and of course, the better benefit for human health. The concentration of polyphenols in the extra virgin olive oil, as well as in table olives, depends on genotype (Ben Othman et al.,

2008; Allalout et al., 2009; Ranalli et al., 2009; Zoidou et al., 2010; Malheiro et al., 2011), location (Therios, 2009), latitude (Garcia-Gonzalez et al., 2010), climate (Garcia-Gonzalez et al., 2010), ripening stage (Jemai et al., 2009b; Ranalli et al., 2009; Ben Youssef et al., 2009; Ortega-Garcia and Peragon, 2009; 2010; Bouaziz et al., 2010), irrigation (Allalout et al., 2009; Gomez-Rico et al., 2009), density of planting (Allalout et al., 2009; Therios, 2009), storage conditions of olive oil (Therios, 2009), and other agronomic and technological factors (Ben Othman et al., 2009; Therios, 2009). In this review, the beneficial role on human health of each of the most important olive oil compounds, as well as of those found in olive leaves, are being presented and discussed under the light of the most recent scientific findings. Furthermore, the influence of different environmental, agronomic and technological factors on the maximum concentration of polyphenols is fully analyzed, in order to help the reader understand their importance on the achievement of the best virgin olive oil quality.

Oleuropein

Oleuropein is the most 'famous' substance of olive oil. It can be also found in olive leaves and green olives together with other closely related compounds, such as 10-hydroxyoleuropein, ligstroside and 10-hydroxyligstroside. All these compounds are tyrosol esters of elenolic acid that are further hydroxylated and glycosylated. Oleuropein gives to olive oil a bitter taste, and has antioxidant, antidiabetic and anti-inflammatory properties. Apart from these beneficial properties of oleuropein, other very important effects for human organism are the increase of high density lipoprotein (HDL) (good cholesterol), as well as the decrease of bad cholesterol (LDL) and blood pressure (Therios, 2009). According to Jemai et al. (2009a), the administration for 4 weeks of oleuropein and hydroxytyrosol rich extracts significantly decreased the serum glucose and cholesterol levels, and restored the antioxidant perturbations, in alloxan-diabetic rats. The authors concluded that the antidiabetic effect of oleuropein might be due to its antioxidant activity restraining the oxidative stress, which is widely associated with diabetes pathologies and complications (Jemai et al., 2009a). Sirianni et al. (2010) found that oleuropein inhibited proliferation of MCF-7 breast cancer cells. According to Bulotta et al. (2011), some oleuropein paracetylated derivatives exerted higher antiproliferative effect than oleuropein, by an arrest of cell cycle progression, associated with a strong antioxidant capacity. So, the conclusion of these authors was that, olive leaves, a by-product of olive manufacture could provide a valuable source of chemical derivatives, obtainable by per-acetylation of oleuropein derivatives, which provided beneficial properties for human health (Bulotta et al., 2011). Oleuropein has not only antioxidant, antidiabetic and anti-inflammatory properties, but also antimicrobial ones. Among some phenolic compounds tested for their antimicrobial activities, oleuropein was found to be the most effective one (Korukluoglu et al., 2010).

Hydroxytyrosol, Tyroxol and Other Antioxidant Compounds of Olive Products- (No capital letters in this subtitle)

Hydroxytyrosol is the second most 'famous', after oleuropein, antioxidant compound. According to Bouallagui et al. (2011), hydroxytyrosol rich extract from olive leaves modulated cell cycle progression in MCF-7 human breast cancer cells. The same authors refer that cytotoxicity assays resulted in a dose dependent growth inhibition of MCF-7 cells. This inhibition was due to the cell cycle arrest in the G0/G1 phase. According to what is referred by many authors, hydroxytyrosol has antidiabetic and anti-tumoral properties and activities, which have been already investigated (Therios, 2009; Bouallagui et al., 2011). However, according to Jemai et al. (2009a), the antidiabetic effect of hydroxytyrosol, as well as that of oleuropein, might be due to its antioxidant activity restraining the oxidative stress, which is widely associated with diabetes pathologies and complications. Ortega-Garcia and Peragon (2010) found that both hydroxytyrosol and tyroxol were present in roots, as well as in stems of *Olea europaea* L. (cv. 'Picual') trees, but their concentration was higher in stems, than in roots. Furthermore, from the middle of September to October the hydroxytyrosol and tyrosol concentration significantly increased in stems.

Oleic acid is another very important compound found in olive oil that has been associated with a reduced risk of human cancer and cardiovascular diseases (Therios, 2009). According to Bouaziz et al. (2010), twenty-six biophenolic compounds were identified in olive oil samples from the Tunisian cultivars 'Zelmati', 'Chemchali', 'Chemlali' and 'Chetoui', but the major ones found were hydroxytyrosol and oleuropein. Furthermore, Hayes et al. (2011) found that in olive leaf extracts were present 6 major polyphenolic compounds: oleuropein, verbascoside, luteolin-7-O-glucoside, apigenin7-O-glucoside, hydroxytyrosol and tyrosol. Cioffi et al. (2010) determined and quantified oleocanthal, one of the main substances responsible for the bitter taste of olive oil.

According to the same authors, the total content of oleocanthal, from Cilento virgin olive oil, expressed as gallic acid equivalent, was 5%, an amount quite comparable to that reported for virgin olive oils coming from other geographical areas (Cioffi et al., 2010). Korukluoglu et al. (2010) found in olive leaf extracts, apart from oleuropein, six other phenolic compounds (4 hydroxybenzoic acid, vanillic acid, p-coumaric acid, tyrosol, caffeic acid, syringic acid) to have antimicrobial activities against different bacteria genus, but those were inferior compared to that of oleuropein. According to the same authors, these phenolic compounds were shown to be more effective against gram positive, than gram negative bacteria. In contrast to those findings, Medina et al. (2007) found that the dialdehydic form of decarboxymethyl elenolic acid, identified for the first time in table olives, and an isomer of oleoside 11-methyl ester were also effective against *Lactobacillus pentosus* and can, furthermore, exert a more potent antibacterial activity than the well studied oleuropein and hydroxytyrosol. Furthermore, according to Malheiro et al. (2011), twelve phenolic compounds were identified and quantified in 'alcaparras' table olives, produced from different olive cultivars.

These phenolic compounds were the following: hydroxytyrosol, tyrosol, chlorogenic acid, vanillic acid, syringic acid, verbascoside, luteolin 7-O-glucoside, oleuropein, rutin, apigenin 7-O glucoside, quercetine and luteolin.

Finally, some of the certain important olive oil minor components, including efficient antioxidant polyphenols, the triterpene hydrocarbon squalene and β-sitosterol, considered as putative nutritional biomarkers, play an important role in the reduction of the incidence of cancer (Sotiroudis and Kyrtopoulos, 2008).

Factors Influencing the Concentration of Phenols in Olive Oil and Table Olives

It is of great importance to know how the genetic, agronomic, climatic and technical factors, analyzed below, affect the concentration of total phenols, so the quality of olive products, and of course, how they maximize, or minimize, the beneficial role of phenols for the human health. The most important of these factors are the following:

a. *Genotype.* The role of genotype (i.e. the genetic factor) is very important in controlling the concentration of total polyphenols. According to the findings of many researchers (Allalout et al., 2009; Therios, 2009; Ortega-Garcia and Peragon, 2009; Ortega-Garcia and Peragon, 2010; Bouaziz et al., 2010), the total phenolic content varied between different olive cultivars. Therefore, by choosing for cultivation the suitable olive cultivars, it can be achieved the production of olive oil, or table olives, with maximum concentration of total antioxidant components, i.e. it can be also achieved the maximum benefit for the human health. According to Malheiro et al. (2011), the cultivar (genotype) affects both quantitative and qualitative phenolic fractions of table olives. Finally, according to Ranalli et al. (2009) and Zoidou et. (2010), the contents of oleuropein were greatly influenced by the olive cultivar (genetic factor) in Italian and Greek olive drupes. Particularly, in the case of 'Throuba Thassos' oleuropein was found in important quantities (1.2 mg/fruit) recorded over a four-year period, so this particular olive type was found to be a nutritional rich source of oleuropein in the usual every-day diet (Zoidou et al., 2010).
b. *Location* (Therios, 2009).
c. *Geographic area.* According to Allalout et al. (2009), the olive cultivar 'Arbosana' produced lower amounts of total phenols when cultivated in Tunisia, as compared to its original growing area (Spain). Moreover, 'Koroneiki' showed a lower amount of total phenols when grown in Tunisia, compared to its original growing area (Greece). It should be pointed out that, not only the concentration of total phenols, but also the fatty acids' composition differed (at least for the main fatty acids, i.e. palmitic, oleic and linoleic acids) for some Spanish olive cultivars between their original geographic area and Tunisia (Allalout et al., 2009).
d. *Climate or latitude.* According to Garcia-Gonzalez et al. (2010), the chemical composition of the oils produced in countries as far distant as Spain and Chile are affected by differences in latitude and climate. Concerning phenol composition, main differences were found in secoiridoids derivatives of oleuropein, ligstroside, apigenin and luteolin.

e. *Ripening stage.* According to Ortega-Garcia and Peragon (2010), the concentration of hydroxytyrosol and tyrosol significantly increased in the stems of the olive cultivar 'Picual' from the middle of September to October. Furthermore, according to the same authors, the oleuropein concentration increased from the middle of September until the end of November. Bouaziz et al. (2010) found that the total phenolic content varied from 3.46 to 4.30 g/kg at the first stage of maturation and from 8.71 to 11.52 g/kg of the fresh weight at the last stage of maturation. Other researchers refer that, as the ripening procedure goes on, the concentration of total phenols, as well as that of oleuropein, is significantly decreased (Ortega-Garcia and Peragon, 2009; Ranalli et al., 2009; Therios, 2009). Ben Youssef et al. (2009) found that total phenols and o-diphenols showed an increase at the early stages followed by a reduction at more advanced stages of maturity. The major phenolic compounds, such as hydroxytyrosol, ligstroside aglycon, elenolic acid, acetoxy-pinoresinol and oleuropein aglycon seemed to have the same behavior (Ben Youssef et al., 2009). Furthermore, according to Jemai et al. (2009b), oleuropein significantly decreased during all the ripeness stages from 3.29 g/kg fresh olive (July) to 0.16 g/kg (October) in Dhokar cv. and from 5.7 g/kg (July) to 3.75 /kg (October) in Chemlali cv. This decrease, according to the same authors, was inversely correlated with hydroxytyrosol concentrations until September. Changes in oleuropein contents during fruit maturity in Dhokar cv. showed a similar pattern reported for other olive cultivars. On the other hand, the enhancement of hydroxytyrosol concentrations could be attributed to the increased activity of hydrolytic enzymes, in particular glycosidases and esterases, which catalyze the hydrolysis of oleuropein (Jemai et al., 2009b).
f. *Irrigation.* It seems possible that, irrigation, especially in high density planting systems, reduces the amount of total polyphenols (Allalout et al., 2009). However, a good agreement between the content of oleuropein and the minimum stem water potential of the olive trees (cvs. 'Cornicabra' and 'Morisca'), measured from the beginning of August to the end of the irrigation period, was found. A lower minimum water potential corresponded, therefore, with a higher biophenol content in the drupe and, consequently, with a superior phenolic content in virgin olive oil (Gomez-Rico et al., 2009).
g. *Density of planting.* Allalout et al. (2009) refer that the lower amount of total phenols of the olive cultivar 'Koroneiki' in Tunisia, compared to that when grown in Greece, is probably attributed to the high density planting systems in Tunisia. According to the same authors, no data are provided under such olive growing systems in Greece.
h. *Storage conditions of olive oil* (Therios, 2009).
i. *Other agronomic and technological factors.* After fermentation in 'Chetoui' table olives, an important loss of total phenolic compounds was observed. Particularly, hydroxytyrosol and caffeic acid concentrations increased, whilst protocatechuic and ferulic acid concentrations, as well as that of oleuropein decreased (Ben Othman et al., 2009).

REFERENCES

Allalout A., Krichen D., Methenni K., Taamalli A., Oueslati I., Daoud D., Zarrouk M., 2009. Characterization of virgin olive oil from super intensive Spanish and Greek varieties grown in northern Tunisia. *Scientia Horticulturae* 120: 77-83.

Ben Othman N., Roblain D., Chammen N., Thonart P., Hamdi M., 2009. Antioxidant phenolic compounds loss during the fermentation of Chetoui olives. *Food Chemistry* 116: 662-669.

Ben Othman N., Roblain D., Thonart P., Hamdi M., 2008. Tunisian table olive phenolic compounds and their antioxidant capacity. *Journal of Food Science* 73: 235-240.

Ben Youssef N., Zarrouk W., Carrasco-Pancorbo A., Ouni Y., Segura-Carretero A., Fernandez-Gutierrez A., Daoud D., Zarrouk M., 2009. Effect of olive ripeness on chemical properties and phenolic composition of Chetoui virgin olive oil. *Journal of the Science of Food and Agriculture* 90: 199-204.

Bouallagui Z., Han J., Isoda H., Sayadi S., 2011. Hydroxytyrosol rich extract from olive leaves modulates cell cycle progression in MCF-7 human breast cancer cells. *Food and Chemical Toxicology* 49: 179-184.

Bouaziz M., Jemai H., Khabou W., Sayadi S., 2010. Oil content, phenolic profiling and antioxidant potential of Tunisian olive drupes. *Journal of the Science of Food and Agriculture* 90: 1750-1758.

Bulotta S., Corradino R., Celano M., D' Agostino M., Maiuolo J., Oliverio M., Procopio A., Iannone M., Rotiroti D., Russo D., 2011. *Food Chemistry* 127: 1609-1614.

Cioffi G., Pesca M.S., De Caprariis P., Braca A., Severino L., De Tommasi N., 2010. Phenolic compounds in olive oil and olive pomace from Cilento (Campania, Italy) and their antioxidant activity. *Food Chemistry* 121: 105-111.

Erbay Z., Icier F., 2010. The importance and potential uses of olive leaves. *Food Reviews International* 26: 319-334.

Fabiani R., De Bartolomeo A., Rosignoli P., Servili M., Selvaggini R., Montedoro G.F., 2006. Virgin olive oil phenols inhibit proliferation of human promyelocytic leukemia cells (HL 60) by inducing apoptosis and differentiation. *The journal of Nutrition* 136: 614-619.

Fabiani R., Rosignoli P., De Bartolomeo A., Fuccelli R., Servili M., Montedoro G.F., 2008. Oxidative DNA damage is prevented by extracts of olive oil, hydroxytyrosol, and other olive phenolic compounds in human blood mononuclear cells and HL60 cells. *The journal of Nutrition* 138: 1411-1416.

Garcia-Gonzalez D.L., Romero N., Aparicio R., 2010. Comparative study of virgin olive oil quality from single varieties cultivated in Chile and Spain. *Journal of Agricultural Food Chemistry* 58: 12899-12905.

Gomez-Rico A., Desmparados-Salvador M., Fregapane G., 2009. Virgin olive oil and olive fruit minor constituents as affected by irrigation management based on SWP and TDF as compared to ETc in medium density young olive orchards (Olea europaea L. cv. Cornicabra and Morisca). *Food Research International* 42: 1067-1076.

Hayes J.E., Allen P., Brunton N., O' Grady M.N., Kerry J.P., 2011. Phenolic composition and in vitro antioxidant capacity of four commercial phytochemical products: Olive leaf extract (Olea europaea L.), lutein, sesamol, and ellagic acid. *Food Chemistry* 126: 948-955.

Jemai H., Bouaziz M., Sayadi S., 2009b. Phenolic composition, sugar contents and antioxidant activity of Tunisian sweet olive cultivar with regard to fruit ripening. *Journal of Agricultural and Food Chemistry* 57: 2961-2968.

Jemai H., El Feki A., Sayadi S., 2009a. Antidiabetic and Antioxidant effects of hydroxytyrosol and oleuropein from olive leaves in alloxan-diabetic rats. *Journal of Agricultural Food Chemistry* 57: 8798-8804.

Korukluoglu M., Sahan Y., Yigit A., Ozer E.T., Gucer S., 2010. Antibacterial activity and chemical constitutions of *Olea europaea* L. leaf extracts. *Journal of Food Processing and Preservation* 34: 383-396.

La Vecchia C., 2004. *Mediterranean diet and cancer.* Public Health Nutrition 7: 965-968.

La Vecchia C., Bosetti C., 2006. Diet and cancer risk in Mediterranean countries: Open Issue. *Public Health Nutrition* 9: 1077-1082.

Lee-Huang S., Huang P.L., Zhang D., Lee J.W., Bao J., Sun Y., 2007. Discovery of small molecule HIV-1 fusion and integrase inhibitors oleuropein and hydroxytyrosol: *Part I. Fusion (corrected) inhibition. Biochemical and Biophysical Research Communication* 354: 872-878.

Malheiro R., Sousa A., Casal S., Bento A., Pereira J.A., 2011. Cultivar effect on the phenolic composition and antioxidant potential of stoned table olives. *Food and Chemical Toxicology* 49: 450-457.

Medina E., Brenes M., Romero C., Garcia A., De Castro A., 2007. Main antimicrobial compounds in table olives. *Journal of Agricultural and Food Chemistry* 55: 9817-9823.

Omar S.H., 2010. Oleuropein in olive and its pharmacological effects. *Scientia Pharmaceutica* 78: 133-154.

Ortega-Garcia F., Peragon J., 2009. Phenylalanine Ammonia-Lyase, Polyphenol oxidase and phenol concentration in fruits of Olea europaea L. cv. Picual, Verdial, Arbequina, and Frantoio during ripening. *Journal of Agricultural Food Chemistry* 57: 10331-10340.

Ortega-Garcia F., Peragon J., 2010. HPLC analysis of oleuropein, hydroxytyrosol, and tyrosol in stems and roots of Olea europaea L. cv. Picual during ripening. *Journal of the Science of Food and Agriculture* 90: 2295-2300.

Ortega-Garcia F., Peragon J., 2010. Phenol metabolism in the leaves of the olive tree (*Olea europaea* L.) cv. Picual, Verdial, Arbequina and Frantoio during ripening. *Journal of Agricultural and Food Chemistry* 58: 12440-12448.

Owen R.W., Giacosa A., Hull W.E., Haubner B., Spiegelhalder B., Bartsch H., 2000. Identification of lignans as major components in the phenolic fraction of olive oil. *Clinical Chemistry* 46: 976-988.

Ranalli A., Marchegiani D., Contento S., Girardi F., Nicolosi M.P., Brullo M.D., 2009. Variations of iridoid oleuropein in Italian olive varieties during growth and maturation. *European Journal of Lipid Science and Technology* 111: 678-687.

Sirianni R., Chimento A., De Luca A., Casaburi I., Rizza P., Onofrio A., Lacopetta D., Puoci F., Ando S., Maggiolini M., Pezzi V., 2010. Oleuropein and hydroxytyrosol inhibit MCF-7 breast cancer cell proliferation interfering with ERK1/2 activation. Molecular *and Nutritional Food Research* 54: 833-840.

Sotiroudis T.G., Kyrtopoulos S.A., 2008. Anticarcinogenic compounds of olive oil and related biomarkers. *European Journal of Nutrition* 47: 69-72.

Therios I., 2009. *Olives*. Crop Production Science in Horticulture. CABI, U.K., p. 303-317.

Trichopoulou A., Lagiou P., Kuper H., Trichopoulos D., 2000. Cancer and Mediterranean dietary traditions. *Cancer Epidemiol Biomarkers Prev 9*: 869-873.

Zoidou E., Melliou E., Gikas E., Tsarbopoulos A., Magiatis P., Skaltsounis A.L., 2010. Identification of Throuba Thassos, a traditional Greek table olive variety, as a nutritional rich source of oleuropein. *Journal of Agricultural and Food Chemistry* 58: 46-50.

In: Olive Consumption and Health
Editors: C. A. Savalas and S. M. Nicolau
ISBN: 978-1-62100-774-6

Chapter 12

HUMAN METABOLISM OF POLYPHENOLS FROM EXTRA VIRGIN OLIVE OIL

Fabiano Jares Contesini*, Ruann Janser Soares de Castro, José Valdo Madeira Júnior and Camilo Barroso Teixeira
Department of Food Science, Faculty of Food Engineering, University of Campinas (UNICAMP), Campinas, SP, Brazil

ABSTRACT

It is well established that food is not considered to be mere nutritional components for maintaining human life. There are a broad number of studies reporting that many foods may provide a health benefit beyond basic nutrition. Within this context, extra virgin olive oil (EVOO) has been related to the prevention of some types of cancers and the reduced risk of coronary heart diseases. This is mainly due to its high concentration of a broad variety of phenolic compounds, such as phenyl ethyl alcohols (tyrosol, hydroxytyrosol), phenolic acids (4-hydroxybenzoic acid, 3,4-dihydroxybenzoic acid, gallic acid, vanillic acid, ferulic acid, caffeic acid), flavonoids (apigenin, luteolin), secoiridoids (oleuropein and ligstroside aglycons) and lignans [(+)-pinoresinol, (+)-acetoxypinoresinol)]. In the human organism these polyphenols are metabolized and form different compounds. Thus the study of their properties is highly important with regards to understanding their functionality. The aglycones can be absorbed from the mall intestine; however, most polyphenols are in the form of esters, glycosides, or polymers that cannot be absorbed in their native form. Thus, these compounds must be hydrolyzed by intestinal enzymes or by colonic microflora in order to be absorbed. During the course of absorption, polyphenols are conjugated in the small intestine and later in the liver, through methylation, sulfation, and glucuronidation reactions. In the blood, polyphenols are conjugated derivatives bound to albumin. They penetrate into tissues where they are metabolized and then eliminated in urine and bile. For example, hydroxytyrosol shows strong antioxidant activity. In spite of this compound's great absorption capacity in the human body, its bioavailability is low. It is reported in the literature that the oleuropeins are not absorbed in the small intestine, but instead, quickly degradated in the large intestine to yield hydroxytyrosol.

Keywords: Metabolism, polyphenols, olive oil

Introduction

Extra virgin olive oil (EVOO) is an important food that is obtained through the mechanical extraction of olive fruit (*Olea europeae* L., *oleacea* family). This oil is found mainly in the diet of the Mediterranean population, who display a greater life expectancy compared to more developed countries in Northern Europe (Trichopoulou & Vasilopoulou). The consumption of olive oil is one of the main reasons to this longevity, whilst taking into account that olive oil presents beneficial health effects in addition to its well-known nutritional properties.

EVOO is composed of 55 to 85% oleic acid, tocopherols (5–25 mg/100 g, 95% - tocopherol), carotenoids (1–2 mg/100 g), phenolic compounds such as oleuropein (20 –500 mg/L), and phytosterols (98–185 mg/100 g). Minor components include • avonids, rutin, leuteolin, and squalene (Boskou et al. 2000).

This oil is produced from the first and second pressings of the olive fruit, using no chemicals; only the cold pressing and a small amount of heat. Olive oil is mainly composed of monounsaturated fatty acid (MUFA), that perform some potent immunoregulatory actions (Yaqoob et al., 1998). An important group of constituents in EVOO is the phenolic compounds, because this oil is not produced by solvent extraction but by a cold-press mechanical process that retains the natural antixodants that are produced by the olive fruits (Visoli & Galli, 2000). They are responsible for distinctive properties of this oil, such as the great oxidative stability, which is very important during processing. In addition, they present several functional properties (Bisignano et al., 1999).

The functional properties of the phenolic compounds in EVOO depend on their absorption and metabolism in the human organism. The consumption of olive oil polyphenols has been estimated to be around 9 mg, based on the consumption of 25–50 mL of olive oil per day. The absorption, metabolism and excretion of these compounds are discussed in this review.

Secoiridoids

General Aspects

The secoiridoids are a large group of naturally occurring terpenoids containing a dimethylcyclopentapyran structure. Most secoiridoids are found in higher plants. Their ecological functions, physiological activity, pharmacology, and significance as chemotaxonomic markers have attracted considerable interest (Perez-Jimenez, 2005).

Secoiridoids occur mainly as glucosides form, but a small number of nonglycosidic occur in the forms of ester, acetal and hemiacetal forms. They are also volatile and are occasionally reported as components of essential oils; mainly olive oil. They are biosynthesized in plants from phenyl-ethyl-alcohol (tyrosol (T) or hydroxytyrosol (HT)) and bound elenolic acid and glucoside residue via secondary metabolism. The great variations of the secoiridoid structures in olive oil are attained by hydrolysis of endogenous β-glucosidases during crushing and malaxation (Bendini et al., 2007).

During the storage of olive oil hydrolytic mechanisms, simple phenols are released, such HT and T, and complex phenols such as secoiridoids may be involved. The most abundant secoiridois of olive oil identified are phenyl-ethyl-alcohols and derivates, dialdehydic forms of secoiridoids and its algycones forms (Figure 1) (Bendini et al., 2007).

Compound	Substituent (MW)	Structure
Phenyl ethyl alcohols		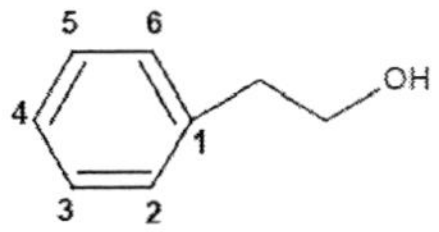
Tyrosol [(*p*-hydroxyphenyl)ethanol] or *p*-HPEA	4-OH (138)	
Hydroxytyrosol [(*3,4*-dihydroxyphenyl)ethanol] or 3,4-DHPEA	3,4-OH (154)	
Other phenolic acids and derivatives		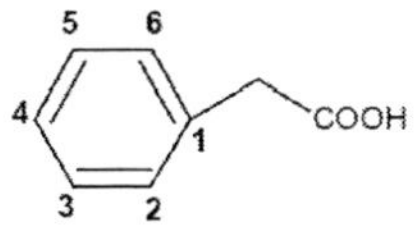
p-Hydroxyphenylacetic acid	4-OH (152)	
3,4-Dihydroxyphenylacetic acid	3,4-OH (168)	
4-Hydroxy-3-methoxyphenylacetic acid	3-OCH_3, 4-OH (182)	
3-(3,4-Dihydroxyphenyl)propanoic acid	(182)	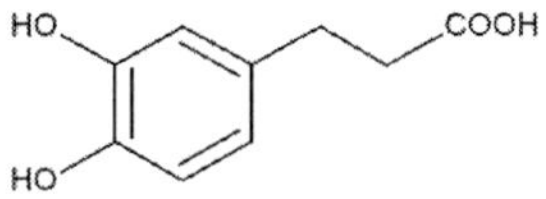
Dialdehydic forms of secoiridoids		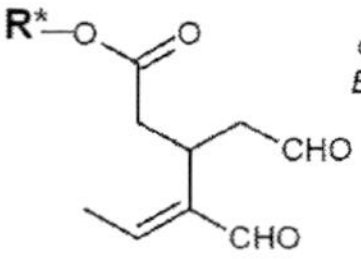 *dialdehydic form of Elenolic Acid (EDA)*
Decarboxymethyloleuropein aglycon (3,4-DHPEA-EDA)	R_1-OH (304)	
Decarboxymethyl ligstroside aglycon (*p*-HPEA-EDA)	R_1-H (320)	
Secoiridoid Aglycons		
Oleuropein aglycon or 3,4-DHPEA-EA	R_1-OH (378)	
Ligstroside aglycon or *p*-HPEA-EA	R_1-H (362)	
Aldehydic form of oleuropein aglycon	R_1-OH (378)	
Aldehydic form ligstroside aglycon	R_1-H (362)	

Structure

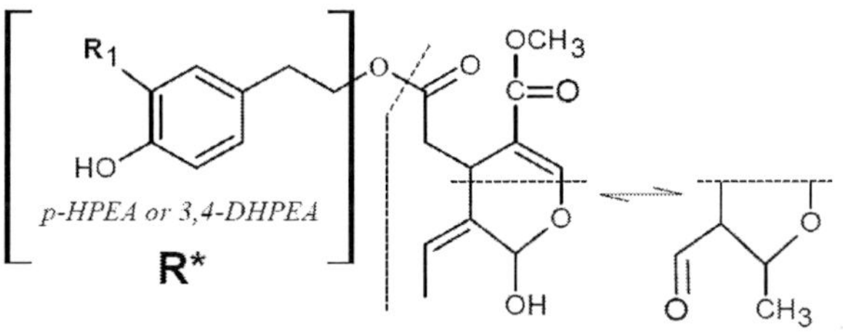

Elenolic Acid (EA) *aldehydic form of Elenolic Acid (EA)*

Bendini et al., 2007.

Figure 1. Classification, name and chemical structure of phenolics present in olive oil.

Pharmacokinetics of Secoiridoids

Absorption

The hydroxytyrosol and tyrosol as well as their derivates (aglycons, glucosides and oleuropein) are hydrolysis under gastric conditions (HCl + pepsin), releasing HT and T, while entering the small intestine (Corona et al., 2006). Figure 2 illustrates the absorption of hydroxytyrosol and oleuropein in the small intestine.

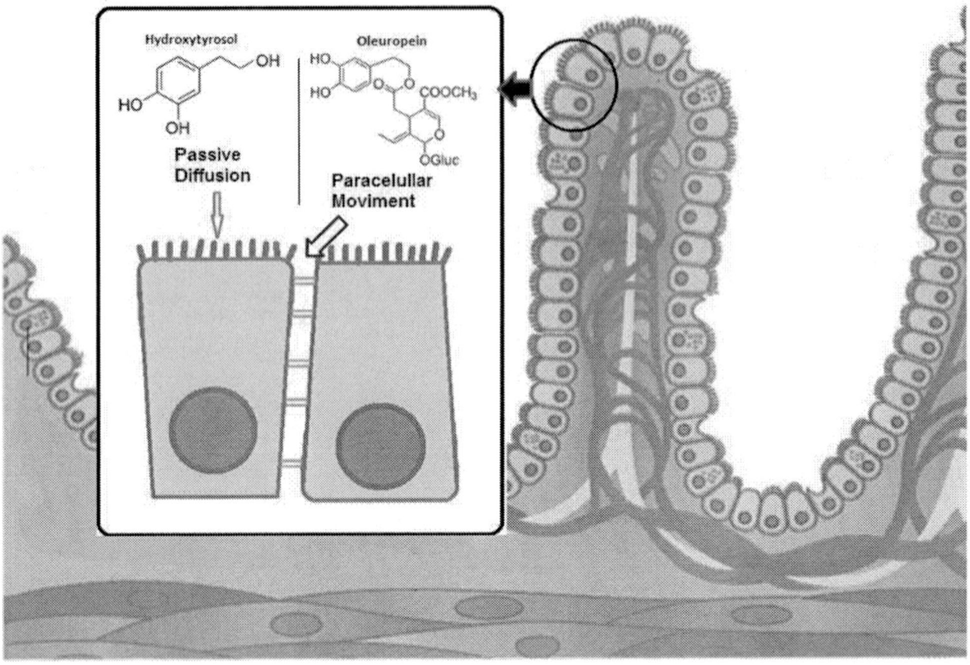

Adapted Townsend, 2006.

Figure 2. Mechanism transport of the hydroxytyrosol (Passive Diffusion) and oleuropein (Paracelullar Moviment) in the epithelium lining the small intestine.

Manna et al., (2000) investigated the transport mechanism and metabolism of olive oil hydroxytyrosol in vitro by human intestinal Caco-2 cells. These studies involving cell culture models suggest that hydroxytyrosol is quantitatively absorbed at the intestinal level and it has been suggested that transepithelial transport can occur by passive and bidirectional diffusion. The absorption of oleuropein has not been clearly identified. However, studies indicate that absorption occurs through the junctions between the epithelial cells lining the intestine; named paracellular movement (Manna et al., 2000; Corona et al., 2006).

Miró-Casas et al., (2003) investigated the absorption of tyrosol and hydroxytyrosol when single (50mL) and sustained doses (25mL/day for a week) were ingested by healthy volunteers. The results showed that the absorption of tyrosol and hydroxytyrosol is dose-dependent. Levels of urinary tyrosol obtained in both intervention periods were similar: after one week of sustained doses (25 mL/day) of virgin olive oil, the urinary recovery (%) is 19,4 ± 12,2 and when a single dose (50mL) was administrated the urinary recovery was 16,9 ± 4,8. The estimated urinary hydroxytyrosol recovery after sustained doses of 25 mL of virgin olive oil was higher than when the single dose (50mL) was administered. In the first case, the recovery of hydroxytyrosol in urine was greater than 100%. The overestimation of hydroxytyrosol recovery can be explained by the endogenous formation of this compound. Some studies showed that hydroxytyrosol has been identified as a metabolite from 3,4-dihidroxyphenylacetaldehyde (a dopamine metabolite) and tyrosine (Mardh & Vallee, 1986; Goldstein et al., 1999).

González-Santiago, Fonollá and Lopez-Huertas (2010) investigated the human absorption of a supplement containing purified hydroxytyrosol (99,5%). Ten healthy volunteers participated in the investigation and ingested the solution. Levels of hydroxytyrosol were measured in plasma and urine. The results showed that the maximal concentration in plasma for hydroxytyrosol was detected at 13.0±1.5 min and 2-h after the administration levels were undetectable. It showed that different metabolites of hydroxytyrosol were detected in the urine collected from the volunteers after the 24 h mark: hydroxytyrosol, homovanillic alcohol, homovanillic acid and 3,4-dihydroxyphenylacetic acid as free forms (44%), as glucuronide (34.4%) and sulphate (21.2%) conjugates. An interesting discovery in this investigation was that the absorption of hydroxytyrosol presented a large variability among the subjects, for example, the maximal concentration (μmol/L) in plasma ranged from 0.17 to 2.24.

Bermúdez et al., (2004) affirms that there are controversial studies about absorption of (extra virgin) olive oil phenolic compounds. Some problems are outlined by several researches: simple phenols can be absorbed in the intestine, however they can suffer degradation by microorganisms in the colon. In addition, some compounds can be derived from endogenous metabolism, resulting in an overestimation of the absorbed amount when faecal and urinary excretion are measured (Scalbert and Williansom, 2000; Miró-Casas et al., 2003).

It was demonstrated that the absorption of hydroxytyrosol is rapid. Some studies showed that the maximum plasma concentration reached 5–15 min after ingestion. While after 1-2h, the concentration was reduced or not detectable (Bai et al., 1998; González-Santiago, Fonollá and Lopez-Huertas, 2010).

The vehicle and form of administration is an important aspect when the absorption of hydroxytyrosol is evaluated. Tuck et al., (2001) studied the absorption of hydroxytyrosol when administered intravenously and orally (in oil- and water-based solutions). The results demonstrated that the absorption of hydroxytyrosol differs according to the vehicle in which it is carried. An oral bioavailability estimate of hydroxytyrosol when administered in an olive oil solution was 99%, and when dosed in an aqueous solution it was 75%. On the other hand, there were no significant differences observed between the intravenous dosing method and the oral oil-based dosing method when levels of hydroxytyrosol were eliminated in urine.

Metabolism and Excretion

There have been several studies that investigated the metabolism of phenolic compounds after ingestion. The main objective of these studies was to find out the mechanisms through which these components exert their activity into the organism. The general mechanism of polyphenols metabolism involves two phases: Phase I) in which they are hydrolysed and Phase II) which conjugated into their glucuronidated, methylated and sulphated forms in order to be absorbed (Suárez et al., 2011).

In a simplified scheme at the process of crossing epithelial cells of the GI tract, Tuck and Hayball (2002) propose four metabolic pathways for phenolics compounds from olive oil: I) oxidation: through the enzymes alcohol dehydrogenase and aldehyde dehydrogenase, resulting to 3,4-dihydroxyphenyl acetic acid (dihydroxyphenylacetic acid); II) methylation: by the enzyme catechol-O-methyltransferase, giving rise to 4-hydroxy-3-methoxy phenylethanol (homovanillic alcohol), about 10% of HT is converted into homovanillyl alcohol (HVAL) by the catechol-O-methyltransferase (Manna et al., 2000); III) glucuronide conjugation by the enzyme glucotransferase and IV) sulfate conjugation by the enzyme sulfotransferase (Figure 3). In addition to the O-methylated derivative of HT, the study found glucuronides of HT and T and a novel glutathionylated conjugate of HT. In contrast, there was no absorption of oleuropein as it was rapidly degraded by the colonic microflora to HT (Corona et al., 2006).

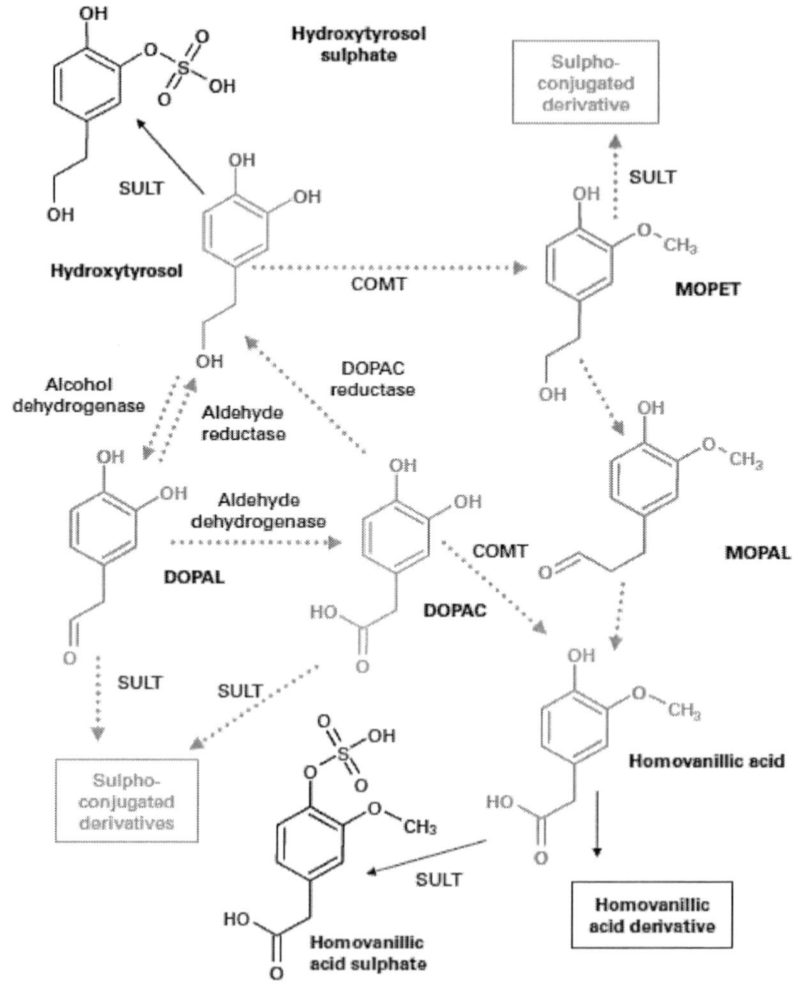

Figure 3.Hydroxytyrosol metabolism (adapted from Suárez *et al*., 2011). Abreviations: MOPET (3-methoxy-4-hydroxy-phenylethanol); SULT (sulphotransferase); COMT (catechol-O-methyltransferase); DOPAL (3,4-dihydroxy phenylacetaldehyde); DOPAC (3,4-dihydroxy-phenylacetic acid); MOPAL (3-methoxy-4-hydroxy-phenylacetaldehyde); homovanillic acid (4-hydroxy-3-methoxy-phenylacetic acid).

The metabolism in the liver of the phenols from olive oil has been studied in human hepatoma HepG2 cells. To measure the concentrations of phenolic compounds a study was carried out on the hydrolysis of the cells with sulfatase and glucuronidase. After 18 hours incubation, the cells, were detected in HT methylated forms, and also glycosylated metabolites methyl-glucuronidated. Hydroxytyrosyl acetate was transformed into free HT and subsequently metabolized, glucuronidated hydroxytyrosyl acetate was detected at low concentrations. Tyrosol showed poor liver metabolization, being below 10% of the phenol glucuronidated. Minor amounts of free or conjugated phenols were detected in cell lysates. No sulfated metabolites were found (Mateos et al., 2005).

According Khymenets et al. (2006), the compounds HT, T and HVAL were mainly glucuronidated in the position 4′ of the benzene ring, a small fraction was conjugated at position 3′ of the ring.

D'Angelo et al. (2001) reported the uptake of the HT by the organs and tissues, mainly renal uptake, administered to rats intravenously. After 5 h, the urine was collected and 90% of the phenolics administered was recovered, and about 5% was detectable in feces and gastrointestinal content. From the HT, four oxidated and/or methylated derivatives were transformed. The author also reported the recovery from HT to sulfo-conjugated forms and subsequently excreted in urine. In excreted product obtained, 6% recovery was HT: 0.3% recovered as HVAL (3-methyl-4-hydroxy-phenylethanol, MOPET), 12.3% as DOPAC (3,4-dihydroxy-phenylacetic acid), 23.6% as homovanillic acid (3-methyl-4-hydroxyphenylacetic acid, HVA), and 26% as DOPAL (3,4-dihydroxy-phenylacetaldehyde).

According to some studies the absence of the 3-O-glucuronide of HT is probably due to the administration route attended. The administration of HT via oral is subject to an extensive first-pass metabolism, where the contribution of intestinal metabolism is quite relevant. Tuck et al. (2002) reported the intravenously administration of HT and concluded that metabolization only occurred in the liver.

Conclusion

Olive oil is known worldwide for its interesting sensory, technological and mainly functional properties. Several phenolic compounds in their composition have considerable antioxidant activity, which results in a higher oxidative stability and therefore a greater shelf life. Several studies in literature report that it has the preventive capacity against several chronic degenerative diseases such as heart diseases, different types of cancer, and Alzheimer's disease, among others. The group of secoroidoids is present in olive oil and is responsible for several functional properties. Within this group the hydroxytyrosol (HT), tyrosol (T) and its derivatives are located. However, their action in the human body depends on several factors such as absorption, metabolism and excretion. Thus, the structure of these compounds is imperative for its' absorption, because both HT and T are, generally, absorbed as aglycone. The glycosidic form is initially hydrolyzed by microbial enzymes in the intestine and then absorbed. Their metabolism involves several steps such as methylation, oxidation and conjugation reactions in the liver. Considering the large number of olive oil compounds and its derivatives, more studies are needed to understand their implications in the human body.

REFERENCES

[1] Bai, C.; Yan, X.; Takenga, M.; Sekiya, K. & Nagata, T. (1998). Determination of synthetic hydroxytyrosol in rat plasma by CG-MS. *Journal of Agricultural and Food Chemistry, v. 46*, 3998-4001.

[2] Bendini, A., Cerretani, L., Carrasco-Pancorbo, A., Gómez-Caravaca, A. M., Segura-Carretero, A., Fernández-Gutiérrez, A. & Lercker, G. (2007). Phenolic Molecules in Virgin Olive Oils: a Survey of Their Sensory Properties, Health Effects, Antioxidant Activity and Analytical Methods. An Overview of the Last Decade. *Molecules, v. 12*, 1679-1719.

[3] Bermúdez, B.; Pacheco, Y. M.; López, S.; Abia, R. & Muriana, F. J. G. (2004). Digestion and absorption of olive oil. *Grasas y Aceites, v. 55*, 1-10.

[4] Bisignano, G., Tomaino, A., Lo Cascio, R., Crisafi, G., Uccella, N. & Saija, A. (1999). On the in-vitro antiomicrobial activity of oleuropein and hydroxytyrosol. *The Journal of Pharmacy and Pharmacology, v. 31*, 971-974.

[5] Boskou, D. (2000). Olive oil. *World Review of Nutrition and Dietetics, v. 87*, 56–77.

[6] Corona, G., Tzounis, X., Assunta-Dessa, M., Deiana, M., Debnam, E.S., Visioli, F., et al. (2006). The fate of olive oil polyphenols in the gastrointestinal tract: implications of gastric and colonic microflora-dependent biotransformation. *Free Radical Research, v. 40*, 647-658.

[7] D'Angelo, S., Manna, C., Migliardi, V., Mazzoni, O., Morrica, P., Capasso, G., et al. (2001). Pharmacokinetics and metabolism of hydroxytyrosol, a natural antioxidant from olive oil. *Drug Metabolism and Disposition, v. 11*, 1492–1498.

[8] Goldstein, D. S.; Swoboda, K. J.; Miles, J. M.; Coppack, S. W.; Nemman, A.; Holmes, C.; Lamensdorf, I. & Eisenhofer, G. (1999). Sources and physiological significance of plasma dopamine sulfate. *The Journal of Clinical Endocrinology & Metabolism, v. 84*, 2528-2531.

[9] González-Santiago, M.; Fonollá, J. & Lopez-Huertas, E. (2010). Human absorption of a supplement containing purified hydroxytyrosol, a natural antioxidant from olive oil, and evidence for its transient association with low-density lipoproteins. *Pharmacological Research, v. 61*, 364-370.

[10] Khymenets, O., Joglar, J., Clapes, P., Parella, T., Covas, M.I. & de la Torre, R. (2006). Biocatalyzed synthesis and structural characterization of monoglucuronides of hydroxytyrosol, tyrosol, homovanillic alcohol and 3-(4′-hydroxyphenyl)propanol. *Advanced Synthesis & Catalysis, v. 348*, 2155–2162.

[11] Manna, C.; Galletti, P.; Maisto, G.; Cucciolla, V.; D'Angelo, S. & Zappia, V. (2000). Transport mechanism and metabolism of olive oil hydroxytyrosol in Caco-2 cells. *FEBS Letters, v. 470*, 341-344.

[12] Mardh, G. & Vallee, B. L. (1986). Human class I alcohol dehydrogenases catalyze the interconversion of alcohols and aldehydes in the metabolism of dopamine. *Biochemistry, v. 25*, 7279-7282.

[13] Mateos, R., Goya, L. & Bravo, L. (2005). Metabolism of the olive oil phenols hydroxytyrosol, tyrosol and hydroxytyrosyl acetate by human hepatoma HepG2 cells. *Journal of Agricultural and Food Chemistry, v. 53*, 9897-9905.

[14] Miró-Casas, E.; Covas, M.; Fitó, M.; Farrá-Albadalejo, M.; Marrugat, J. & Torre, R. (2003). Tyrosol and hydroxytyrosol are absorbed from moderate and sustained doses of virgin olive oil in humans. *European Journal of Clinical Nutrition, v. 57*, 186-190.

[15] Perez-Jimenez, F. (2005). International conference on the healthy effect of virgin olive oil. *European Journal of Clinical Investigation, v. 35*, 421-424.

[16] Scalbert, A. & Williamson, G. (2000). Dietary intake and bioavailability of polyphenols. *Journal of Nutrition, v. 130*, 2073-2085.

[17] Suárez, M.; Valls, R. M.; Romero, M.; Macià, A.; Fernández, S.; Giralt, M.; Solà, R. & Motilva, M. (2011). Bioavailability of phenols from a phenol-enriched olive oil. *British Journal of Nutrition*, 1-11.

[18] Townsend, C. M. Sabiston – Tratado de Cirurgia. 17ª Edition, v. 2. Brazil; 2006.

[19] Trichopoulou, A. & Vasilopoulou, E. (2000). Mediterranean diet and longevity. *The British Journal of Nutrition*, *v. 84*, 205-209.

[20] Tuck, K. L. & Hayball, P. J. (2002). Major phenolic compounds in olive oil: metabolism and health effects. *Journal of Nutritional Biochamistry, v. 13*, 636-644.

[21] Tuck, K. L.; Freeman, M. P.; Hayball, P. J.; Stretch, G. L. & Stupans, I. (2001). The in vivo fate of hydroxytyrosol and tyrosol, antioxidant phenolic constituents of olive oil, after intravenous and oral dosing of labeled compounds to rats. *The Journal of Nutrition, v. 131*, 1993-1996.

[22] Visioli, F. & Galli, C. (2000). Olive oil: more than just oleic acid. *The American Journal of Clinical Nutrition, v. 72*, 853.

[23] Yaqoob, P., Knapper, J. A., Webb, D. H., Williams, C. M., Newsholme, E. A. & Calder, P. C. (1998). Effect of olive oil on immune function in middle-aged men. *The American Journal of Clinical Nutrition, v. 67*, 129-135.

INDEX

B

C

D

E

F

G

H

I

J

K

L

M

N

O

P

Q

R

S

V

W

X

Y